MC
Neuro-radiology

Self-assessment
For
DM(Neuroradiology)
DM(Neurology)
MCh(Neuro-surgery)
FRCR Part 2A
American Board of Radiology

DR.NAGENDRA KUMAR SINHA
MD(Radio-diagnosis)

Copyright © 2016
Dr.Nagendra Kumar Sinha
All rights reserved.

DEDICATED
TO
MY TEACHERS

DR N GOGOI
&
DR R K GOGOI

CONTENTS

      Acknowledgments   x

01)   **Test Paper 1**   11
02)   Test Paper 1 Answer   21
03)   **Test Paper 2**   31
04)   Test Paper 2 Answer   40
05)   **Test Paper 3**   49
06)   Test Paper 4 Answer   59
07)   **Test Paper 4**   67
08)   Test Paper 4 Answer   77
09)   **Test Paper 5**   87
10)   Test Paper 5 Answer   97

11)	**Test Paper 6**	**107**
12)	Test Paper 6 Answer	116
13)	**Test Paper 7**	**125**
14)	Test Paper 7 Answer	135
15)	**Test Paper 8**	**144**
16)	Test Paper 8 Answer	153
17)	**Test Paper 9**	**163**
18)	Test Paper 9 Answer	173
19)	**Test Paper 10**	**181**

20) Test Paper 10 Answer 191

21) **Test Paper 11** 201
22) Test Paper 11 Answer 211
23) **Test Paper 12** 219
24) Test Paper 12 Answer 229
25) **Test Paper 13** 238
26) Test Paper 13 Answer 248
27) **Test Paper 14** 257
28) Test Paper 14 Answer 267
29) **Test Paper 15** 277

30) Test Paper 15 Answer 286

31) **Test Paper 16** **295**
32) Test Paper 16 Answer 309

PREFACE

MCQ is a standard format to assess the conceptual and factual knowledge.DM(Neuro-radiology),DM(Neurology),MCh(Neuro-surgery),FRCR and American board of radiology have adopted the MCQ approach of testing knowledge.But there is a dearth of MCQ on NEURO—RADIOLOGY.So, I have made an humble endeavor to fill that void.

This MCQ book on neuro-radiology contains 16 TEST PAPERS.Each Test Paper consists of approx.60 MCQs ,so this book contains approx.995 MCQs.Each test paper is designed to cover all the different topics of neuro-radiology.Some questions are deliberately repeated.Each test paper is followed by answer with detailed explanations .Most of MCQs answer and explanation can be seen in **MRI of The Brain And Spine ,3rd edition,--S.Atlas** and **Diagnostic neuroradiology ,Annie Osborn**

I believe this book will be a perfect tool for students in sitting in DM ,FRCR 2A (Neuro-radiology module)and Amercan board of radiology exams .This book will also be useful as a sharpening tool for radiologists and residents and all doctors who wish to make concept of neuro-radiology more clear .

Wishing you all the best

Nagendra Kumar Sinha

ngdrkus@yahoo.co.in

ACKNOWLEDGEMENTS

I am grateful to ALMIGHTY GOD who inspired me to write this book.

I am grateful to all my teachers ,especially Dr N K Gogoi and Dr R K Gogoi who chided me for my ignorance and who prodded me towards excellence .

I am grateful to my father Late Dwarika Prasad and mother Smt Kaushalya Devi for their constant blessings.

I really feel privileged to extend my gratitude to my brother Er S K P Sinha who taught me 'Never To Quit' and sister-in-law Manjula Rani Renu.

I am thankful to my wife Mrs Rina Sinha who constantly inspired me to complete the book. I am indebted to my son Rajat Kumar Sinha who gave his valuable time to write manuscript,edit and format this book.It is beyond my word to acknowledge patience of my younger son Anmol Kumar Sinha.

It is of great pleasure to acknowledge the contribution of nephews Naveen,Praveen,Sachin and niece Avanti.

I am highly indebted to my father-in-law R A Roy and B N ROY and mother-in-law Aruna Roy and sister-in-law Nina,Manju , Rachna and Pinki

I am grateful to my colleagues and seniors for their support,cooperation and suggestions,to name a few :Dr Akshay Dharmah ,Dr Naveen Niraj,Dr Rajnish ,Dr Pawan Pandey,Dr Mukesh Verma,Dr Vidya Nandan,Dr Jyotsana Rani Malik,Dr Jitendra Dahiya ,Dr Bhupender singh ,Dr Surendra Singh,Dr Suman Bharati,Dr Dhruv Pathak,Dr Anil Shahni,Dr D K Jha,Dr Mukesh Prasad,Dr Mukesh Singh, Dr Sanjay Mintoo,Dr Lokesh,Dr Ansari,Dr Sharaf,Dr Yogesh,Dr K K Sinha,Dr Purvey,Dr Permanand,Dr B P Sharma,Dr MM Mehra, Dr C L Verma,Dr. Vinay Mohan,Dr.Rajesh Ranjan,Dr.Babbar,Dr.Kameshwar ,Dr.Ray,Dr.Raj Mehta ,Dr.Sunil,Dr.Anuj Bhatnagar,Dr.Arun Choudhary,Dr.Suresh ,Dr.Diwakar and Dr.Jitendra ,Dr.Sharad

I am grateful to Mrs Sunita R George,Mr. Pawawn ,Mrs Manju ,and Ved Pal.

I am grateful to Facebook and Nagendra 's radiology blog fraternity who responded and appreciated the questions posted during manuscript preprations

My special thanks to my friends Sanjay Jayaswal ,Ashok kumar and Sanjay Bharati.

Last but not the least ,I am indebted to Pothi.com for providing me plateform to publish this book.

Nagendra Kumar Sinha

TEST PAPER 1

1. All are true regarding lacunar infarctions except
a. involve deep subcortical structures
b. generally involve perforating arteries
c. generally less than 1 cm and are not larger than 1.5 cm in diameter
d. no role of Diffusion-weighted MR
e. the prognosis better than large-vessel infarctions

2. All are true regarding cerebral circulation except
a. the recurrent artery of Huebner is a perforating branch from the MCA
b. ACA supply the head of the caudate and the anterior portions of the putamen
c. ACA supply the medial portions of the parietal lobe
d. MCA supply much of the globus pallidus and putamen and the internal capsule.
e. MCA supply the lateral portions of the frontal and parietal lobes

3. All are true regarding periventricular infarction except
a. common in the preterm infant (25-40%)
b. m/c common site --- white matter adjacent to the trigones of the lateral ventricles and that to the foramina of Monro
c. ventricular margins may be wavy and follow the contour of the cortical gray matter
d. the sulci may be deep and in close proximity to the ventricles
e. compensatory markedly thick corpus callosum

4. All are disorder of secondary neurulation except
a. diastematomyelia
b. meningocoele
c. myelomeningocoele
d. dermal sinus
e. lipoma

5. All are true regarding chronic subdural hematoma except
a. low attenuation on CT
b. hyperintense on T1 MR because of methemoglobin content
c. FLAIR easily differentiate it from a subdural hygroma
d. gradual decrease in intensity on T1-weighted images
e. Hemosiderin accumulation in the adjacent dural structures is a consistent feature

6. All are features of AVMs on MRI except
a. cluster of focal round, linear, or serpentine areas of signal void on FSE
b. enlargement of deep veins may be the only clue to the diagnosis
c. high intensity in areas of flowing blood may be due to flow related enhancement
d. AVM nidi can partially enhance after gadolinium
e. arterial feeding vessels generally enhance

7. MR features of cavernous angioma are all except
a. focal central heterogeneity corresponding to subacute-chronic hemorrhage
b. circumferential complete

hyperintense rings around low - intensity central areas
c. no mass effect or edema
d. no demonstrable feeding arteries or draining veins a
e. contrast enhancement

8. The most sensitive imaging method for the detection of acute subarachnoid blood is
a. CT
b. MRI
c PET
d. USG
e. nuclear scan

9. All are true regarding cortical contusion except
a. primarily involve the superficial gray matter of the brain
b. the underlying white matter usually spared
c. less likely to be hemorrhagic than DAI lesions
d. tend to be multiple and bilateral
e. Contusions most commonly involve the temporal (46%) and frontal (31%) lobes

10. All are true regarding multiple sclerosis except
a. Charcot type ---most common form
b. most patients initially present in the third and fourth decades
c. two to three times higher incidence in females than in males
d. impaired or double vision--- often the first clinical symptom
e. primary-progressive MS relapsing – the most common (80-85%) temporal patterns

11. All are true regarding Hurst disease except
a. strictly non- hemorrhagic
b. coma and death within 1 to 5 days of onset
c. tonsillar and transtentorial herniation
d. Multifocal asymmetric areas of high signal intensity in white matter son the T2W
e. strict sparing of the subcortical U fibers.

12. All are true regarding Alexander disease except
a. enlarged brain
b. substantial accumulation cf Rosenthal fibers
c. The basal ganglia and cortex usually relatively preserved
d. sparing of the subcortical U fibers
e. Cavitation common

13. The most common lesions in patients undergoing neurosurgical treatment of epilepsy is
a. hippocampal sclerosis (50% to 70%)
b. perinatal hypoxia or other insult (13% to 35%)
c. tumors (15%)
d. vascular malformations (3%)
e. traumatic gliosis (2%)

14. All are true regarding hippocampal sclerosis except
a. The amygdala remains superior to temporal horn
b. the CSF signal in the uncal recess of temporal horn / the alveus seprate amygdale from hippocampus
c. Both amygdala and hippocampus are hypointense to gray matter on almost all MR pulse sequences.
d. The hippocampus may be slightly hyperintense to gray matter on FLAIR images

e. the posterior hippocampal boundary for volumetry extend to the crus of the fornix

15. All are true regarding intracranial tumour in adult except
a. 80% to 85% of all intracranial tumors occur in adults
b. most of intracranial tumors are situated in the supratentorial compartment
c. the most common primary intraaxial supratentorial neoplasm is the glioblastoma
d. meningioma is the most common intraaxial tumor of the posterior fossa
e. MR imaging is more sensitive for brain tumors than CT

16. All are true regarding tumour except
a. malignant gliomas enhance because of formation of fenestrated endothelium
b. Metastatic lesions virtually always enhance due to presence of non-CNS capillaries in the lesion
c. Extraaxial tumors arise from tissues with capillaries lacking tight junctions leading to enhancement
d. there is discordance between MR imaging and angiographic findings of hypervascularity
e. there is concordance between contrast enhancement and perfusion MR techniques

17. Feature favouring astrocytoma over oligodendroglioma is
a. usually more heterogenous b. more frequently calcified,
c. often deeper in the hemisphere
d. less peritumoural edema
e. relatively of lower intensity on T2-W

18. The most common pineal mass is
a. germinoma
b. teratoma
c. pineoblastoma
d. pineocytoma
e. glioma

19. All are true regarding meningioma except
a. About 40% of the meningiomas demonstrate a vascular marginal interface with high-resolution MR.
b. CSF interfaces are identifiable in about 80% of meningiomas on MR
c. vascular rims and CSF clefts are both present at the brain–tumor interface in approx. two thirds of meningioma
d. The dural margin interface is seen primarily in meningiomas of the cavernous sinus.
e. arcuate bowing and compression of adjacent cortical convolutions in an onion skin–like configuration noted in meningioma

20. All are true regarding subarachnoid lipoma except
a. due to differentiation of incomplete reabsorption of the meninx primitiva
b. most frequently found in the cerebellopontine angle
c. pericallosal cistern lipoma frequently associated with corpus callosum agenesis
d. hyperintense on T1-weighted images
e. chemical shift artifact noted

21. All are true regarding choroid plexus tumour except
a. 80% occur in patients less than 2 years of age
b. Forty percent arise in the fourth ventricle
c. Choroid plexus carcinomas more common in the lateral ventricles
d. usually hypodense on CT
e. cluster-of-grapes morphology

22. All are true regarding imaging of CNS infection except
a. T1W with contrast is the most sensitive MR sequence for meningitis
b. Diffusion-weighted imaging characteristically shows restricted diffusion
c. HSV-1 is the causative agent in 95% of herpetic encephalitis
d. HSV-1 is the most common cause of fatal sporadic encephalitis
e. HSV-2 account for 80% to 90% of neonatal herpes virus infections

23. A 60 yrs old patient presents with rapidly progressive dementia, myoclonic jerks, and periodic sharp-wave EEG tracing. CJD is suspected. MR of brain was advised as MR is highly sensitive and specific for the detection of CJD abnormalities. All are true regarding CJD except
a. Lesions do not enhance and do not demonstrate mass effect
b. DWIs is superior to over any T2-weighted images in the assessment of CJD
c. DWI changes have been observed as early as 1 month after the onset of symptoms
d. hyperintensity is noted in the cortex and basal ganglia on DWI
e. primary sensorimotor cortex is almost always involved

24. All are true regarding space of Virchow-Robin (VRS) except
a. isointense to CSF on all pulse sequences
b. type 2 lacunae
c. lack mass effect
d. round, oval, or curvilinear with well-defined, smooth margins
e. common in relation to anterior commissure

25. All are true regarding neuroimaging of Wilson disease except
a. diffuse or focal atrophy of the cerebrum, brainstem, and/or cerebellum
b. Gray matter nuclei involvement is usually bilateral and symmetric
c. lenticular nucleus typically involved
d. Cerebral lesions are hyperdense on CT
e. variable signal on MRI.

26. All are true regarding cranial nerve schwannomas in NF 2 except
a. Multiple cranial nerve schwannomas are the hallmark of NF2
b. The most common site for cranial nerve schwannomas is the vestibulocochlear cranial nerve
c. Deformity and/or enlargement of the internal auditory canal in Vestibular schwannomas noted on CT
d. Vestibular schwannomas present in 5nd decade
e. prominent contrast

enhancement in Vestibular schwannomas

27. All are true regarding von Hippel-Lindau Disease except
a. an autosomal dominant disorder without any racial or sexual predilection
b. gene located on chromosome 3p25.5
c. VHL with pheochromocytoma reffered as type 1
d. the hemangioblastoma-- The hallmark lesion of VHL
e. cerebellar hemangioblastomas ----considerably more predictive of the presence of VHL

28. All are true regarding Kallmann Syndrome except
a. hypogonadotropic hypogonadism
b. KAL2 ---X-linked
c. the olfactory bulbs are most likely to be absent
d. may be associated with facial anomalies
e. High-resolution, coronal, fast spin-echo T2-weighted sequences are the preferred method

29. All are true regarding dermoids except
a. nonneoplastic developmental mass
b. derived from ectodermal rests
c. may cause chemical meningitis
d. usually situated off the midline
e. most often involve the basal surface of the brain

30. All are features of persistent trigeminal artery except
a. vessel arising from the cavernous (or precavernous) carotid artery
b. an abrupt lateral bend in posterior fossa to communicate with the basilar artery
c. small caliber of the basilar artery caudal to the trigeminal artery
d. small ipsilateral PComA
e. vessel appearing to penetrate the dorsum sellae

31. All are true regarding nerve sheath tumour except
a. posterior scalloping of the vertebral bodies and widening of the neural foramina
b. increased signal intensity compared with muscle on noncontrast T1-weighted images
c. markedly increased signal intensity on T2W
d. Schwannomas displace encase nerve fibers to appear fusiform
e. usually enhance intensely and fairly homogeneously

32. All are true regarding Spinal cord arteriovenous malformations (SCAVM) except
a. congenital lesions
b. nidus of the SCAVM is located on or within the substance of the spinal cord itself
c. most frequently occur in the thoracolumbar region
d. the arterial supply to SCAVMs arises from only anterior spinal arteries
e. dilated venous drainage -- usually present on both dorsal and ventral to the spinal cord.

33. All are true regarding molecular signaling in neurulation except
a. Hensen's node secretes molecules that lead to neural induction.
b. noggin, follistatin, and chordin

are neural inducers
c. BMP-4 promote formation of neural ectoderm
d. the notochord secretes the signaling molecule sonic hedgehog (SHH)
e. floor plate produces SHH and the winged helix transcription factor hepatocyte nuclear factor (HNF)-3β

34. All are true regarding diastematomyelia except
a. coronal clefting of spinal cord
b. 80 % cases in female
c. 45% cases in lumbar/lumbosacral area
d. the smaller hemicord often lies ventral to the larger hemicord
e. conus medullaris usually low

35. All are true regarding pituitary adenoma except
a. slow-growing benign neoplasms of epithelial origin
b. invasion of adjacent tissue regarded as unequivocal proof of malignancy
c. pseudocapsule of compressed tissue containing condensed reticulin
d. those less than 10 mm in diameter are considered micro adenomas
e. the prolactinoma accounts for approximately 50% of hormonally active adenomas

36. All are true regarding intracranial germinoma except
a. the pineal region is the most frequent site
b. Germinomas are tumors of children or young adults.
c. Suprasellar germinomas are encapsulated
d. suprasellar germinomas are typically centered at or just behind the pituitary infundibulum
e. the posterior pituitary bright spot is absent in most cases

37. All are true regarding orbital meningiomas except
a. isointense to muscle on T1W and isointense/hyperintense to fat on T2W
b. use of fat suppression technique is useful
c. CT is the most sensitive imaging technique for the detection of intraorbital meningioma
d. en-plaque meningiomas involving orbital walls are most definitively evaluated with fat suppression and contrast-enhanced studies
e. tram track sign of perineural enhancement

38. All are true regarding chemical exchange saturation transfer (CEST) agent except
a. make use of the phenomenon of magnetization transfer between water protons and protons in other molecules
b. used to detect endogenous species that are abundant in vivo, such as amide groups in tumors
c. offer unique approaches to obtaining MR contrast from physiologic changes such as pH
d. acquisition of two data sets is required
e. rely on the same principles of relaxation as simple paramagnetic ions

39. commonly calcified brain tumours are all except
a. Oligodendrogliomas (90%)
b. Choroid plexus tumours
c. Ependymoma

d. Metastases
e. Central neurocytoma

40..All are true regarding pineal region tumours, germinoma except
a. often grey matter isointensity on standard MRI
b. poor contrast enhancement
c. virtually never calcify.
d. the hypothalamic region ----the second commonest site of germinoma
e. show diffuse subependymal and subarachnoid spread

41.All are true regading pathophysiology of stroke except
a. A CBF of around 23 ml 100 g^{-1} min^{-1} causes a reversible neurological deficit.
b. electrical activity ceases below about 18–20 ml 100 g^{-1} min^{-1} of CBF
c. cytotoxic edema develops at 10–15 ml 100 g^{-1} min
d. Most carotid territory infarcts involve the middle cerebral artery.
e. The commonest cause of ACA infarcts is embolism

42.All are true regarding aneurysm except
a. 30 per cent arise from vertebral or basilar arteries
b. giant aneurysms account for approximately 5 per cent of all cerebral aneurysms
c. clot in the septum pellucidumis is virtually diagnostic of an aneurysm of the anterior communicating artery
d. the basilar artery bifurcation aneurysm rupture with blood in the interpeduncular fossa, brainstem or thalamus
e. the posterior inferior cerebellar arteries aneurysm often haemorrhage into the ventricular system.

43..All are white matter disease in HIV-related CNS disease except
a. Small nonspecific focal white-matter hyperintensities on T2W
b. HIV encephalopathy
c. PML
d. viral encephalitis—CMV
e. CJD

44.All are true regarding spinal cord supply except
a. supplied by the midline anterior spinal artery and two posterolateral spinal arteries
b. artery of Adamkiewicz is found in the thoracolumbar region
c. artery of Adamkiewicz is usually on the left side, between T8 and L1–2
d. The anterior spinal artery supplies the major portion of the cord substance
e. posterolateral spinal arteries supply the motor cells of the anterior horns

45.All are true regarding normal gyration except
a. the interhemispheric fissure and Sylvian fissures is formed by 16 weeks gestation
b. the callosal sulcus and parieto-occipital fissure are recognizable at 22 weeks gestation
c. The central sulcus is seen in most infants by 32 weeks
d. The slowest regions of gyration are the frontal and temporal poles
e. the gyral pattern becomes adult like by the term of gestation

46.All are true regarding spine except

a. The spinal cord termination ---- abnormal if seen at or below L3
b. myelomeningoceles are virtually always associated with Chiari II malformation
c. The filum terminale lipoma is considered to arise from a disturbance of caudal regression
d. The 'tight' filum terminale is a short, thick filum greater than 2 mm in diameter
e. dermal sinus is typically seen in the thoracic region

47. All are true regarding Vein of Galen aneurysmal malformations (VGAMs) except
a. account for 3% of vascular malformations in children
b. hydrocephalus
c. focal infarctions and generalized cerebral atrophy
d. Angiography the gold standard of diagnosis
e. a persistent embryological remnant

48. All are true regarding cerebral vasospasm except
a. one-third of patients with subarachnoid haemorrhage develop symptomatic vasospasm
b. Medical treatment consists of hypertension, hypervolaemia and haemodilution (triple H therapy).
c. Intracranial balloon angioplasty is suitable for treatment of spasm of the proximal segments of intracranial vessels
d. intra-arterial NTG infusion is used to treat vasospasm
e. Papaverine may be useful to facilitate access for endovascular treatment of a ruptured aneurysm

49. .All are true regarding vein og Galen aneurismal malformation (VGAM) except
a. arteriovenous shunts at the choroidal level within the subarachnoid space
b. abnormal persistence of the median vein of the prosencephalon,
c. absent falcine sinus
d. may be agenesis of the straight sinus
e. present in the fetal period

50. Multiple small rounded and clear-cut defects.in the skull is seen in
a. multiple myeloma
b. haemangioma
c. chordoma
d. epidermoid
e. none

51. All are true regarding radionuclide imaging except
a. proximity to a cyclotron is essential in case of use of carbon-11 and oxygen -15
b. Krypton-81m requires delivery by intracarotid infusion for cerebral blood flow measurement
c. A rebreathing method using xenon-133 offers a noninvasive method for assessment of regional blood flow
d. iodoamphetamine labelled with iodine-123 (]"I-IMP) cross blood brain barrier
e. exametazime (`°I"Tc-HMPAO) has low extraction efficiency by brain tissue

52. All are true regarding following lesions except
a. pseudolaminar cortical infarction typically affect the middle layer
b. venous infarction primarily affect the white matter

c. the anterior circulation is particularly prone to develop hypertensive encephalopathy – related lesions
d. SAH visualised on CT more than 1 week after the initial hemorrhage suggests rebleeding
e. cavernous hemangioma typically have a popcorn-like appearance

53. the feature that favour infarction over tumour is/are
a. sudden onset
b. gray and white matter involvement
c. wedge-shaped or gyriform involvement
d. vascular distribution
e. all

54. All are true regarding temporal lobe lesions except
a. Gradenigo 's syndrome – osteomyelitis of the apex
b. cholesterol granuloma---hypointense on T2W
c. paraganglioma---derived from neural crest cell derivatives
d. malignant otitis externa—osteomyelitis of temporal bone
e. glomus tympanicum tumours---paraganglioma localized to the chochlear promontory

55. All are true regarding Lhermitte –Duclos disease except
a. anbormal population of large neurons in the granular layer
b. aberrant myelination of neurons in Purkinje layer
c. cerbellar cortex dysplastic
d. laminated, increased signal on T2W
e. progressive hypertrophy of the cerebellar cortex

56. All are true regarding congenital herpes simplex except
a. limbic system localization
b. relative hyperdensity of cortical gray matter
c. thrombosis/haemorrhagic infarction
d. HSV-2 causes 75% to 90% cases
e. CNS manifestation 2 to 4 weeks after birth

57. Strokes are seen in all except
a. ALD
b. Leigh syndrome
c. MELAS
d. MERRF
e. Homocystinuria

58. All are features of normal aging brain except
a. scattered WMHs on T2W
b. moderate enlargement of sulci
c. periventricular high signal rim on PD, T2W
d. decreasing iron deposition in globus pallidus and putamen
e. moderate enlargement of ventricles

59. All are true regarding spine cyst except
a. synovial cyst is located adjacent to degenerated facet joints
b. arachnoid cyst is located ventral to cord
c. lateral meningocele is most common in thoracic region
d. Tarlov cyst is located at root sleeve at dorsal root ganglion
e. intraosseous meningocoel is located in sacrum

60. All are true regarding Wyburn –Mason syndrome except
a. unilateral AVMs of visual pathways and midbrain seen in Wyburn –Mason syndrome
b. Progressive cerebellar hypertrophy is seen in Louis-Bar

synsrome
c.Multiple AVMs are found in Rendu-Osler-Weber Disease
d.soft issue or bone hypertrophy is seen in Klippel-Trenaunay-Weber Syndrome
e.Gorlin syndrome shows medulloblastoma

TEST PAPER 1 (ANSWER)

1-----d
Diffusion-weighted MR has been useful in confirming the neuroanatomic location of infarctions in patients presenting with lacunar syndromes.Lacunar infarction involve deep subcortical structures (basal ganglia, the white matter of the internal capsule, the brainstem, and the deep white matter of the hemispheres).It generally involve perforating arteries (the lenticulostriate arteries, thalamoperforating arteries and small perforating arteries from the main stem of the basilar artery)

2---a
The recurrent artery of Huebner is generally the largest perforating branch from the proximal anterior cerebral artery. ACA supply the head of the caudate and the anterior portions of the putamen and globus pallidus and the anterior limb of the internal capsule , supply the inferior and medial portions of the frontal lobe and medial portions of the parietal lobe. MCA supply the lateral portions of the frontal and parietal lobes and the anterior and lateral portions of the temporal lobe.

3---e
The posterior periventricular white matter adjacent to the trigones of the lateral ventricles and the white matter adjacent to the foramina of Monro—m/c site of periventricular infarction
Markedly thin corpus callosum is feature of periventricular infarction.(

4.---c
Myelomeningocoele is a disorder of primary neurulation
The average packing density of coils with GDC coil within the aneurysm is approx.20 to 40% ,there is relatively high long term recanalisation and there is little healing response.
Polyglycolic lactic acid copolymer-coated cells is an example of polymer –enhanced coils.Ethylene vinyl alcoholbcoplymer –Onyx is an example of liquid polymer.

5 ---e
Hemosiderin and other iron storage from accumulation in the adjacent dural structures is not a consistent feature of subdural and epidural hemorrhage presumably because of the absence of a blood–brain barrier in dura.
Rebleeding into a subdural collection should be suspected if irregular hypointense membranes loculating areas of different ages of subdural are found or if there are debris–fluid levels seen within the collection
An important role in MR of extraaxial hemorrhage, with its unique ability to stage intracranial hemorrhage temporally, lies in

the documentation of suspected child abuse because the depiction of multiple sites of intracranial hemorrhage at different stages of evolution can be an important clue to this diagnosis

6---e
Gadolinium enhancement of the enlarged vessels occurs in those vessels with relatively slow flow, that is, mainly the venous side of the lesion. AVM nidi can partially enhance after gadolinium but the rapidly flowing blood within arterial feeding vessels generally does not enhance.

Certain MR sequences can result in high intensity in areas of flowing blood because of either flow-related enhancement or even echo rephasing or because of the now routine incorporation of gradient moment nulling into SE imaging.

7—b
Cavernous angioma shows circumferential complete rings of markedly hypointense iron-storage forms around high-intensity central areas

8---a

9----c
Because gray matter is much more vascular than white matter, contusions are much more likely to be hemorrhagic than are DAI lesions (52% vs. 19%)

10.-----e
Most patients (80% to 85%) experience a relapsing-remitting course of exacerbations (attacks) and remissions of neurologic deficits separated by stable periods

About 10% to 15% of the cases have a nonremitting progressive course and have been termed primary-progressive MS . Less than 5% of patients start off with a primary progressive course but develop discrete exacerbations and are categorized under the progressive- relapsing MS.

In addition, many patients initially presenting with the relapsing-remitting form (up to 50% to 60%)worsen steadily in their clinical baseline between exacerbations and are categorized in the secondary progressive MS group.

In addition to these clinical patterns, patients may be monosymptomatic, in which the presentation consists of a single episode of a neurologic deficit, and these patients are included in the clinically isolated syndrome category, such as optic neuritis, transverse myelitis, or brainstem syndrome.

11.---a
Hurst disease is considered a hyperacute or fulminant form of ADEM , also known as Acute hemorrhagic leukoencephalitis. High fatality is seen due to respiratory paralysis secondary to tonsillar and transtentorial herniation

Postmortem examination of the brain usually shows multifocal areas of acute perivascular demyelination and hemorrhage confined to the cerebral white matter (especially in the central part of the centrum semiovale, internal capsule, and convolutional white matter of the cingulate gyrus) with strict sparing of the subcortical U fibers.

12.---d
There is no sparing of the subcortical U fibers in Alexander disease. The cerebellum is less often affected than in other leukodystrophies. MR findings classically demonstrate increased signal intensity on the T2-weighted images in the frontal white matter .The occipital white matter and cerebellum are usually spared.

13.---a

14.----c
Both amygdala and hippocampus are isointense to gray matter on all MR pulse sequences. The hippocampus, however, may be slightly hyperintense to gray matter on fluid attenuated inversion recovery (FLAIR) images due to incomplete suppression of CSF

15.---d
Metastasis is the most common intraaxial tumor of the posterior fossa

16.---e
There is discordance between contrast enhancement and perfusion MR techniques.Several precursors are necessary for contrast enhancement to occur: absence of the blood–brain barrier, adequate delivery of the contrast agent (i.e., perfusion), extracapillary interstitial space for the accumulation of contrast agent, appropriate contrast agent dosage, spatial resolution and imaging parameters to allow its detection, and time for the contrast agent to accumulate in the region in question. The formation of tumor capillaries deficient in blood–brain barrier constituents(rather than active destruction of the blood–brain barrier) is presumed to be the explanation for tumor enhancement.Permeability imaging quantifies the rate of contrast agent extravasation (e.g., k_{trans}), providing a measure of blood–brain.

17.-----c
Oligodendrogliomas are usually heterogeneous but are of relatively lower intensity than astrocytomas (i.e., isointense to gray matter) on T2-weighted images because they are typically hypercellular.
Astrocytomas usually are more homogeneous, not as frequently calcified, and often are deeper in the hemisphere, arising within the white matter.relative to oligodendroglioma

18.---a
Germinomas are the most common germ cell tumor and also are the most common pineal mass.

19.---a
About 80% of the meningiomas demonstrate a vascular marginal interface with high-resolution MR.

20---b
Subarachnoid lipoma are usually located in the subarachnoid space and are most frequently found in the pericallosal cistern.

21.----d
The tumor is usually of uniform

increased density on CT and enhances intensely and homogeneously . The choroid plexus papilloma typically on T1 is a hypointense mass, and it is usually somewhat hyperintense on T2 with focal hypointensities

22.---a
FLAIR is the most sensitive MR sequence for meningitis

23.----e
Symmetric increased signal in T2-weighted images in the caudate nuclei , putamen, thalamus and cortex , basal ganglia , periventricular white matter , and occipital lobes are noted in CJD. Primary sensorimotor cortex is almost always spared, even when extensive abnormalities are found in the frontal and parietal cortex.

The mechanism of hyperintensity on DWI found in the cortex and basal ganglia is poorly understood, although it correlates with deposition of abnormal prion protein, vacuolation, neuronal loss, and gliosis. DWI changes have been observed as early as 1 month after the onset of symptoms and may show modifications 6 months prior to T2-weighted images and 4 months prior to FLAIR images

24.---b
Type I lacunae are small infarcts, type II are small hemorrhages, and type III are dilated VRS
Perivascular space of Virchow-Robin (VRS) is an extension of the subarachnoid space that accompanies penetrating vessels into the brain to the level of the capillaries. The VRS at the base of the brain follow the lenticulostriate arteries as they enter the basal ganglia through the anterior perforated substance. On axial images they are typically adjacent to the anterior or posterior surface of the lateral portion of the anterior commissure . In the coronal or sagittal plane they are adjacent to the superior surface of the commissure or just lateral to the putamen.

Those in the high convexity follow the course of the penetrating cortical arteries and arterioles from the high-convexity gray matter into the centrum semiovale.

High signal intensity (i.e., higher intensity than CSF, most notably on proton density–weighted or FLAIR images) foci in the midbrain can be seen from enlarged perivascular spaces(along branches of the collicular and accessory collicular arteries)

25.---d
Cerebral lesions are hypodense on CT but show variable signal on MRI. Lesions are hyperintense, hypointense, or both on long-TR sequences.

Gray matter nuclei involvement is more common and is usually bilateral and symmetric; white matter lesions usually are asymmetric. In a recent investigation of 100 patients with WD , signal abnormalities were present in the putamen in 72%, caudate nuclei in 61%, thalami in 58%, midbrain in 49%, cerebral white matter in 25%, pons in 20%, medulla in 12%, cerebellum in 10%, and cerebral cortex in 9%.

26.---d

Vestibular schwannomas present as solitary lesions in the fifth decade; with NF2 they present as bilateral masses in the second and third decades.**27.---e**

The hallmark lesion of VHL is the hemangioblastoma. These are most common in the cerebellum but occasionally present in the medulla oblongata (the most common brainstem site), pons, spinal cord, and supratentorially in the optic nerves and cerebral hemispheres

Spinal hemangioblastomas are considerably more predictive of the presence of VHL. Any patient with multiple hemangioblastomas should have a thorough evaluation (including abdominal imaging) because of the high likelihood of having VHL.

27.---e

The hallmark lesion of VHL is the hemangioblastoma. These are most common in the cerebellum but occasionally present in the medulla oblongata (the most common brainstem site), pons, spinal cord, and supratentorially in the optic nerves and cerebral hemispheres

Spinal hemangioblastomas are considerably more predictive of the presence of VHL. Any patient with multiple hemangioblastomas should have a thorough evaluation (including abdominal imaging) because of the high likelihood of having VHL.

28.----b

Kallmann syndrome may be of X-linked, autosomal dominant, or autosomal recessive inheritance . It can be divided by genotype into four different types: KAL1 (X-linked) and the autosomal types KAL2, KAL3, and KAL4.

29.----d

Dermoids are usually situated in the midline.

30.---b

Three specific features help to make the diagnosis of the trigeminal artery. First is the presence of a vessel that arises from the cavernous (or precavernous) carotid artery and courses directly posteriorly into the posterior fossa, where an abrupt medial bend is noted, and communication with the basilar artery is established.

The second feature is that the basilar artery will typically be of small caliber caudal to the trigeminal artery, and the ipsilateral PComA will also be small.

A variant trigeminal artery arises medially and courses through the sella and directly through the dorsum to reach the basilar artery . Thus, the third diagnostic feature is the identification of a vessel that appears to penetrate the dorsum sellae.

31.---d

Schwannomas appear as masses that project from one side of the nerve . Because they arise from a single focus, they displace normal nerve fibers to appear as lobulated, rather than fusiform,

tumors. Cyst formation is common, although gross hemorrhage is not.
Neurofibromas consist of mixtures of fibroblasts and proliferated Schwann cells between dispersed nerve fibers. The matrix of a neurofibroma contains acid mucopolysaccharides and large amounts of tissue fluids with numerous fibrous strands. The matrix spreads apart the axons to produce the fusiform shape of the neurofibroma.

32----d
The arterial supply to SCAVMs arises from anterior or posterior spinal arteries.
In contrast to SDAVF, spinal hemorrhage constitutes a prominent feature in the clinical course of greater than half of patients with SCAVM.
SCAVM may represent part of a more widespread systemic vascular disorder such as Rendu-Osler-Weber or Klippel-Trenauney syndrome . A complex metameric vascular malformation, Cobb syndrome, involves all embryonic layers from the spinal cord to the skin and may be present in 5% of SCAVM patients.
The prochordal plate establishes the cranial end of the bilaminar disk

33.---c
The ventral mesoderm and the early ectoderm itself produce BMPs, especially BMP-4, which inhibit formation of neural ectoderm and promote differentiation of epidermal ectoderm.

34.----a
Diastematomyelia signifies a sagittal clefting of the spinal cord, conus medullaris, and/or filum terminale into two hemicords
The two hemicords are each narrower than normal and nearly always (91%) reunite distally into a re-formed cord below the cleft . In 30% of cases the hemicords are grossly asymmetric in size. When the hemicords are asymmetric, the cord above and below the cleft is usually asymmetrically smaller on the side of the smaller hemicord, and the smaller hemicord often lies ventral to the larger hemicord. The filum terminale is usually-perhaps always-thickened and may itself tether the reunited cord.
Hydromyelia is present in up to 50% of cases of diastematomyelia. It may affect the cord above the cleft and extend into one or both hemicords.

35.---b
Invasion of adjacent tissue is not regarded as unequivocal proof of malignancy. Conventionally, the diagnosis of carcinoma is used only when distant metastases occur.
Elevated prolactin levels are not always due to increased production by a hormonally active adenoma. Any process that interferes with the production, release, or pituitary portal venous transport of prolactin-inhibiting factors from the hypothalamus will result in hyperprolactinemia because of disinhibition of normal

prolactin cells. This is most commonly due to suprasellar tumors that compress the hypothalamus or pituitary stalk ("stalk section effect"), certain drugs (particularly phenothiazines), and primary hypothyroidism. Nevertheless, the degree of hyperprolactinemia caused by these latter processes is at most moderate; serum prolactin levels above 150 ng/mL are almost always due to an underlying autonomously secreting adenoma (normal serum prolactin less than 20 ng/mL). However, the converse is not true because many patients with prolactinomas have serum prolactin levels between 20 and 150 ng/mL.

36.---c

Suprasellar germinomas are not encapsulated. They are very infiltrative, adherent to the ventral surface of the brain, and often closely related to the optic nerves. They have a propensity to spread through the subarachnoid space with metastatic deposits to the walls of the ventricles and the basal cisterns.

37.---c

CT is the most sensitive imaging technique for the detection of intraorbital meningioma.
En plaque meningiomas involving orbital walls are most definitively evaluated with fat suppression and contrast-enhanced studies. Despite the fact that MR is not sensitive to the calcification often found in these lesions, most perioptic meningiomas enhance with IV contrast. In conjunction with fat suppression, gadolinium-enhanced MR is clearly the most sensitive imaging technique for the detection of intraorbital meningioma, regardless of whether it is perioptic.

38.---e

CHEMICAL EXCHANGE AGENTS is a different class of contrast agents that does not rely on the same principles of relaxation as simple paramagnetic ions but instead make use of the phenomenon of magnetization transfer between water protons and protons in other molecules, such as in amide groups, which have a different resonant frequency. These so-called chemical exchange saturation transfer (CEST) agents produce contrast in appropriate imaging sequences as a result of magnetization transfer between water protons and protons in the agent that may dissociate and thereby undergo "chemical exchange."

By applying saturating radiofrequency energy at the precise frequency of the labile proton while it is chemically associated with the agent (which is different from the frequency of the solute water), one causes the MR signal from the water to decrease when the exchange occurs. The magnitude of the effect on the MR signal intensity depends strongly on the rate at which the protons exchange between the agent and the water. Moreover, the effect of the agent is visible only when the saturating

RF pulse is applied to induce the effect.
In simple CEST experiments, acquisition of two data sets is required; in one, an RF pulse is applied at the frequency of the agent-bound proton, and in a second, the applied RF is set symmetrically on the other side of the water resonance. The signal from the first data set contains a combination of the CEST effect and direct saturation of the water, whereas the second acquisition measures only the latter. Subtraction of these two sets results in signal changes due to the CEST effect alone. CEST techniques have been used to detect endogenous species that are abundant in vivo, such as amide groups in tumors (36) and -OH groups in glycogen in perfused liver

39---d
Commonly calcified lesions --- Oligodendrogliomas (90%),Choroid plexus tumours,Ependymoma,Centralneurocytoma,Meningioma,Craniopharyngioma,Teratoma,Chordoma
Commonly haemorrhagic lesions----GBM (grade 4 glioma),Oligodendroglioma,Metastases (Melanoma,Lung,Breast)
40.----b
Germinoma show marked, homogeneous contrast enhancement and virtually never calcify.
41---e
The commonest cause of ACA infarcts is vasospasm following subarachnoid haemorrhage.
. Brainstem infarcts are commonly due to occlusion of short perforating vessels. A combination of infratentorial, thalamic and occipital infarcts suggests an occlusion of distal basilar artery, or 'top of the basilar' syndrome. Multiple infarcts in different arterial territories suggest a cardiac rather than a carotid source of emboli, or haemodynamic strokes due to hypotension if the distribution conforms to the arterial border zones.
42.----a
Around 90 per cent of intracranial aneurysms arise from the carotid circulation, the remaining 10 per cent from vertebral or basilar arteries. The anterior and posterior communicating arteries give rise to approximately one-third each of all intracranial aneurysms, with another 20 per cent from middle cerebral arteries and 5 per cent from the basilar termination. The remainder arises from other vessel origins and bifurcations.
Aneurysms of the posterior communicating artery can present with isolated third nerve palsy
43..---e
44..---e
The anterior spinal artery is the most important of supply because it supplies the major portion of the cord substance, including the motor cells of the anterior horns. It gives off tiny sulcocommissural arteries that

run into the cord; they are not visible at angiography unless pathologically enlarged.

45.---c
The central sulcus is seen in most infants by 27 weeks

46..----e
Dermal sinus is typically seen in the lumbosacral region

47.---a
Vein of Galen aneurysmal malformations (VGAMs) are a rare cause of paediatric stroke but have a wide range of clinical presentations and account for 30% of vascular malformations in children.

48.---d
Intra-arterial papaverine infusion is used to treat vasospasm in distal branches of cerebral arteries that are not suitable for balloon dilatation. Papaverine may be useful to facilitate access for endovascular treatment of a ruptured aneurysm if this is impeded by vasospasm.

49..---c
In VGAM, there is associated aneurysmal dilatation and abnormal. persistence of the median vein of the prosencephalon, an embryological midline venous structure and precursor of the vein of Galen. The malformation often drains into a persistent falcine sinus and there may be agenesis of the straight sinus and anomalies of other dural venous.
VGAM and dural sinus malformations are the only intracranial AVMS, demonstrated to have been present in the fetal period.

50.----a

51.---e
Exametazime (`°I"Tc-HMPAO) and ethylcysteinedimer (`fI"Tc-ECD) has high extraction efficiency by brain tissue.
About 5% of the injected dose is taken up by brain tissue and only a small proportion of this is washed out in the first few hours after injection, giving an ample time window for imaging. ECD has some practical advantages in that it is more stable in vitro and its extraction efficiency is slightly better than HMPAO, but the kinetics of ECD in abnormal brain are as yet less well established than those of HMPAO.

52----c
The posterior circulation is particularly prone to develop hypertensive encephalopathy – related lesions

53.---e

54.---b
Cholesterol granuloma---hyperintense on both T1W and T2W image

55.---b
Aberrant myelination of neurons is noted in molecular layer.

56.---a
Limbic system localization does not occur in congenital herpes simplex

57.—a

58.---d
Increasing iron deposition in globus pallidus and putamen is a feature of normal aging of brain

59.---b
Arachnoid cyst is located dorsal to

cord
60.---b
Progressive cerebellar atrophy is seen in Louis-Bar synsrome

TEST PAPER 2

1. Which cause should be actively sought as an etiology in any young adult with infarction (particularly posterior fossa infarctions)
a. vasculopathy
b. aortic dissection
c. fibromuscular dysplasia (FMD)
d. collagen vascular diseases
e. lupus erythematosus, and scleroderma

2. All are true regarding DWI-PWI except
a. the perfusion deficit is measured as a prolonged mean transit time or time-to-peak delay
b. PWI deficits > DWI deficit within the first 6 hours of stroke is noted in 70% to 80% of patients
c. PWI > DWI on the initial scan predict DWI expansion into the surrounding lesion
d. the PWI deficit < DWI deficit , reperfusion significantly reduce the eventual infarction size
e. the DWI lesion is due to cytotoxic edema

3. The most common area to undergo ischemic injury in the premature infant is
a. the periventricular white matter
b. thalamus
c. basal ganglia
d. cerebellum
e. frontal cortex

4. All are true regarding forbrain formation except
a. the germinal matrix forms at about 7 weeks
b. neurones that form the deepest cortical layer (6) migrate first
c. neuronal migration and layering process occurs from weeks 6 to 7 through 24 to 26 weeks
d. the corpus callosum forms from back to front except for rostrum
e. cerebral commissure develop between approx. 8 to 17 weeks gestation

5. All are true regarding subdural and epidural hematomas except
a. easily identified by T1- and T2- weighted MR images
b. Traditional morphologic criteria applied to MR images
c. hypointense on MR
d. may be confused with marrow fat
e. pulse sequence used is important

6. The definitive method for fully characterizing the vascular supply and venous drainage of intracranial AVMs
a. MRA
b. CTA
c. catheter angiography
d. doppler study
e. All

7. All are true regarding MRS of Inborn Errors of Metabolism except
a. abnormal accumulation of NAA in the brain in Canavan disease
b. increased lactate in MELAS
c. increase in PDE and PME on ^{31}P MRS in demyelinating disorders
d. increase of Glycine in Nonketotic hyperglycinemia

e. presence of branched-chain amino acids and oxo-acids in maple syrup urine disease

8. All are CT features of cavernous angioma except
a. focal high-attenuation lesion
b. variably present calcification
c. no edema or mass effect
d. strong enhancement
e. less sensitivity than MR for its the detection

9. All are true regarding saccular aneurysm except
a. usually occur at vessel bifurcations
b. typically on the convexity of a curve in the parent vessel
c. multiple in 20% to 25% of aneurysms
d. sylvian fissure hemorrhage typically indicates ICA bifurcation aneurysm rupture
e. anterior interhemispheric blood correlates with ruptured anterior communicating aneurysms

10. All are true regarding duffuse axonal injury except
a. severe loss of consciousness at the moment of impact
b. stage 3 DAI involves the dorsolateral aspect of the midbrain and upper pons
c. Most callosal lesions occur anteriorly
d. Stage 1 DAI typically involves the parasagittal regions of the frontal lobes
e. The corpus callosum is the second-most-common area involved with DAI

.11. The most common demyelinating disease is
a. multiple sclerosis
b. Acute disseminated encephalomyelitis
c. nutritional/vitamin deficiency
d. physical/chemical agents or therapeutic procedures
e. Binswanger disease

12. A child undergoes vaccination for measles and develops fever, headache, meningeal signs and seizure and focal neurological deficit after about three weeks of vaccination. Multifocal areas of high signal intensity are seen on the T2-weighted images in the supratentorial white matter, brainstem, and cerebellum, The masslike lesion show mild mass effect ant there is no enhancement. Follow-up MR demonstrated complete resolution of the lesions on steroid treatment. The most likely diagnosis is
a. multiple sclerosis
b. ADEM
c. Hurst disease
d. Subacute Sclerosing Panencephalitis
e. Progressive Multifocal Leukoencephalopathy

13. All are true regarding Canavan disease except
a. involve both gray and white matter
b. centripetal distribution beginning in the subcortical white matter of the cerebrum and cerebellum
c. relative sparing of the internal and external capsules and corpus callosum
d. characteristic increase in the NAA peak
e. microcrania

14. Radial T2 hypointense bands/stripes are seen in
a. Metachromatic leukodystrophy and Pelizaeus-Merzbacher disease
b. MELAS and Fabry disease
c. CADASIL and Amyloid angiopathy
d. Canavan disease and Pelizaeus-Merzbacher disease
e. Adrenoleukodystrophy and Alexander disease

15. All are true regarding imaging of hippocampus except
a. best performed in a slightly oblique coronal plane, perpendicular to the long axis of hippocampus
b. FLAIR is optimal for quantitative volumetry
c. high-resolution fast spin echo and inversion recovery sequences are important for depiction of hippocampal architecture
d. Conventional / fast spin echo T2-weighted acquisitions are sensitive for assessing hippocampal signal changes
e. Enhancement with intravenous gadolinium has been shown to be of no value in hippocampal sclerosis

16. .All are true regarding magnetic resonance spectroscopy except
a. Reduced N-acetylaspartate (NAA) has been the most important finding in temporal lobe epilepsy.
b. Bilaterally decreased NAA ratios have been associated with surgical failure.
c. abnormally elevated apparent diffusion coefficients (ADCs) is noted in hippocampal sclerosis
d. DTI has been useful in assessing the integrity of the white matter adjacent to the FCD
e. Choline has been suggested to be a dynamic marker of epileptic activity and neuronal function

17. Blood–brain barrier interfaces are seen in
a. the choroid plexus
b. pituitary gland
c. tuber cinereum
d. area postrema
e. basal ganglia

18. All are true regarding imaging of oligodendroglioma except
a. usually heterogeneous but are of relatively lower intensity than astrocytomas (i.e., isointense to gray matter) on T2W
b. the cortical infiltration and marked cortical thickening
c. Diffusion MR imaging highly sensitive to calcification of tumour
d. edema is not usually a significant feature of lower-grade oligodendrogliomas
e.. Contrast enhancement in about one half of cases

19. All are components of Perinaud syndrome of tectal compression except
a. palsy of upward gaze
b. pupillary reflex impaired with light
c. pupillary reflex preserved with accommodation
d. failure of convergence
e. palsy of upward and downward gaze

20. All are true regarding meningioma except
a. mostly in the middle and late decades of life

b. strong male predilection, with a male-to-female ratio of about 2:1
c. Multiple meningiomas are often associated with neurofibromatosis
d. close relationship between the location of the arachnoid granulations and the prevalent sites of origin for meningiomas
e. Approximately 50% of convexity meningiomas are parasagittal / attached to the sagittal sinus

21. All are true regarding dermoid cyst except
a. marked hypointensity on T1W due to triglycerides and unsaturated fatty acids
b. inhomogenous hyperintensity similar to epidermoid tumors on T2W
c. droplets and streaks of high intensity within the subarachnoid cisterns
d. a fat–fluid level in the anterior superior portions of ventricle
e. chemical shift artifact

22. All are true regarding imaging of ependymoma except
a. The mixed higher densities seen within the tumor due to calcification or hemorrhage
b. inhomogenous Contrast enhancement on CT and MRI
c. frequent presence of hydrocephalus
d. elevation of creatine, elevation of choline, and decrease in NAA
e. both the brain and the spinal canal are examined preoperatively

23. All are true regarding hypothalamic hamartoma except
a. present with precocious puberty and/or gelastic seizures
b. uniformly isointense to white matter on T1-weighted imaging
c. do not show enhancement
d. hyperintense or isointense to gray matter on T2-weighted imaging
e. nonneoplastic in nature

24. Kuru disease is characterized by all except
a. progressive cerebellar ataxia
b. dementia a prominent feature.
c. high incidence in Fore linguistic group
d. due to ritual cannibalism
e. high prevalence in Papua New Guinea

25. The sine qua non of pyogenic abscess is
a. smooth ring enhancement of capsule
b. hypointense rim on T2-weighted images
c. hyperintense center
d. daughter abscess
e. hyperintense rim on T1W

26. All are true regading brain abscess except
a. an abscess often exhibit mesial thinning of the ring
b. Abscesses tend to demonstrate high signal intensity on DWI
c. lactate and pyruvate are fairly specific markers for pyogenic abscesses
d. an amino acid peak (valine, leucine, and isoleucine) at 0.9 ppm are seen in necrotic/cystic tumour
e. The spectra of S. aureus abscesses donot demonstrate increased peaks of succinate and acetate or amino acid resonance

27. All the parts of brain shows

hyperintense signal normally on T2W except
a. the parietopontine tracts of the posterior limb of the internal capsule
b. Triangular-shaped regions posterior and superior to the trigones
c. anterior and lateral to the frontal horns
d. ependymitis granularis
e. periaqueductal areas

28. All are true regarding Wilson disease except
a. abnormal copper deposition
b. most pronounced involvement in the liver and brain
c. results from excessive function of the copper transport protein
d. autosomal recessive
e. peak age at presentation is between 8 and 16 years

29. All are true regarding NF1 except
a. dehiscence and dysplasia of the sphenoid bone
b. intra- and extracranial arterial dysplasia
c. moyamoya disease
d. dysplastic neural foraminal enlargement
e. acquired meningoceles.

30. Unenhanced fluid-attenuated inversion recovery sequence in a child reveals a bright pial signal, the "Ivy" sign. This sign is noted in
a. tuberous sclerosis
b. SWS
c. NF1
d. NF2
e. VHL

31. All are true regarding corpus callosum agenesis except
a. colpocephaly
b. a crescentic shape of lateral ventricle in the coronal plane view
c. medial convexity of the frontal horns
d., parallel lateral ventricles
e. secondary interdigitation of gyri across the midline

32. All are true regarding the developmental venous anomaly (DVA) except
a. The most common sites of DVA are the temporal lobes and the posterior fossa
b. may be associated with the Sturge-Weber syndrome
c. sinus pericranii may be seen
d. the caput medusae is usually seen within the deep white matter
e. DVAs may drain to the superficial or deep venous system

33. All are true regarding nerve sheath tumour except
a. the most common intraspinal lesion in the general population
b. Schwannomas generally are solitary
c. neurofibromas envelop in the dorsal sensory root
d. neurofibromas frequently are multiple
e. Schwannomas usually are associated with neurofibromatosis

34-. All are true regarding Spinal Dural Arteriovenous Fistula(SDAVFs) except
a. acquired lesions
b. present after the fourth or fifth decade
c. most commonly occur at cervical level
d. dilated pial veins of the cord,

most commonly along the dorsal surface
e. spinal angiographic remains the gold standard for confirming the diagnosis,

35. All are true regading embryogenesis except
a. The epiblast give rise to all future ectoderm, mesoderm, and endoderm of the embryo
b. The hypoblastic cells form the extraembryonic tissues
c. The prochordal plate establishes the caudal end of the bilaminar disk
d. The thickening at the cephalic end of the primitive streak is designated as Hensen's node
e. At about day 13 the primitive streak forms in the midline at the caudal end of the epiblast

36. Scimitar sacrum is seen in
a. anterior sacral meningoceles
b. sacral agenesis
c. sacral chordoma
d. sacral fusion
e. sacrum variant

37. All are true regarding neuroenteric cyst
a. wide spinal canal with widened interpediculate distance noted in neuroenteric cyst
b. Persistence of a patent neurenteric canal (canal of Kovalevsky) lead to neurenteric cysts.
c. Neurenteric cysts exhibit a definite connection with the spinal cord and/or vertebrae
d. Spina bifida and segmentation anomalies of the bodies are common in neuroenteric cyst
e. the neurenteric cysts shows contrast enhancement

38. All are true regarding "empty sella turcica" except
a. severely flattened pituitary gland
b. the superior portion of the sella turcica filled with CSF
c. the diaphragma sella thin
d. enlargement of the sella turcica
e. abnormally positioned stalk

39. All are true regarding meningioma except
a. most frequently isointense relative to gray matter on unenhanced T1-weighted images
b. 50% remain isointense on the T2-weighted images
c. Vascular encasement is common, particularly with meningiomas in the cavernous sinus
d. the "dural tail sign" together with the characteristic wide dural base is the most distinctive feature
e. phosphorus MR spectroscopy is of no use in distinguishing pituitary adenomas from meningiomas

40. All are true regarding optic nerve lesions except
a. perioptic (optic sheath) meningiomas most common in men (80%) in their third to fifth decades
b. CT demonstrate intense enhancement, calcifications, and adjacent hyperostosis of bone in perioptic (optic sheath) meningiomas
c. MR easily distinguishing optic nerve lesions from sheath lesions
d. MR is superior to CT for visualizing the intracanalicular

portion of the optic nerve
e. direct oblique parasagittal MR imaging provide exquisite anatomic delineation of the course of the optic nerve through the orbital apex

41. All are true regarding MRS of Inborn Errors of Metabolism except
a. abnormal accumulation of NAA in the brain in Canavan disease
b. increased lactate in MELAS
c. increase in PDE and PME on ^{31}P MRS in demyelinating disorders
d. increase of Glycine in Nonketotic hyperglycinemia
e. presence of branched-chain amino acids and oxo-acids in maple syrup urine disease

42. All are true regarding the great vein of Galen except
a. formed by the confluence of internal cerebral and basal veins
b. unpaired
c. lies in the quadrigeminal cistern
c. show upward concavity delineating the posterior end of the corpus callosum
e. discharge into the lateral sinus.

43. All are true regarding Dysembryoplastic neuroepithelial tumours (DNETs) except
a. preferentially located in the supratentorial cortex
b. usually hypodense on CT
c. 'bubbly' appearance due to small intratumoural cyst
d. Calcification -- seen in about 25 per cent
e. enhancement noted as a rule

44. Blistering of sphenoid sinus is seen in
a. suprasellar meningioma
b. parasellar meningioma
c. craniopharyngioma
d. optic nerve glioma
e. Rathke cleft cyst

45. Which lesions in HIV-related CNS disease cause masss in basal ganglia
a. Cryptococcomas
b. Lymphoma
c. PML
d. Tuberculosis
e. Candida

6. All are true regarding anatomy of spine except
a. fatty marrow constitute up to 50 per cent of spinal marrow volume in adults
b. the spinal canal is widest and almost circular at C1
c. an AP diameter of 15 mm plus seems ideal in the lumber spine
d. disc margins may normally bulge up to 2–3 mm beyond the vertebral margins
e., posterior surface of disc is normally convex

47. All are true regarding normal myelination except
a. corpus callosum is myelinated completly at 4 months
b. internal capsule demonstrate T1 shortening within the anterior limb by 3 months
c. the peritrigonal areas may show persistent hyperintensity on T2W well into adulthood
d. fronto-temporal subcortical white matter may persist as regions of signal hyperintensity beyond 2 years
e. the brain is fully myelinated by T1 criteria after 10 months

48. All are true regarding Sturge–Weber syndrome except

a. leptomeningeal angiomas with a primarily fronto –parietal distribution
b. abnormal venous drainage with chronic ischaemia
c. involved hemisphere progressively becomes atrophied
d. enlargement of the ipsilateral choroid plexus
e. 'tramline calcifications' on x ray of skull by the age of 2yrs

49. All are true regarding pediatric stroke except
a. Sickle cell disease is the most common cause of ischaemic stroke in children worldwide
b. sickle cell disease may cause infarction typically in MCA territory
c. progressive stenosis of the terminal ICA and proximal segments of the major intracranial arteries in Moya-Moya disease
d. multiple small flow voids within the basal ganglia in Moya-Moya disease
e. Moya moya accounts for up to 30% of cerebral vasculopathy in paediatric stroke

50. Intravenous thrombolysis with recombinant tissue plasminogen activator (rTPA) has been approved for the treatment of acute ischacmic stroke
a. within 2 hours of onset
b. within 3 hours of onset
c. within 4 hours of onset
d. within 5 hours of onset
e. within 6 hours of onset

51. All increases risk of hemorrhage of cerebral AVM except
a. false aneurysms
b venous ectasias
c. multiple draining vein
d. deep venous drainage
e. venous stenosis

52. Rounded lucent area with a characteristic stippled appearance in the skull is seen in
a. dermoid cyst
b. epidermoid
c. haemangioma
d. chordoma
e. meningioma

53. All are causes of basal ganglia calcification except
a. Toxoplasmosis
b. Fahr's syndrome
c. Cockayne's syndrome
d. Carbon dioxide poisoning
e. Mitochondrial cytopath

54. All are true regarding hypertensive intracerebral haemorrhage except
a. predilection for areas supplied by penetrating branches of the middle crebral artery and basilar arteries
b. prefentially involves the external capsule and putamen
c. poor prognosis when haemorrhage dissects into fouth ventricle
d. most common cause of lobar white haemorrhage
e. cerebellum relatively rarely involved

55. All are features of lateral medullary syndrome on ipsilateral side except
a. Horner syndrome
b. atxia
c. facial pain
d. dysphagia
e. decreased pain and temperature in trunk and extremities

56. All are true regarding CPA masses except
a. acoustic swannoma ---Ice cone appearance
b. meningioma ---strong enhancement
c. epidermoid ---insinuates along cisterns
d. epidermoid cyst ---strong enhancement
e. meningioma ---calcification common

57. All are true regarding ganglioglioma except
a. most common location --- temporal lobe
b. cyst with non-calficied mural nodule
c. scalloped appearance of calvarium
d. strong enhancement
e. most patients under 30yrs

58. All are true regarding congenital infection of brain except
a. CMV—predilection for germinal matrix
b. Toxoplasmosis ----neuronal migrational abnormalities
c. Toxoplasmosis---multifocal and scattered lesions
d. Toxoplasmosis ---hydrocephalus
e. Rubella –micocephaly

59. Macrocephaly is seen in all except
a. Alexander disease
b. Canavan disease
c. Hurler disease
d. Hunter disease
e. ALD

60. All are true regarding white matter hyperintensities (WMHs) except
a. subcortical WHMs may be due to myelin pallor
b. the extent and frequency of central WMHs are closely related to age
c. "caps" adjacent to the frontal horns are normal finding in patients of all ages
d. thin smooth periventricular rims are indicative of NPH
e. patchy periventricular hyperintensities are more common in hypertension

TEST PAPER 2(ANSWER)

1.----b
2.----d
DWI-PWI mismatch criteria may identify patients who will benefit from early reperfusion with acute stroke therapies. In those patients in whom the PWI deficit is already smaller than the DWI deficit, reperfusion is not likely significantly to affect the eventual infarction size.
3.----a
Periventricular white matter ------ the vascular watershed zone in developing fetus and has a relatively high metabolic demand.

4.—d
The corpus callosum forms from front to back except for rostrum., which forms in the last
5.---e
Subdural and epidural hematomas can be easily identified by T1- and T2-weighted MR images, because the contrast between calvarium (marrow and cortical bone) and blood is high regardless of what pulse sequence is used. Perhaps the most common pitfall of evaluating extraaxial hematomas by MR is potential confusion of marrow fat with hyperintense blood.
6.---a
Associated hemorrhage and other parenchymal changes and posttherapy follow-up of AVMs are best evaluated with the use of MR in conjunction with supplemental MRA.
7.---c

In demyelinating disorders, ^{31}P MRS has been shown to be a helpful tool because the loss of membrane phospholipids leads to decreases in PDE and PME that are readily detected.
8.---d
Enhancement of cavernous angima is typically mild on CT but may not be identifiable.
9.—d
Sylvian fissure hemorrhage typically indicates MCA bifurcation aneurysm rupture
10.---c
The corpus callosum is the second-most-common area involved with DAI (21% of DAI lesions). DAI of the corpus callosum invariably occurs in conjunction with DAI of the lobar white matter (stage 2 DAI). Most callosal lesions (72%) occur in the posterior body and splenium.
11---a
12.----b
13----e
Canavan disease is seen predominantly in children of Ashkenazi Jewish decent. It is due to deficiency of NAA acylase with excessive accumulation of NAA Macrocrania is seen in Canavan disease.
The signal abnormality in Canavan disease has a centripetal distribution beginning in the subcortical white matter of the cerebrum and cerebellum. Typically, there is diffuse, symmetric increased signal intensity on the T2-weighted

images throughout the white matter, with relative sparing of the internal and external capsules and corpus callosum . High signal intensity is always seen within the globus pallidus, with frequent involvement of the thalamus and relative sparing of the putamen and caudate nucleus

14.---a
Subcortical U fiber involvement is noted in Canavan disease, Pelizaeus-Merzbacher disease

15.----b
Coronal, T1-weighted, three-dimensional volume gradient echo is optimal for quantitative volumetry

16.---e
Reduced N-acetylaspartate (NAA) has been the most important finding in temporal lobe epilepsy. NAA is a marker of metabolically active neurons, and decreased NAA:creatine or decreased NAA:(creatine + choline) ratio signifies neuronal loss and/or metabolic dysfunction. A decrease in these ratios has been shown to lateralize temporal lobe epilepsy in 65% to 96% of patients with bilateral temporal lobe structural abnormalities on MR . In cases of temporal lobe epilepsy with normal MR studies, NAA ratios can provide lateralizing evidence in at least 20% of patients .
Bilaterally decreased NAA ratios have been associated with surgical failure.
NAA has been suggested to be a dynamic marker of epileptic activity and neuronal function and not simply a reflector of decreased neuronal number.

17.----e
Blood–brain barrier interfaces are not found in some regions of the brain, notably the choroid plexus, pituitary gland, tuber cinereum, area postrema, and pineal gland.

18.---c
Gradient echo imaging (not Conventional spin echo and diffusion) MR imaging is highly sensitive to calcification .Linear or nodular tumoral calcification on CT has been reported in 50% to 90% of oligodendrogliomas, which are the intracranial tumors with the highest frequency of calcification .
Pronounced thickening of cortex in a heterogeneous intraaxial mass should prompt the consideration of oligodendroglioma.
Calvarial erosion is seen

19---e
Parinaud syndrome of tectal compression comprises of palsy of upward gaze, pupillary reflex impaired with light but preserved with accommodation, and failure of convergence.

20.----b
There is a strong female predilection, with a female-to-male ratio of about 2:1. Approximately 50% of convexity meningiomas are parasagittal or attached to the sagittal sinus. Other favorite sites include the dura adjacent to the anterior sylvian fissure region, the sphenoid wings, tuberculum sellae, perisellar region, and olfactory grooves.

They may also arise from the optic nerve sheath intraorbitally or extend into the optic foramen from a tuberculum sella tumor.
In the posterior fossa they frequently arise from the petrous bone in the cerebellopontine angle, the clivus, the tentorial leaf, and the tentorial free margin.
Meningiomas are usually broad based and firmly attach to the adjacent dura but can arise without any dural attachments apparently from pial meningeal cells. These pial-based meningiomas may be found in the depths of the sylvian fissure or may present intraventricularly, usually in the lateral ventricle but occasionally in the third and fourth ventricles arising from either the tela choroidea or arachnoidal cell rest within the stroma of the choroid plexus.

21.---a

Marked hyperintensity on T1W is noted in dermoid cyst due to triglycerides and unsaturated fatty acids

A chemical shift artifact is frequently projected into the lesion on long-TR sequences. On T1-weighted sequences a high-intensity fluid level is present anterior to the hypointensity of CSF, whereas on long-TR sequences an intermediate and low-intensity fluid collection is observed anterior to the high intensity of the CSF.

22.---d

Proton spectroscopy is a useful adjunct to the imaging studies because ependymomas have a different spectrum than do astrocytomas and PNETs, with preservation of creatine, elevation of choline, and decrease in NAA . The creatine is not preserved in PNET and astrocytoma.
Ependymomas are known for the production of calcification and for a tendency to bleed.

23.----b

Hypothalamic hamartomas are uniformly isointense to gray matter on T1-weighted imaging, and in two thirds of cases they are slightly hyperintense or isointense to gray matter on T2-weighted imaging . They do not show enhancement.

24----b

Kuru is clinically characterized by progressive cerebellar ataxia, and, in contrast to CJD, dementia is not a prominent feature. The human prion disease syndrome most often associated with dementia is CJD

25.---a

The sine qua non of abscess—smooth ring enhancement of an abscess capsule on postgadolinium MR images—is the most important part of distinguishing a nonneoplastic from a neoplastic brain mass because nearly all enhancing brain lesions can present with ring enhancement.

MR enhancement parallels the enhancement seen on postcontrast CT images . The abscess ring is most commonly very smooth, regular in thickness, and thin walled (approximately 5 mm in thickness),although it may

be thinner along its medial margin, possibly due to variations in perfusion of gray and white matter. Only infrequently, nodular or solid enhancement, incomplete thin rings, or thick and irregular rings may be observed, and these should make the radiologist consider other diagnoses.
Daughter abscesses appear as adjacent smaller enhancing rings, often along the medial margin of the parent abscess, and can masquerade as a thick irregularity in the abscess wall at cursory inspection

The evolution to abscess is a continuous process and has been characterized by four stages: early cerebritis, late cerebritis, early capsule formation, and late capsule formation. The early stage of cerebritis (3 to 5 days) is characterized by a focal infection with a variable number of microorganisms, associated with the presence of polymorphonuclears, edema, and petechial hemorrhage.

In the later phase of cerebritis (4 to 5 days up to 2 weeks), the necrotic foci coalesce; a rim of mononuclear inflammatory cells surrounds the necrotic area. The next stage is the early capsule (about 2 weeks), with a well-defined collagenous capsule involving the necrotic core surrounded by reactive astrocytosis and edema in the adjacent brain. In the final stage, the late capsule (weeks to months), the collagen capsule is complete and the surrounding area of cerebritis extends only minimally beyond the capsule, which is less well developed on its ventricular side than on its cortical side, probably related to slight differences in perfusion. Daughter abscesses become apparent during this stage. The length of time required to form a mature abscess varies from 2 weeks to several months. Most patients present in the late cerebritis or mature abscess stage.

26.---d
The differential diagnosis for a ring-enhancing lesion includes primary brain tumor (high-grade astrocytoma), metastasis, infarction (bland or septic), resolving hematoma, thrombosed aneurysm, arteriovenous malformation, radiation necrosis, AIDS-related lymphoma, and other inflammatory conditions (e.g., demyelinating disease, granulomata, etc.)

Abscesses tend to demonstrate high signal intensity on DWI, with a corresponding reduction in the apparent diffusion coefficient values This is directly related to the cellularity and viscosity of the pus contained within an abscess cavity. In contrast, high-grade gliomas and metastases with central necrosis have a low signal on DWI and high apparent diffusion coefficient values .Nonbacterial abscesses often do not show restricted diffusion.
The MR spectroscopy (MRS) pattern derived from the central portion of an abscess appears to be fairly characteristic. Thus, MRS

seems to contribute to distinguishing an abscess from a necrotic brain tumor and a tuberculoma
. In an untreated abscess, resonances may be seen corresponding to acetate (1.92 ppm), lactate (1.3 ppm), alanine (1.5 ppm), succinate (2.4 ppm), and pyruvate, as well as a complex peak at 0.9 ppm indicating amino acids valine, leucine, and isoleucine .
Acetate, lactate, succinate, and pyruvate are metabolic end products arising from microorganisms .
Acetate and succinate are not seen in association with necrotic tumors and are therefore fairly specific markers for pyogenic abscesses. However, these two resonances are not consistently identified in all abscess cavities
In vivo MRS does reveal an amino acid peak (valine, leucine, and isoleucine) at 0.9 ppm, which can be found in all abscesses but not in necrotic/cystic tumors .
The central portion of a necrotic/cystic tumor often reveals only a lactate resonance peak. Thus, the presence of amino acid inverted peak at 0.9 ppm seems to be a reliable indicator of a pyogenic abscess
MRS can also be of some use in the etiologic classification of brain abscesses because different MR spectra can be obtained from specific underlying agents .
It could be possible to differentiate an anaerobic from a pyogenic brain abscess, as well as from aerobic and sterile lesions. The selective presence of succinate and acetate in the anaerobic abscess is probably the result of the involvement of alternative anaerobic pathways for energy demands, enhancing glycolysis and the fermentative pathways for energy generation .
The spectra of S. aureus abscesses do not demonstrate increased peaks of succinate and acetate or amino acid resonance.
Resonances of lipids and lactates dominate the MR spectra of such lesions.

27.-----e
Posterior and superior to the trigones that are variably hyperintense on T2-weighted images are normal in patients in their first and second decades. Hyperintense foci on T2-weighted images exist in virtually all normal patients anterior and lateral to the frontal horns. This region displays ependymitis granularis, which refers to a focal breakdown of the ependymal lining with adjacent astrocytic gliosis.

28.---c
The Wilson results from loss of function of the copper transport protein ATP7B.
The differential diagnosis of unexplained hepatic disease in a young patient should include WD .
Neurologic and/or psychiatric manifestations more commonly present in young adults aged 19 to 20 years.
The Kayser-Fleischer ring, a granular deposit of copper in Descemet's membrane of the

cornea, is virtually diagnostic of WD . The definitive diagnosis is made biochemically, with low levels of serum ceruloplasmin, increased rate of urinary copper excretion, and elevated hepatic copper levels

once the diagnosis is established in symptomatic patients with WD, screening of all first-degree relatives (siblings and children) is necessary to detect presymptomatic patients who would benefit from treatment to prevent hepatic and cerebral disease and to detect asymptomatic carriers who would benefit from genetic counseling.

29.----e

Dysplastic neural foraminal enlargement, and acquired meningoceles are seen in NF1.The lateral thoracic meningocele is strongly suggestive of NF1. These lesions represent a pulsion diverticulum of the spinal subarachnoid space. This occurs in the thorax because there are no paravertebral muscles overlying the neural foramina and because there is a larger pressure difference between the negative intrathoracic pressure and normal cerebrospinal fluid (CSF) pressure of the subarachnoid space.

Bony spinal abnormalities include kyphoscoliosis, which may involve a short segment and be acutely angled, progressive vertebral scalloping, and enlargement of the spinal canal

30.---b

31.---c

The corpus callosum is the most concentrated bundle of axons in the brain

The bundles of Probst invaginate the medial borders of the lateral ventricles to give them a crescentic shape when viewed in the coronal plane .The features that are well seen on axial images include the characteristic lateral convexity of the frontal horns, parallel lateral ventricles, colpocephaly, upward extension of the third ventricle between the lateral ventricles , and secondary interdigitation of gyri across the midline owing to partial absence of the falx in the interhemispheric fissure . Midline sagittal images on MRI reveal the full extent of the features of callosal dysgenesis.

32.----a

The most common sites of DVA are the frontal lobes and the posterior fossa .The final periods of intracranial venous development described by Padgett are stages 7 and 7a, referring to the "threshold of fetal period" and "fetus at the third month" . These periods are of particular interest because it is at this time that much of the definitive cerebral venous system appears

33.—e

Schwannomas do not envelop the adjacent nerve root, which usually is the dorsal sensory root, generally are solitary, and clinically are not typical of neurofibromatosis . In contrast, neurofibromas envelop the dorsal sensory root, frequently are multiple, and usually are associated with neurofibromatosis, even when single.

34---c
Spinal Dural Arteriovenous Fistula(SDAVFs) is the most common spinal vascular malformation.
It most commonly occur at thoracolumbar levels, usually between T5 and L3
The pathology of Spinal Dural Arteriovenous Fistula(SDAVFs) cause the disorder referred to as Foix-Alajouanine syndrome
The presence of symptoms in SDAVF is an indication for treatment because the benefits are multiple and the risks minimal .
First-line treatment of SDAVF is usually accomplished with endovascular techniques. Endovascular occlusion of SDAVF is possible in greater than 80% of cases and can be accomplished at the same time as the diagnostic angiogram by using permanent liquid embolic agents such as N-butylcyanoacrylate
In contrast, the use of particulate emboli for occlusion of SDAVF results in nearly 100% recanalization with progression of neurologic deficits and is contraindicated . If endovascular therapy is unsuccessful or contraindicated, surgical coagulation or resection of the nidus and
surrounding dura can be safely performed in nearly all cases

35.----c
The prochordal plate establishes the cranial end of the bilaminar disk

36.---a

37.—e
The neurenteric cysts doesnot shows contrast enhancement

38.---e
It is the deficiency of the diaphragma that is the primary defect in "empty sella turcica". This allows the suprasellar cistern to herniate into the sella, exposing it to CSF pulsation and eventually resulting in enlargement of the sella turcica. The only differential diagnosis is that of an arachnoid cyst occupying the superior portion of the sella turcica. It is important to determine the position of the pituitary stalk to distinguish these entities. In the empty sella, the stalk is normal in position, whereas space-occupying cysts cause it to be obliterated or displaced

39.---e
It has been reported that phosphorus MR spectroscopy may be used in distinguishing pituitary adenomas from meningiomas because pituitary adenomas have a much higher phosphate monoester peak than meningiomas.

40.----a
Perioptic (optic sheath) meningiomas most common in women (80%) in their third to fifth decades

41.---c
In demyelinating disorders, ^{31}P MRS has been shown to be a helpful tool because the loss of

membrane phospholipids leads to decreases in PDE and PME that are readily detected.

42.---e
The confluence of both internal cerebral and both basal veins gives rise to the unpaired great vein of Galen, which lies in the quadrigeminal cistern and shows a characteristic upward concavity as it delineates the posterior end of the corpus callosum before discharging into the straight sinus.

43.----e
DNETs are usually hypodense on CT and T1-hypointense and T2-hyperintense on MRI. Thinning of the overlying bone is present in approximately half of the cases, reflecting the extremely slow growth of these tumours, which allows bone remodelling to occur

44.---a
Suprasellar meningiomas often show a forward extension along the dura mater of the anterior cranial fossa and are associated with dilatation ('blistering') of the sphenoid sinus
Parasellar meningiomas are strongly enhancing masses that expand the cavernous sinus and frequently encase and narrow of the cavernous portion of the internal carotid arteries..
Intracranial extension of optic nerve sheath meningiomas characteristically involves the planum shenoidale.

45.---a
Toxoplasmosis produce mass in basal ganglia

46.----e
The disc margins may normally bulge up to 2–3 mm beyond the vertebral margins, especially in children. The posterior surface is normally flat or concave, not convex (except at L5/S1).

47.----a
The splenium of the corpus callosum on T2-weighted images becomes hypointense at 3 months of age. The hypointense signal extends anteriorly along the body and genu, and the complete corpus callosum is myelinated at 6 months.
Regions of persistent hyperintensity on T2-weighted sequences known as the 'terminal myelination zones' may be seen within the peritrigonal areas well into adulthood, and can be distinguished from white matter disease by the presence of a rim of normal myelinated brain between these areas and the ventricular margin

48.---a
Sturge–Weber syndrome is a congenital syndrome characterized by a port-wine naevus on the face and ipsilateral leptomeningeal angiomas with a primarily parieto-occipital distribution

49.----b
The imaging pattern of infarction in Sickle cell disease is typically of arterial watershed infarction between the major cerebral arterial territories. A fifth of strokes in sickle cell disease may be haemorrhagic.

50.----b
51.----c

Single draining vein is the risk factor.
52.---c
53.----d
Idiopathic,Familial,Hypoparathyroidism,Pseudohypoparathyroidism,Fahr's syndrome,Cockayne's syndrome,Carbon monoxide poisoning,Lead poisoningToxoplasmosis,Mineralising microangiopathy,Secondary hyperparathyroidism.Mitochondrial cytopathy are causes of basal ganglia calcification
54.---e
Cerebellum is ralatively commonly involved ,the midbrain,medulla and spinal cord are rarely involved.
55.---e
Decreased pain and temperature in trunk and extremities occurs on contralateral side
56.---d
Enhancement in epidermoid is rare
57.---b

Mural nodule in ganglioglioma is often calcified
58.---b
Toxoplasmosis is not associated with neuronal migrational abnormalities.CMV is associated with neuronal migrational abnormalities
59.---e
ALD and Alexander disease show contrast enhancement
60.---d
Thin, smooth periventricular rims are not indicative of NPH.. Patchy periventricular hyperintensities are more common in hypertension or NPH.

TEST PAPER 3

1. The most common site for atherosclerotic plaque formation in the carotid circulation is
a. at the carotid bifurcation with involvement of the distal common carotid artery and the first 2 cm of the internal carotid artery.
b. at the carotid bifurcation with involvement of the distal common carotid artery and the first 2 cm of the external carotid artery.
c. at the carotid bifurcation with involvement of the distal common carotid artery and the first 4 cm of the internal carotid artery.
d. the carotid siphon region and the proximal portions of the anterior and middle cerebral arteries.
e. origin of common carotid artery and the first 2 cm of the internal carotid arter

2. All are true regarding diffusion imaging in stroke except
a. DWI changes have been observed in less than 1 hour after the onset of ischemia
b. the ADC map shows hyperintensity beyond 10 days of stroke
c. Infarcts with greater percentages of low ADC values have higher rates of hemorrhagic transformation
d. Enhancement and restricted diffusion often coexist in arterial infarction.
e. DWI of lesion volumes enlarge over time after the acute stroke.

3. Investigation that provides greater sensitivity for the detection of infarction in children
a. USG
b. CT
c. MRI
d. PET
e. x ray

4. All are true except
a. methemoglobin contain the ferrous state of iron with five d electrons.
b. too high or too low O_2 retard conversion to methemoglobin
c. the hemichromes is a state of iron
d. methemoglobin enhance relaxivity effects on T1 and T2 relaxation
e. Glial cells show phagocytic activity

5. MRI of brain shows parenchymal siderosis. All are true except
a. marked hypointensity along the parenchymal surfaces on T2-weighted images.
b. The cerebrum is a particularly common site for hemosiderin deposition in siderosis
c. Intracranial hemorrhage from tumors that continue to bleed can result in superficial hemosiderosis.
d. Intraventricular siderosis is a common sequela of neonatal intraventricular hemorrhage
e. intraventricular siderosis in an adult is usually from vascular malformations and aneurysms.

6. All are true regarding treatment of AVMs except
a. untreated case shows grim prognosis

b. the goal of management is complete obliteration of the nidus for cure
c. the nidus less than 3.5 cm suitable for radiosurgery
d. the effect of radiosurgery takes months to years
e. Endovascular treatment is usually primary treatment

7. Angiographically "occult cerebrovascular malformations" refers to
a. AVMs
b. cavernous angioma
c. capillary telangiectasia
d. venous angioma
e. developmental venous anomaly

8. All are true regarding saccular aneurysm except
a. most common variety
b. mostly isolated
c. Hemodynamic stresses -- the most likely cause
d. typically at circle of Willis in case of septic emboli
e. usually occur at vessel bifurcations.

9. All are true regarding diffuse axonal injury (DAI) except
a. usually ovoid to elliptical with the long axis parallel to the direction of the involved axonal tracts
b. multiple, small (5 to 15 mm) focal lesions
c. Most lesions spare the overlying cortex
d. frequently located at the gray–white matter interface
e. usually (80%) hemorrhagic in nature

10. All are true regarding MR spectroscopy except
a. NAA peak is a marker of normal neuronal adult tissue
b. reduction of NAA suggests neuronal damage
c. choline peak is prominent early in brain development
d. choline is considered a glial cell marker
e. progressive reduction of myo-inositol and choline with progressing fetal development

11. All are true regarding optic neuritis except
a. routine spin echo sequences highly sensitive
b. optic neuritis is often the first evidence of MS
c. MR appears to be important in prognosis of optic neuritis.
d. 45% to 80% of isolated case develop MS during the next 15 years
e. most of isolated case optic neuritis MS within the first 5 years

12. All are correctly matched imaging finding except
a. multiple strokelike lesions primarily in the parietal and occipital cortex - MELAS
b. calcification of the dentate nucleus and globus pallidus---MERRF
c. predilection for involvement of the peripheral U fibers and sparing of the periventricular white matter ---KSS
d. high signal in bilateral symmetric basal ganglia (particularly putamen)--- Leigh
e. Prominent extraaxial spaces----Maple syrup urine disease

13. Macrocephaly is seen in
a. Alexander disease and MELAS
b. Alexander disease and Canavan

disease
c. Krabbe disease and Canavan disease
d. Alexander disease and ALD
e. ALD and Canavan disease

14. All are true regarding hippocampal formation except
a. infolding of hippocampal components occurs around the hippocampal sulcus.
b. Obliteration of the hippocampal sulcus starts from its lateral side
c. infolding of hippocampal components occurs due to unequal growth within the hippocampus.
d. fusion of the molecular strata of the dentate gyrus with the subiculum results in the obliteration of the hippocampal sulcus
e. The alveus and fimbria changes orientation from horizontal to vertical course

15. All are true related to epilepsy except
a. hippocampal sulcus remnant is a normal variation
b. asymmetry of calcar avis can be misinterpreted as cortical dysplasia
c. in cortical dysplasia, cortical thickening persists in its orthogonal plane
d. hippocampus body usually has elongated shape in the coronal plane.
e. In Rasmussen encephalitis, signal changes may be transient and shift in location

16. All are true regarding blood brain barrier except
a. Endothelial cells of cerebral capillaries have fused membranes
b. Endothelial cells of cerebral capillaries have continuous basement membranes
c. Endothelial cells of cerebral capillaries have wide intercellular gaps
d. a paucity of pinocytosis
e. cerebral capillary endothelium closely surrounded by a sheath of astrocytic foot processes

17. All are true regarding oligodendroglioma except
a. The peak incidence in the fourth to fifth decades
b. mostly located superficially in the frontal and frontotemporal cortex
c. densely cellular, with only minimal acellular stroma
d. the "fried egg" artifact---the presence of perinuclear halos
e. calcification ---extremely rare

18. All are true regarding imaging of haemangioblastoma except
a. frequently cystic
b. avascular solid nodules
c. a peripheral pial-based mural nodule of solid tissue
d. enhancement of mural nodule after intravenous contrast
e. large vessels within and/or at the periphery of the mass

19. The most common primary nonglial intracranial tumor is
a. meningioma
b. schwannoma
c. arachnoid cyst
d. medulloblastoma
e. dermoid cyst

20. All are true regarding dermoid cyst except
a. usually present in the third decade

b. most commonly located in the anterior fossa in the midline
c. mar contain hair follicles ,sebaceous, sweat, and apocrine glands.
d. Calcification may develop in the portion of the walls,
e. may be bone and cartilage within some of the cysts

21. All are true regarding imaging of ependymoma except
a. The mixed higher densities seen within the tumor due to calcification or hemorrhage
b. inhomogenous Contrast enhancement on CT and MRI
c. frequent presence of hydrocephalus
d. elevation of creatine, elevation of choline, and decrease in NAA
e. both the brain and the spinal canal are examined preoperatively

22. All are true regarding craniopharyngioma except
a. The cyst fluid is of lower density than that of CSF
b. 90% are partially cystic
c. 90% are suprasellar
d. 90% enhance
e. hyperintense on T2

23. All are true regarding brain development except
a. Neural plate forms at about 2 weeks
b. proximal two third of the neural tube forms the future brain
c. closure of the neural tube begins in the midbrain
d. diencephalon forms from mesencephalon
e. psosencephalon give rise to telencephalon

24. All are true regarding the parietopontine tracts of the posterior limb of the internal capsule except
a. On axial images at the level of the velum interpositum
b. medial to the distal putamen near the junction of the posterior limb and retrolenticular portion of the internal capsule
c. oval, and symmetric low signal intensity on T2W
d. do not demonstrate intravenous contrast enhancement .
e. not seen in patients younger than the age of 10 years

25. All are true regarding the "eye-of-the-tiger" sign except
a. coined by Sethi et al
b. low signal intensity surrounding a central region of high signal intensity on T2W
c. in the anteromedial globus pallidus
d. mutation-negative, NBAI-1 patients
e. Abnormal iron deposition within the globus pallidus

26. All are true regarding optic nerve glioma (ONG) in NF1 except
a. The chiasma are more likely to be involved in NF1
b. the shape of the optic pathways is preserved in NF1
c. the tumor is smaller in NF1
d. extension beyond the optic pathway at diagnosis is uncommon in NF1
e. cystic components are less common in the NF1

27. The most sensitive test for revealing the full extent of the lesions in SWS

a. CT
b. MRI
c. USG
d. PET-CT
e. x ray

28. All are true regarding cortical dyplasia of Tylor(CDT) except
a. CDT-D has balloon cells within dysplastic areas
c. CDT resembles the cortical tubers of tuberous sclerosis
d. common cause of epilepsy attributable to focal cerebral dysgenesis
e. blurring of the gray–white matter junction
e. High-resolution imaging useful

29. All are true regarding callosal malformations except
a. the bundles of Probst run parallel to and indent the medial walls of the lateral ventricles
b. persistent eversion of the cingulate gyrus in absence of corpus callosum
c. The third ventricle and foramina of Monro are usually widened in callosal agenesis
d. the third ventricle often extends superiorly between the bodies of the lateral ventricles in callosal agenesis
e. dilation of the trigones, occipital horns, and posterior temporal horns

30. All are true regarding Vein of Galen Malformation except
a. Newborns with choroidal malformations typically develop signs of congestive heart failure and multiorgan failure within hours of birth
b. changes of cerebral ischemia including encephalomalacia and dystrophic parenchymal calcification are common in choroidal type
c. venous outflow restriction is noted in mural type
d. The development of hydrocephalus secondary to venous hypertension is noted in choroidal type
e. The goals of embolization is decreasing the severity of congestive heart failure in neonates

31. All are true except
a. The brain is the most-common location for metastatic disease
b. breast and lung tumors metastasize more frequently to the thoracic spine
c. small neuromas and meningiomas is easily detected on T2W images
d. leptomeningeal tumor is difficult to visualize on noncontrast MR images
e. The enhancement of intradural extramedullary disease generally is most prominent on the immediate postcontrast scans

32. All are true regarding vascular anatomy of spinal cord except
a. The radicular artery supplies the root sleeve and spinal dura
b. Radicular artery branches contributing to the ASA are referred to as "radiculopial arteries
c. From six to eight radiculomedullary arteries arise from radicular arteries along the length of the cord
d. Hemodynamic watershed areas occur at the margins of each region

e. the artery of Adamkiewicz is radiculomedullary artery of thoracolumber region

33. All are true regarding sacral agenesis except
a. association of with maternal diabetes mellitus
b. defects in the HLXB9 homeobox gene
c. OEIS complex, VATER syndrome association
d. Sirenomelia (sympodia)
e. the conus always ends cephalic to the lower border of L-1

34. All are true regarding imaging of pituitary gland except
a. Immediately after contrast injection, most adenomas appear as relatively nonenhancing (dark) lesions within an intensely enhancing pituitary gland
b. dynamic scanning has shown that the contrast enhancement behavior of microadenomas is inconsistent from case to case.
c. Delayed scans (i.e., longer than 30 minutes after contrast injection) occasionally may demonstrate a reversal of image contrast of adenoma
d. The MTR of the normal pituitary varies with age
e. The MTR has been shown to be lower in prolactin-secreting or growth hormone–secreting adenomas compared to normals

35. All are true regarding Rathke Cleft Cyst except
a. predominantly intrasellar in location in the centre of pituitary gland
b. share a common origin with some craniopharyngiomas
c. Calcification in the cyst wall is rare
d. The cyst contents are typically mucoid
e. constant enhancement of cyst wall

36. All are true regarding retinoblastoma except
a. hyperintense signal to the vitreous on T1W and hypointensity on T2W
b. mild to intense enhancement on postcontrast MR images
c. shares histopathologic features of medulloblastoma and pineoblastoma
d. fat-suppressed, T2W with IV contrast is the best technique for documenting sign of spread
e. rubeosis iridis correlate significantly with extension into the choroid and prelaminar segment of the optic nerve

37. All are true regarding spectroscopy except
a. The decline in Cho is typically more abrupt with metastasis than that of primary neoplasm
b. low CBV in perfusion MRI and only a slight elevation of Cho/Cr in the MR spectrum suggest radiation necrosis
c. in true necrosis, there is an absence of the typical brain metabolite signals and an increase in the signal from lipids
d. very high elevation of the choline (Cho) resonance is characteristic of medulloblastomas.
e. meningiomas and choroid plexus papillomas can have very low levels of Cho

38. All are true regarding vertebro-basilar system except

a. vertebral arteries usually arise from subclavian arteries
b. vertebral arteries enters the foramen transversarium of the fifth cervical vertebra
c. the left vertebral artery is usually the larger than right
d. The anterior inferior cerebellar arteries loop in the cerebellopontine angle
e. the P3 refers to 'ambient' segment of posterior cerebral artery

39. All are true regarding tumour except
a. WHO grade II oligodendrogliomas have significantly higher rCBV than WHO grade II astrocytomas
b. rCBV measurements significantly increased the sensitivity and positive predictive value of conventional MR imaging in glioma grading
c. In radiation necrosis the enhancing lesion has a lower rCBV than recurrent tumour
d. ADC measurements of the enhancing components in recurrent tumour are significantly lower than in radiation necrosis
e. peritumoural regions in metastases show increase in rCBV or decrease in FA

40. All are true regarding intracranial tumour except
a. schwannomas usually grow on the sensory nerves, most frequently from the superior vestibular division of the vestibulocochlear nerve
b. 'pearly tumours' result from inclusion of ectodermal elements during the closure of the neural tube
c. epidermoid cysts are non-enhancing lesions of similar density to CSF.
d. water diffusion is markedly restricted in epidermoid tumours (dark on DWI)
e. arachnoid cysts cause bone thinning.

41. All are tue regarding role of MRI in SAH except
a. $T2^*$ gradient-echo has sensitivities of 94–100 per cent in the acute (less than 4 d) SAH
b. FLAIR has sensitivities of 80 per cent in the acute (less than 4 d) SAH
c. FLAIR may remain positive for at least 45 d after a haemorrhage
d. SAH appear as low signal on gradient echo sequences
e. the CSF appears high signal on FLAIR

42. Which lesions in HIV-related CNS disease cause neither masss nor enhancement
a. Cryptococcomas
b. Lymphoma
c. PML
d. Tuberculosis
e. Candida

43. All are true regarding spine except
a. 'swimmer's view is for thoracic spine
b. midline defect of the posterior arch of the atlas occurs in 6 per cent of the normal population
c. intervertebral fusion usually occur only in the cervical region
d. Complete or partial fusion of L5 with the sacrum is seen in more than 6 per cent of the normal population

e. Cervical ribs involving the seventh cervical vertebra occur in about 6 per cent of the normal population

44. All are true regarding tuberous sclerosis except
a. subependymal giant cell tumour is associated with reduced life expectancy
b. SENs are the most common lesion (88–95% of individuals)
c. SENs are hyperintense on T1W and hypointense on T2W in infants in older children and adults
d. calcification in SENs increase with age
e. infantile spasms or myoclonic seizures are the presenting symptom in 80% of patients with TS

45. All are true regarding pediatric stroke except
a. restricted diffusion may occur for a shorter time in younger children
b. pseudonormalization may occur earlier than in adults
c. intracranial vascular abnormality more frequent than extracranial
d. involve the posterior circulation more than anterior circulation
e. typically consist of occlusion of proximal large arteries

46. Endovascular techniques for lumen restoration (recanalisation) is /are
a. dilatation balloons
b. stents
c thrombolysis
d. vasodilatatory drugs
e. All

47. All are true regarding endovascular treatment of cerebral AVMs except
a. aim is the prevention of cerebral haemorrhage or re-haemorrhage
b. the most commonly used approach is venous embolisation using a permanent fluid agent
c. may be used to reduce the size of the AVM prior to radiosurgery
d. partial AVM embolisation can be effective in improving the control of epileptic seizures
e. partial AVM embolisation bring relief of symptoms related to venous hypertension

48. The commonest cause of pathological vascular markings in the skull vault is
a. meningioma
b. angiomatous malformation
c. NF I
d. Sturge weber syndrome
e. tuberous sclerosis

49. All are true except
a. cyst of the cavum vergae is reactangular on axial CT
b. velum interpositum lies below the third ventricle
c. velum interpositum is .triangular on axial CT with apex anteriorly
d. velum interpositum contains internal cerebral vein
e. .velum interpositum is normal condition

50. All are true regarding anastomoses of maxillary artery to internal carotid artery except
a. middle meningeal artery and ophthalmic artery
b. artery of foramen Rotandum to inferolateral trunk of ICA
c. accessory meningeal artery to

inferolateral trunk
d.Vidian artery to intratemporal ICA
e.ascending pharyngeal artery to ICA

51.All are true regarding cerebral infarction except
a.hyperdense artery in 25% to 50% within 12 hrs
b.insular ribbon sign in acute case
c.obscuration of lentiform nuclei (1 to 2 days)
d.wedge-shaped low density (1to 3 days)
e.gyral enhancement (4 to 7 days)

52.All are common CPA cisterm masses except
a.acoustic swannoma
b.meningioma
c.epidermoid
d.arachnoid cyst
e.metastases

53..All are true regarding ependymoma except
a.more tha 90% in fourth ventricle
b.extrudes through outlet foramina
c.spinal seeding common
d. 50% calcify
e.mostly isodense on NECT

54.All are true regarding brain parenchymal metastases except
a.the most common primary is in lung
b.the most common site –gray -white junction
c.strong solid /rim enhancement
d.high dose contrast –more sensitive for detection
e.mets from mucin secreting tumour –hyperntense on T2W

55.All are true regarding leucodystrophy except
a.complete or near complete lack of mylination is seen Pelizaeus-Merzbacher disease
b.temporal lobe white matter is most involved in Alexander disease
c.occipital lobe white matter is most involved in adrenoleukodystrophy
d.thick meninges are seen in Hurler syndrome
e.high density basal ganglia is seen in Krabbe disease

56.All are true except
a.bilateral high intensity on NECT in globus pallidus and substantia nigra noted in Hallervorden-Spatz Disease
b.pallodonigral low intensity on T2W image in Hallervorden-Spatz Disease
c.Eye –of-the –tiger sign is noted in Hallervorden-Spatz Disease
d.basal ganglia and dentate nucei calcification is seen in Fahr disease
e.bilateral putaminal low intensity on NECT is seen in Wilson disease

57.All are true regarding anaplastic astrocytoma except
a.absent necrosis
b.presence of at least 20% gemistocytes in a glial neoplasm is a poor prognostic sign
c.protopplasmic astrocytoma is located superficially in the cerebral cortex
d.spread through the extracelluar space and along compact white matter tracts
e.uniform strong enhancement

58..All are true regarding epidermoid tumour except

a. mother pf pearl appearance
b. lobulated cauliflower like mass
c. 40 % to 45 % in middle fossa
d. insinuates in CSF spaces
e. TIW and T2W image like CSF

59. All are true regarding CNS tuberculosis
a. the most common acute presentation ---meningitis
b. the most common parenchymal presentation---tuberculomas
c. the most common parenchymal site of infection in children---basal ganglia
d. tuberculomas typically larger than cysticercosis
e. central tuberculomas are typically isointense to brain on T1W

60. All are true regarding lipidoses except
a. lysosomes referred to as 'Darth Vaders" of cells
b. lysosomal disorders primarily affect the gray matter
c. hypodense thalmi in Tay-Sach disease
d. enlarged caudate nuclei in early stage of Tay-Sachs disease
e. no white matter changes are seen in Neuronal ceroid-lipofuscinosis

TEST PAPER 3(ANSWER)

1.-----a
In the carotid circulation (and the entire cerebrovascular circulation), the most common site for atherosclerotic plaque formation is at the carotid bifurcation with involvement of the distal common carotid artery and the first 2 cm of the internal carotid artery. .

2---d
Enhancement and restricted diffusion are not generally found coexisting in arterial infarction. ADC values is seen low within hours after the stroke and continue to decline for the next few days. They remain reduced through the first 4 to 5 days after stroke and then undergo pseudonormalization between 4 and 10 days . After this the ADC subsequently has been found to rise in the lesion (i.e., the ADC map shows hyperintensity) beyond 10 days.
DWI has been shown to improve lesion localization and detect the age of the infarction more accurately, DWI has also been shown more accurately to detect and size ischemic lesions.

3.---c

4.----a
In Methemoglobin, the iron is in the ferric state with five d electrons.

5.---b
The cerebellum is a particularly common site for hemosiderin deposition in siderosis and is typically more severely affected with hypointensity and concomitant parenchymal loss (cerebellar atrophy) on MR. In the absence of an intracranial cause for the siderosis, an ependymoma of the conus medullaris or other spinal source of bleeding should be explored as the etiology of the recurrent hemorrhage.

6.---e
Endovascular treatment is usually an adjunctive measure to either surgery or radiation
Radiosurgery or stereotactic external beam radiation therapy uses focused irradiation directed at the AVM nidus. Radiosurgery is usually pursued in those cases considered unsuitable for resection because of either location of the AVM nidus or overall operative risk.
The efficiency of AVM obliteration is low when the AVM nidus exceeds 3.0 cm when treated with (radiation ("gamma knife") or x-ray photon radiation ("LINAC radiosurgery"). Large AVMs greater than 3.0 cm may benefit from stereotactic heavy-charged-particle Bragg-peak radiation.

7.----b

8.—d
In less than 5% of cases, aneurysms are associated with septic emboli, head trauma, or neoplasia. In these instances, aneurysms are typically at peripheral sites or in regions other than branch points.

Saccular aneurysms usually occur at vessel bifurcations
Larger arteries in the region of the circle of Willis are most frequently involved.
More than 90% of saccular aneurysms originate at one of the following five locations: the junction of the anterior cerebral and anterior communicating arteries, the ICA at the origin of the posterior communicating artery, the bifurcation of the MCA, the tip of the basilar artery, and the bifurcation of the ICA . In approximately 20% to 25% of cases, aneurysms are multiple.

9.---e
DAI lesions are usually (80%) nonhemorrhagic in nature

10.---d
Myo-inositol is considered a glial cell marker.The NAA peak is a marker of normal neuronal adult tissue, and the increase in NAA early in development reflects the normal neuronal maturation. Because NAA is a metabolite present within neurons, it has been widely studied in a variety of contexts to document neuronal viability and density, with reduction of NAA suggesting neuronal damage.

11.---a
Routine spin echo sequences, even with high resolution, often fail to detect optic nerve involvement in clinically affected MS individuals. STIR and fat-suppressed fast spin echo, show promise in detecting optic neuritis with a high degree of sensitivity . With these techniques, optic neuritis appears as abnormal high signal intensity within the affected nerves .. High-resolution T2-weighted fast spin echo MR with fat suppression and high-resolution postcontrast enhanced T1-weighted images also can often detect intraneural signal abnormalities.

12.----e
Prominent extraaxial spaces---is seen in Glutaric aciduria type I.GM2 gangliosidosis and Krabbe disease show hyperdense basal ganglia and thalami

13.---b

14.---e
The alveus and fimbria changes orientation from vertical to horizontal course

15.---d
The hippocampus body usually has an oval or round shape in the coronal plane.

16.----c
The blood–brain barrier, a concept was postulated first by Goldmann in 1913. Endothelial cells of cerebral capillaries have fused membranes, termed tight junctions, which are probably the most important feature in regulating capillary permeability in the brain. Other unique characteristics of brain capillaries include continuous basement membranes, narrow intercellular gaps, and a paucity of pinocytosis . All of these structures act together to function as the blood–brain barrier.
Capillaries of tissues outside the nervous system typically have discontinuities in their basement

membranes with wide intercellular gaps, permitting the free passage of protein molecules from the lumen of the capillary into the extravascular space. Besides tight junctions between cerebral capillary endothelium, these cells are also closely surrounded by a sheath of astrocytic foot processes

17.----e

Calcification is extremely common, being associated with the walls of intrinsic blood vessels. The calcification can be within the tumor tissue or separate in the surrounding brain parenchyma, especially in the cortical gray matter.

18.---b

The most important imaging features of hemangioblastoma are (a) the cystic nature of the mass, (b) a peripheral pial-based mural nodule of solid tissue that enhances markedly with intravenous contrast, and (c) large vessels within and/or at the periphery of the mass. Approximately two thirds of cerebellar hemangioblastomas are at least partially cystic.

Cysts of hemangioblastoma are commonly of high signal intensity relative to CSF on T1-weighted, proton density–weighted, and FLAIR images. The mural nodule (or solid portion of the tumor) is usually only slightly hyperintense or isointense to gray matter on T2-weighted image.

High rCBV is a typical feature of hemangioblastomas and may help to differentiate hemangioblastomas from metastases. In patients with von Hippel-Lindau disease, the presence of multiple enhancing lesions in the cerebellum is pathognomonic for hemangioblastomas, with lesions often of varying sizes.

19.----a

20.----b

Dermoid cyst are most commonly located in the posterior fossa in the midline but may occur in the cisterns about the sella turcica and elsewhere. They may also have an intraventricular location arising within the cisterns of the tela choroidea in the lateral, third, or fourth ventricular region.

21.—d

Proton spectroscopy is a useful adjunct to the imaging studies because ependymomas have a different spectrum than do astrocytomas and PNETs, with preservation of creatine, elevation of choline, and decrease in NAA. The creatine is not preserved in PNET and astrocytoma. Ependymomas are known for the production of calcification and for a tendency to bleed.

22.---a

The 90% rule implies that 90% are partially cystic, 90% are suprasellar, and 90% enhance. The most common MR picture of a craniopharyngioma is that of a cystic mass that is hypointense on T1, hyperintense on T2, and enhances in the cyst wall or the mural tissue.

The cyst fluid is of higher density than that of CSF

23.---c
Closure of the neural tube begins in the hindbrain

24.---c
In certain locations, elevated signal intensity on conventional and FLAIR T2-weighted images is a normal finding even in young individuals .The parietopontine tracts of the posterior limb of the internal capsule is one such location.Here foci are well circumscribed, round or oval, and symmetric, and they appeared comparable to cortical gray matter on T2 and iso- or hypointense on proton-density images.

25.—d
Both PKAN-classic and PKAN-atypical patients showed the "eye-of-the-tiger" sign on long-TR/TE MRI studies .In contrast, mutation-negative, NBAI-1 patients do not show the "eye-of-the-tiger" sign .

26.---b
The primary findings of ONG include abnormal optic nerve elongation, thickening, kinking, and abnormal enhancement . In addition, dural ectasia of the optic nerve sheath, without a neoplasm, can mimic the enlargement and beaded configuration of an optic glioma. The orbital nerves are more likely to be involved in NF1 while chiasm is the most common site of involvement in non-NF1 patients

27.---b

28.---a
The cortical dysplasias of Taylor (CDTs) are characterized by the presence of abnormal neurons and glia within localized regions of the cerebral cortex.
At least two types of CDT are recognized: CDT with dysplastic neurons only and no balloon cells (CDT-D), and CDT with giant so-called balloon cells (BC) that are found within the area of dysplasia (CDT-BC)
The most common features seen in CDT in the series by Lawson et al. were blurring of the gray–white matter junction (80%), thick cortex (70%), and elevated signal on T2-weighted images in the affected gray matter (70%).
In the study by Lawson et al. both CDT-D and CDT-B most often involved the frontal lobe . In a study by Yagishitia et al., however, 60% of CDT was found within the temporal lobes.

29.---b
A characteristic of the absence of the corpus callosum is persistent eversion of the cingulate gyrus. In the normal patient, the crossing callosal fibers result in a superomedial displacement of the cingulate gyri, the end result being a cingulate gyrus that is oriented roughly perpendicular to the interhemispheric fissure. This normal inversion of the cingulate gyrus results in the formation of the cingulate sulcus . When the corpus callosum is absent, the cingulate gyri remain everted and the cingulate sulci remain unformed . As a result, the mesial hemispheric sulci course uninterrupted in a radial manner

all the way into the third ventricle .There may be associated hypogenesis of the hippocampal formations

30.---d

The mural type of Galenic malformation has fewer arteriovenous shunts than the choroidal type and is often associated with venous outflow restriction.

Because the degree of shunting is less severe in mural malformations, infants with this lesion do not usually develop congestive heart failure. In fact, infants with mural malformations are often asymptomatic in the newborn period, and the malformation may only come to attention when hydrocephalus or neurologic symptoms develop later in infancy. The development of hydrocephalus is secondary to venous hypertension resulting from the arteriovenous shunting coupled with venous outflow obstruction. Compression of the aqueduct of Sylvius by a large varix may contribute to the hydrocephalus. Because the blood flow to the brain parenchyma is better preserved in mural malformations than in choroidal malformations, the early onset of cerebral ischemia is uncommon

31.—c

Primary tumors, such as meningiomas and neurofibromas, generally are well seen on noncontrast MR images . These tumors tend to be compact and to stand out against the lower intensity surrounding CSF on T1-weighted sequences. On T2-weighted sequences, contrast is reversed and the tumors often appear of lower signal intensity against the high intensity of CSF. Small neuromas and meningiomas may be difficult to visualize without contrast.

In case of intradural extramedullary disease , T1-weighted sagittal sequences before and after the administration of gadolinium is sufficient. T2-weighted scans may not be necessary.

32.---b

Radicular artery branches contributing to the ASA are referred to as "radiculomedullary" arteries, and those giving supply to a PSA are known as "radiculopial" arteries

33.---e

The position of the conus defines two distinct groups of patients with sacral agenesis. The conus doesnot always ends cephalic to the lower border of L-1, it may end lower, below L-1.

Sirenomelia (sympodia) is a condition characterized by fusion of the pelvic girdle and the lower extremities into a single conical structure . The distal end of this fused structure may exhibit no feet (sirenomelia apus) (35%), one foot (sirenomelia monopus) (26%), or two feet (sirenomelia dipus) (29%) . The lower extremity is always inverted and externally rotated, so that the knee is situated posteriorly, the leg flexes forward on the thigh, and the foot points posteriorly . Rare sirens exhibit two separate lower extremities, each flexed and rotated externally (anchipod form).

34.---e
The MTR has been shown to be higher in prolactin-secreting or growth hormone–secreting adenomas compared to normals and lower in nonsecreting adenomas compared to normals.

35.---e
Rathke cleft cysts do not typically enhance. However, occasionally there may be thin marginal enhancement of the cyst wall. This feature (lack of enhancement) can be used to advantage to separate these cysts from craniopharyngiomas in difficult cases. Another distinguishing feature of Rathke cyst from craniopharyngioma can be found on CT because calcification, frequently found in craniopharyngiomas, is not commonly a feature of Rathke cyst.

The cysts with mucoid fluid are indistinguishable from cystic craniopharyngiomas on MR: Both are hyperintense on both T1- and T2-weighted images. The serous cysts match the signal intensity of CSF and are the only subtype that has the typical imaging features of benign cysts. Those containing cellular debris pose the greatest difficulty in differential diagnosis because they resemble solid nodules

36.---d
Episcleral and optic nerve extension of retinoblastoma is critical to exclude, and fat-suppressed, T1-weighted MR with the use of IV contrast is the best technique for documenting this ominous sign of spread.

37.---e
Tumors such as meningiomas and choroid plexus papillomas can have very high levels of Cho even when these tumors are low grade by histologic criteria and clinical behavior. The reasons behind such an observation are unclear.

38.----b
The right and left vertebral arteries usually arise as the first branches of the corresponding subclavian arteries. Each then enters the foramen transversarium of the sixth cervical vertebra.

The basilar artery runs superiorly on the anterior surface of the pons and gives off anterior inferior cerebellar, superior cerebellar and posterior cerebral arteries on both sides.

After bifurcating, the basilar artery gives rise to the two posterior cerebral arteries, each of which has four segments. P1 is the precommunicating segment before which it joins with the posterior communicating arteries to become the P2 or 'ambient' segment and P3 or 'quadrigeminal' segment, named after the basal cistern in which it runs. The P4 segment is the terminal segment of the posterior cerebral artery, which includes the occipital and inferior temporal branches. There is reciprocity in calibre of the precommunicating

(P1) segments of the posterior cerebral arteries and the posterior communicating arteries

39.----e
The peritumoural regions of high-grade gliomas show a more marked decrease in ADC, fractional anisotropy and NAA and increase in rCBV compared to low-grade tumours. This is a reflection of the more invasive nature of these tumours, which infiltrate the adjacent brain tissue along vascular channels, leading to an rCBV increase; destroy ultrastructural boundaries with a consequent decrease in ADC and FA; and replace normal brain tissue, resulting in a drop of NAA. Metastases on the other hand are surrounded by 'pure' vasogenic oedema, which contains no infiltrating tumour cells. These peritumoural regions in metastases therefore show no increase in rCBV or decrease in FA.

40.---d
On CT and standard T1W and T2W images, epidermoid cysts are non-enhancing lesions of similar density or signal intensity to CSF. They have to be differentiated from arachnoid cysts, which have better defined margins and cause bone thinning. DWI is very helpful to distinguish epidermoid tumours from arachnoid cysts : water diffusion is markedly restricted in epidermoid tumours (which appear bright on DWI) but not in arachnoid cysts, which have similar signal characteristics to CSF.

41.----b
Spin-echo MRI sequences are unreliable in SAH but using a $T2^*$ gradient-echo or FLAIR sequence, sensitivities of 94–100 per cent and 81–87 per cent can be achieved in the acute (less than 4 d) and subacute (more than 4 d) periods, respectively. However FLAIR is less sensitive at low CSF red blood cell concentrations following normal CT. The susceptibility effects of para-magnetic iron cause low signal on gradient echo sequences; on FLAIR the CSF appears high signal due to the presence of increased protein. FLAIR may remain positive for at least 45 d after a haemorrhage, at a time when the blood has long since become invisible on CT.

42.----c

43.----a
Lateral view of cervical spine is best obtained as a 'swimmer's view' with one arm elevated above the head and the other down by the side.
Intervertebral fusion usually occur only in the cervical region, C2/3 being the commonest

44.----c
SENs and linear parenchymal tuberous sclerosis lesions in infants under 3 months old are hyperintense on T1-weighted images and hypointense on T2-weighted images as opposed to the reverse pattern of signal intensity in older children and adults

45.---d
Vascular abnormalities in

paediatric ischaemic stroke are common. These are more frequently intracranial than extracranial, involve the anterior rather than posterior circulation and typically consist of occlusion of proximal large arteries, i.e. middle cerebral artery (MCA), anterior cerebral artery (ACA) and terminal internal carotid artery (ICA).
46.---e
47.-----b
The most commonly used endovascular approach is arterial embolisation using a permanent fluid agent such as NBCA
48.----a
49.---b
Velum interpositum lies above the third ventricle
50.---e
51.----c
Obscuration of lentiform nucei noted within 12 hrs of infarction.
52.---d
53.---c
Spinal seeding is relatively uncommon
54.----e
Mets from mucin secreting tumour is hypointense on T2W
55.---b
Frontal lobe white matter is most involved in Alexander disease
56.—a
Bilateral low intensity on NECT in globus pallidus and substantia nigra noted in Hallervorden-Spatz Disease
57.---e
Anaplastic astrocytoma enhance strongly but nonuniformly
58.---c
40 % to 45 % in CP angle
59.—c
The most common parenchymal site of infection in childrenis cerebellum andin adult basal ganglia and the cerebral hemishphere
60.---c

TEST PAPER 4

1. All are true regarding edema and stroke except
a. Cytotoxic edema develops with water accumulation in the intracellular environment.
b. tissue water content increases by 3% to 5% with the development of cytotoxic edema
c. Loss of integrity of the blood–brain barrier is generally believed to begin 1 to 2 hours after the ischemic insult
d. proteins and water flood into the extracellular space from the intracellular environment in vasogenic edema
e. cerebral infarction is generally associated with decreased cerebral blood flow and cerebral blood volume

2. All are true of perfusion-weighted imaging except
a. gadolinium-DTPA used as contrast
b. contrast induce a T2* lengthening
c. cause transient signal loss in perfused tissue with intact BBB
d. can be performed by magnetically labeling water protons
e. Spin tagging methods are more readily quantifiable

3. All are true regarding Virchow-Robin spaces except
a. refers to dilated perivascular spaces
b. prominent Virchow-Robin spaces is referred as état-criblé
c. Virchow-Robin spaces tend to be smaller (2 × 2 mm or less by MR)
d. the signal intensity of lacunae virtually always similar to that of CSF
e. classically situated at the anterior commissure or radiating out from the ventricles

4. All are features of acute haematoma except
a. usually isointense with brain on T2-weighted images under low-field conditions
b. intracellular deoxyhemoglobin cause T2 shortening
c. The signal intensity influenced only to a minor extent by the protein content
d. Fibrin clot formation and retraction affect significantly in vitro the appearance
e. GRE imaging is very useful, particularly on low-field systems

5. All are true regarding subarachnoid hemorrhage except
a. the sensitivity for acute SAH is believed to approach 100% on CT scan
b. MRI is superior to CT for suspected acute SAH
c. FLAIR imaging has been used to evaluate acute, subacute, and chronic SAH
d. marked hypointensity along the parenchymal surfaces on T2W noted in superficial hemosiderosis
e. The cerebellum is a particularly common site for hemosiderin deposition in siderosis

6. All are true regarding AVM grading system (proposed by Spetzler and Martin)

a. higher grades lesions indicate that lesions are more surgically difficult
b. evaluates the size of the nidus, the location of the nidus, and the arterial feeders
c. "eloquent" areas AVMs is is given score of 1
d. large or diffuse AVMs encompassing the entirety of critical structures are classified as grade VI
e. large AVMs with eloquent cortex involvement, deep drainage belongs to grade V

7. All are true regarding cavernous angioma except
a. encapsulated
b. no muscularis /elastic in sinusoidal vascular channels
c. the absence of interposed brain tissue
d. a rim of gliotic brain with hemosiderin pigment
e. subacute-to-chronic clotted blood

8. Morbidity and mortality of SAH is
a. morbidity (20% to 25%) and mortality (50% to 60%)
b. morbidity (15% to 20%) and mortality (40 % to 50%)
c. morbidity (10% to 15%) and mortality (30% to 40%)
d. morbidity (5% to 10%) and mortality (20% to 30%)
e. morbidity (0% to 5%) and mortality (10% to 20%)

9. All are true regarding shear-strain deformation in head injury except
a. change in shape
b. change in volume
c. cause of most mechanically induced lesions
d. greatest at the junction of tissues of different density and rigidity
e. rotationally induced shear-strain lesions are typically bilateral and multiple

10. All are true regarding Newer Techniques for Imaging Brain Development except
a. diffusion MR has the potential to be very useful in assessing both the normal development and the disease states of cerebral white matter.
b. Diffusion tensor imaging (DTI) is not useful for characterization of the early laminar microarchitecture of the developing white matter tracts prior to full myelination in premature infants
c. Three-dimensional (3D) fiber tractography allows the three-dimensional analysis of the white matter pathways and their possible aberrant development.
d. MR spectroscopy techniques may be useful for documentation of normal fetal brain maturation,
e. Proton (^{1}H) MR spectroscopy is a noninvasive technique that allows for the in vivo measurement of various brain metabolites.

11. All are true regarding spinal cord lesions in multiple sclerosis except
a. are usually found in combination with lesions in the brain
b. cord abnormalities may be found in approx. 75% of MS

patients
c. Most lesions are found in the thoracic region
d. peripheral location of MS lesions,commonly the dorsolateral aspect of the cord
e. multifocal lesions

12. Hypointense subependymal germinolytic cysts ,typically involving the caudothalamic grooves is seen on MR imaging of
a. mucopolysaccharidoses
b. Zellweger Syndrome
c. Fabry Disease
d. Krabbe disease
e. MLD

13. Hyperdense basal ganglia and thalami is seen In
a. Mucopolysaccharidoses
b. Zellweger syndrome
c. Alexander disease
d. MELAS
e. Krabbe disease

14. All are true regarding development of hippocampus except
a. At 13 to 14 weeks, the unfolded hippocampus is situated on the medial surface of the temporal lobe
b. infolding of the dentate gyrus and cornu ammonis starts by 15 to 16 weeks
c. The CA1, CA2, and CA3 fields of the cornu ammonis are arranged non-linearly .
d. the hippocampus begins to resemble the adult hippocampus by 20 weeks,
e. an unfolded (vertical) hippocampal configuration and hippocampal sulcal cyst are aberrations of development.

15. All are true imaging finding except
a. neurocysticercosis is one of the most common causes of new-onset partial seizures in developing countries
b. Widespread cerebral gliosis and atrophy are seen in infantile hemiplegia
c. Rasmussen encephalitis usually presents in adult
d. Sturge-Weber syndrome shows tram-track gyriform calcification on CT
e. MR is usually normal in paradoxical medial temporal lobe epilepsy

16. All of following tumour shows relatively low intensity on T2-weighted images except
a. medulloblastoma and pineoblastomas
b. neuroblastomas and most lymphomas,
c. Metastases from small-cell lung cancer and mucinous adenocarcinomas
d. amelanotic melanoma metastases
e. ependymoma and meningioma

17. All are true regarding gliomatosis cerebri except
a. diffusely infiltrative glioma involving large portions of the nervous system
b. relative preservation of the underlying neural structures
c. The peak incidence is in the second to fourth decades
d. lack of definite focal mass production
e. Contrast enhancement is a typical feature

18. All are true regarding heamangioblastoma except

a. benign neoplasm
b. The cerebellum is their most frequent site
c. peak incidence during the fifth and sixth decades
d. present in older adults in von Hippel-Lindau syndrome
e. Multiplicity more common when they arise within the spinal cord

19. All are true regarding metastases except
a. regular, thin, even and smooth enhancing ring enhancement /nodular enhancement
b. The major causes of multiple enhancing lesions are metastases, abscesses, multifocal glioma, and radiation necrosis
c. causes of the solitary enhancing neoplastic posterior fossa mass of an adult are metastasis, hemangioblastoma, lymphoma
d. most metastases enhance dramatically on the immediate postcontrast scan
e. immediate postcontrast scan is probably the most practical method for detecting metastases

20. All features favour epidermoid cysts over arachnoid cyst except
a. lobulated in configuration
b. tend to engulf and surround vessels and cranial nerves
c. virtually always isointense to CSF on FLAIR
d. reduced diffusion within epidermoids
e. focal calcifications in their walls

21. All are true regarding ependymomas of the posterior fossa except
a. arises within the fourth ventricle
b. extending into and through the foramina of Luschka and the foramen Magendie
c. the initial peak age incidence is between 3 and 6 years
d. lateral location of tumor –a good prognostic feature
e. surveillance imaging recommended after the postoperative study

22. All are true regarding craniopharyngioma except
a. arise from Rathke's pouch
b. suprasellar location in three-fourth
c. Mean age at presentation for children is late first decade.
d. Mostly both solid and cystic
e. no Calcification

23. All are true regarding brain development except
a. Neural plate forms at about 2 weeks
b. proximal two third of the neural tube forms the future brain
c. closure of the neural tube begins in the midbrain
d. diencephalon forms from mesencephalon
e. prosencephalon give rise to telencephalon

24. All are true regarding fungal infection of CNS except
a. Cryptococcus result in acute or chronic leptomeningitis less frequently than parenchymal lesions
b. the candida abscess has "target appearance" on T2W image
c. "gelatinous pseudocysts" primarily in the basal ganglia and midbrain is noted in CNS Cryptococcosis
d. an acute hemorrhagic

infarction is seen in aspergillosis
e. the trehalose resonance at 5.19 ppm noted in cryptococcoma

25. All are true regarding risk factor of Alzheimer disease except
a. increasing age and positive family history
b. Carriers of the apolipoprotein e2 allele
c. the amyloid precursor protein gene on chromosome 21
d. the presenilin-1 gene on chromosome 14
e. the presenilin-2 gene on chromosome 1

26. All are true regarding Huntington disease except
a. repeating CAG triplet on chromosome 4 (>36 or more) noted in Hallervorden-Spatz Syndrome
b. atrophy of the caudate and putamen(striatum) noted in Huntigton disease
c. the "eye-of-the-tiger" sign is noted in Hallervorden-Spatz Syndrome
d. Selective bilateral pallidal necrosis ---- an organic hallmark of hypoxic-hypotensive insults
e. Lesions of the subthalamic nucleus typically result in contralateral hemiballistic movements

27. All are true regarding optic nerve glioma (ONG) in NF1 except
a. The presence of bilateral ONGs is considered specific for NF1
b. ONGs in NF1 are almost invariably juvenile pilocytic astrocytomas in childhood.
c. 20% of the patients with ONGs have NF1
d. 50% of childhood juvenile pilocytic astrocytoma present in the optic chiasm and hypothalamus
e. 5% to 40% of patients with NF1 develop ONGs

28. The secondary changes seen in Sturge-Weber Syndrome are all except
a. cerebral cortical atrophy
b. gyriform cerebral calcification
c. ventricular enlargement
d. "angiomatous" enlargement of the contralateral choroid plexus
e. asymmetric sinus enlargement ipsilateral to the cortical atrophy

29. All are true regarding heterotopias except
a. focal collections of ectopic neurons in the cerebral hemispheres
b. MRI is far more sensitive than CT in the detection of subependymal heterotopias
c. isointense with gray matter on all imaging sequences.
d. perilesional edema / contrast enhancement present as a rule
e. DD of subependymal heterotopia ---tuberous sclerosis and ependymal metastases

30. All are true regarding corpus callosum malformation except
a. the axons normally constituting the the corpus callosum arise from layer 3 of the cerebral cortex
b. the corpus callosum develops during about 8 and 20 weeks of gestational
c. the development of the corpus callosum is bidirectional and proceeds in a largely

anteroposterior fashion
d. The anterior genu forms around the time of formation of the posterior body and splenium (according to Rakic)
e. posterior genu and anterior body of the CC is absent or small in true callosal hypogenesis

31.-All are features of persistent trigeminal artery except
a. vessel arising from the cavernous (or precavernous) carotid artery
b. an abrupt lateral bend in posterior foss to communicate with the basilar artery
c. small caliber of the basilar artery caudal to the trigeminal artery
d. small ipsilateral PComA
e. the identification of a vessel that appears to penetrate the dorsum sellae

32. All are true regarding Vein of Galen Malformation (Vein of Galen Aneurysm) except
a. the venous sac represent a varix of the persistent median prosencephalic vein (of Markowski)
b. absence of a straight sinus in many cases
c. presence of falcine sinus
d. mural type-----numerous arteriovenous connections with no venous obstruction
e. The choroidal type accounts for the majority of symptomatic Galenic malformations in the neonatal period

33. All are true regarding
a. The adrenal medulla and upper abdominal parasympathetic chain are the primary sites of 65% of neuroblastomas
b. Ganglioneuroma is composed almost entirely of mature ganglia cells
c. neuroblastoma is the most common solid tumor of children, excluding central nervous system (CNS) tumors
d. ganglioneuroma and ganglioneuroblastoma tend to present later than neuroblastomas
e. relatively high intensity on T2-weighted images

34. All are true regarding vascular anatomy of spinal cord except
a. receives its blood supply from the paired anterior spinal artery and posterior spinal arteries
b. anterior spinal artery (ASA) originates from the intradural vertebral arteries at the cervicomedullary junction
c. Anterior spinal artery is the longest artery in the body
d. size of the ASA in the lower cervical and lumbosacral regions, often exceed 1 mm in diameter
e. The ASA often narrows to less than 0.5 mm in diameter in the thoracic region between T2 and T9

35. All are true regarding spinal cord infection except
a. Tubercular Spinal Arachnoiditis is frequently associated with radiculomyelitis
b. paravertebral abscesses in blastomycosis frequently erode the neighboring ribs
c. The use of CISS sequence increases the conspicuity of lesions in the subarachnoid space
d. Vacuolar myelopathy is the

most common chronic myelopathy associated with HIV infection
e. polio attacks principally sensory neurons of the spinal cord and brainstem

36. All are true regading Terminal Myelocystocele (Syringocele) except
a. typically associated with the OEIS constellation
b. related to the teratogen retinoic acid
c. posterior spina bifida, tethered cord
d. meningocele communicate with the terminal ventricle
e. No spinal nerves traverse the cyst

37. All are true regarding imaging technique of pituitary gland except
a. use a high-resolution MR protocol
b. coronal plane is the most useful plane
c. the use of thin (3 mm or smaller) slices
d. high-resolution T2-weighted images standard for pituitary pathology
e. 2-D FT GE images produce the marked susceptibility artifacts

38. All are true regarding papillary craniopharyngioma except
a. typically found in the adult patient
b. solid with extensive calcification
c. often found within the third ventricle
c. encapsulated
d. typically enhance

39. All are true regarding retinoblastoma except
a. the most common intraocular malignancy of childhood
b. trilateral" retinoblastoma ---- bilateral retinoblastoma with associated pontine tumor
c. bilateral tumors occur in up to one third of patients
d. The majority of tumors contain calcification
e. MR is a more sensitive evaluation for extraocular tumor along the optic nerve

40. All are true regarding ^{1}H MRS Changes in Neoplasia except
a. the hallmark of neoplasia --- elevation of the Cho
b. a reduction of NAA
c. little or minor changes in Cr
d. low Cho/NAA ratio --a strong indicator of a higher-grade neoplasm
e. A Cho/NAA ratio of greater than 1.3 ---high accuracy for detection of neoplasm

41. All are true regarding MCA except
a. opercular segment refers to M4 segments
b. The M1 segment runs in the Sylvian fissure
c. inferior border of the 'Sylvian triangle' is formed by main middle cerebral artery trunk
d. supply the basal ganglia and capsular region.
e. supply most of the lateral surface of the cerebral hemisphere

42. All are true regarding oligodendroglioma except
a. found almost exclusively in the cerebral hemispheres
b. chicken wire' appearance

c. case with 1p/19q loss shows a better response to chemotherapy
d. Up to 90 per cent contain visible calcification on CT
e. contrast enhancement is a reliable indicator of tumour grade

43. All are true regarding pituitary adenoma except
a. Prolactinomas are the most common functioning microadenomas
b. Microadenomas are best shown on contrast-enhanced images
c. Most macroadenomas are hypointense with brain parenchyma on unenhanced T1W images and hyperdense on CT
d. pituitary apoplexy is due to acute haemorrhage into a pituitary
e. the role of imaging in cases of hyperprolactinaemia is mainly to exclude macroadenoma

44. All are true regarding SAH except
a. no underlying cause is found on angiography in 30% cases
b. nonaneurysmal perimesencephalic SAH have a very good long-term prognosis
c. CT is positive for SAH in 98 per cent within 12 h of onset
d. A lumbar puncture should be performed in case of strong clinical suspicion of SAH and negative CT
e. Spin-echo MRI sequences are unreliable in SAH

45. Which lesions in HIV-related CNS disease cause masss with enhancement
a. Cryptococcomas
b. Lymphoma
c. Tuberculosis
d. Candida
e. Toxoplasmosis

46. All are true regarding epilepsy except
a. the most common of the partial epilepsies –temporal lobe epilepsy
b. hippocampal sclerosis is associated with temporal lobe epilepsy (TLE)
c. MRI in the axial plane is mandatory to detect hippocampal sclerosis
d. The signs of hippocampal sclerosis on MRI are volume loss and increased signal on T1W
e. C-flumazenil PET may be useful in investigation of epilepsy

47. At full term, T1-weighted images should show high signal in all except
a. the dorsal medulla and brain stem
b. the cerebellar peduncles
c. about a third of the anterior limb of the internal capsule
d. the central corona radiate
e. the deep white matter in the region of the pre- and post-central gyrus

48. All are true regarding NF1 except
a. thickening of long bone cortices
b. lambdoid sutural dysplasia
c. lateral meningoceles
d. 'empty' or 'bare' orbit
e. dural ectasia with vertebral scalloping

49. All are true regarding dysembryoplastic neuroepithelial tumour (DNT) except

a. Most tumours enhance
b. well-defined cortically based lesion
c. 'bubbly' internal structure
d. minimal mass effect and no associated vasogenic oedema
e. a third of lesions demonstrate calcification

50. All are true regarding endovascular procedure except
a. The femoral approach is almost exclusively used
b. Microcatheters are used to ensure stable access
c. Angiography must he repeated as often as is necessary to monitor the effects of treatment
d. Heparin is used to decrease the risk of thrombosis
e. used to restore narrowed or obliterated endovascular lumen supplying normal tissue

51. All are true regarding endovascular therapy of aneurysm except
a. the aim is total exclusion of the aneurysm lumen with preservation of the parent artery and its branches.
b. most reliably achieved in narrow-necked saccular aneurysms
c. Aneurysms with wide necks amenable to endovascular treatment by balloon remodelling and stenting
d. Potential complications include aneurysm perforation or rupture, inadvertent occlusion of the parent or branch arteries and thromboetnbolic events
e.. preservation of patency of the parent vessel is easily assured in fusiform or serpentine aneurysm

52. Tram-like occipital cortical calcification is seen in
a. neurofifbromatosis typeI
b. Sturge-Weber syndrome
c. tuberous sclerosis
d. lissencephaly
e. neurofifbromatosis type II

53. All are true regarding HU except
a. The baseline Hounsfield number for plasma is 24 HU
b. each gram percent of haemoglobin adds 4 HU
c. A blood specimen with 15 g haemoglobin has a Hounsfield number of approximately 50 units
d. contracted clot has Hounsfield number of aprox. 80HU
e. high HU of contracted clot is mainly due to iron

54. All are true regarding Vein of Galen except
a. formed by basal veins of Rosenthal and internal cerebral vein
b. runs under the splenium of corpus callosum
c. unite with inferior saggital sinus to form the straight sinus
d. also known as great cerebral vein
e. receive Vein of Trolard

55. All are true regarding cavernous angioma except
a. low hemosiderin rim
b. angiographically occult
c. 50% to 80% multiple
d. haemorrhage risk −0.5 % to 1% per year
e. blooming on T1

56. All are true regarding cerebellopontine angle masses except

a. CPA cistern contain 5th and 7th nerve
b. majority of CPA tumours are intra-axial in adult
c. Acoustic schwannoma account for about 75 % of CPA masses
d. epidermoid cyst has pearly surface
e. braod flat base towards dural surface is noted in meningioma

57. All are true regarding brainstem glioma except
a. nonifiltrating neoplasm
b. relatively late onset hydrocephalus
c. may encase basilar artery
d. hypointense on T1W
e. poor prognosis

58. All are true regarding craniopharyngioma except
a. most common nonglial brain tumour in children
b. 50%--combined suprasellar /intrasellar lesion
c. 90%---partially cystic
d. 90%--calcification
e. 90% --nodular enhancement

59. All athe structures show normal myelination at birth
a. optic nerve tract
b. medulla and dorsall midbrain
c. superior and inferior cerebellar peduncle
d. posterior limb of internal capsule
e. venterolateral thalamus

60. All are cacauses of bilateral basal ganglia calcification except
a. TB
b. cysticercosis
c. tuberous sclerosis
d. Down syndrome
e. Canavan disease

TEST PAPER 4 (ANSWER)

1. ----c
Loss of integrity of the blood–brain barrier is generally believed to begin 4 to 6 hours after the ischemic insult and lasts for approximately 3 to 5 days after the start of the infarction.

2----c
Magnetic susceptibility contrast agents such as dysprosium-diethylene triamine pentaacetic acid (DTPA)-bis(methylamide) or gadolinium-DTPA induce a T2* shortening and produce a signal loss in perfused tissue.

3.---d
Signal intensity of lacunes virtually always differ somewhat from that of CSF.

4.---d
Fibrin clot formation and retraction have not been shown to affect significantly the in vitro appearance of the acute hematoma at 1.5 T

5.---b
Brain MR has clearly replaced, or at least obviated, CT for most neurologic diseases. one of the sole indications for head CT is in suspected acute SAH. The most important exception to the superiority of MR over CT in neuroradiology has been in setting of ACUTE SAH.

6.---b
Spetzler and Martin grading of AVMs involves evaluation of three features: the size of the nidus, the location of the nidus, and the venous drainage pattern.

7.—a
On microscopic examination, cavernous angioma shows a honeycomb of multiple, partially collagenized, endothelial-lined sinusoidal vascular channels that varies in caliber. The walls of these channels may be thin, irregularly thickened and hyalinized or partially calcified Although virtually always well demarcated by a rim of gliotic brain stained by hemosiderin pigment from prior hemorrhages or diffusion of red cell pigment from prior intracavernous sequestration , the lesions are not encapsulated
Absent muscularis /elastica in vessel walls and the absence of interposed brain tissue in the lsion differentiate cavernous angioma from AVMs.
Adjacent parenchymal atrophy and gliosis may be found

8.---a

9.---b
Shear-strain deformation is characterized by a change in shape without a change in volume and is responsible for most mechanically induced lesions. Because of their inherently low rigidity, neurons are extremely susceptible to shear-strain deformations. These shear-strains develop because of differential movements of one portion of the brain with respect to another. Shear-strain forces are greatest at the junction of tissues of different

density and rigidity (CSF–brain, gray–white matter, brain–pia-arachnoid, pia-arachnoid–dura, skull–dura).

10.----b
Diffusion tensor imaging (DTI) is useful for characterization of the early laminar microarchitecture of the developing white matter tracts prior to full myelination in premature infants

11.---c
Most lesions are found in the cervical region.
MR studies have shown that cord abnormalities may be found in approximately 75% of MS patients and in an even higher proportion of patients with spinal cord symptoms . If a patient is shown to have an intramedullary lesion that is suspected to represent MS, an MR of the brain should always be performed to screen for asymptomatic multifocal disease , with the caveat that a normal brain MR in no way excludes MS as the diagnosis.
Gadolinium contrast administration frequently demonstrates enhancement of acute spinal cord lesions.
Enhancing MS plaques can be virtually indistinguishable from neoplastic lesions and other inflammatory lesions of the spinal cord

12.---b
Hypointense subependymal germinolytic cysts (typically involving the caudothalamic grooves) is noted on on MR imaging of Zellweger Syndrome.Other associated MR finding are microgyria (predominantly in the frontal and perisylvian cortex), polymicrogyria, and pachygyria (particularly in the perirolandic and occipital regions).

13.---e
GM2 gangliosidosis and Krabbe disease show hyperdense basal ganglia and thalami

14.---c
The CA1, CA2, and CA3 fields of the cornu ammonis are arranged linearly .
By 18 to 20 weeks, the hippocampus begins to resemble the adult hippocampus. Disorders arising from aberrations of hippocampal development include an unfolded (vertical) hippocampal configuration and hippocampal sulcal cyst remnants due to incomplete closure of the hippocampal sulcus .

15.---c
Rasmussen encephalitis usually presents in children younger than the age of 15 years.

16.---e

17.----e
MR imaging of gliomatosis cerebri shows extensive parenchymal involvement, especially of the white matter, as manifested by ill-defined regions of high intensity on T2-weighted images . Contrast enhancement is not believed to be a typical feature unless dedifferentiation has occurred
On pathologic studies, involved portions of the brain typically include nearly the extent of the cerebral hemispheres, with both

gray and white matter affected and the distinction between these regions lost

18.----d

Heamangioblastoma present in younger adults in von Hippel-Lindau syndrome. .
Hemangioblastomas are usually solitary lesions; multiplicity is said to occur in 20% of patients with von Hippel-Lindau syndrome and only rarely in otherwise healthy patients. Multiple hemangioblastomas are more common when they arise within the spinal cord .

19.----a

Malignant neoplasms, but not all neoplasms, demonstrate thick, irregular, or nodular enhancement, as opposed to the regular, thin, even, and smooth enhancing wall of the benign conditions.
Metatstases from melanoma, small cell lung carcinoma, thyroid cancer, choriocarcinoma, and renal cell carcinoma have a particular tendency to bleed.
High doses of MR imaging contrast agents appear to allow the detection of more metastatic lesions

20.---c

On MRI, epidermoids are distinctly different from arachnoid cysts, in that epidermoid tumors are virtually never isointense to CSF on MR images when using FLAIR . In addition, diffusion-weighted imaging demonstrates reduced diffusion within epidermoids.
On T1-weighted MR images, epidermoid tumors demonstrate subtle hypointensity compared to CSF. There is usually mild inhomogeneity of low intensity, with some patchy regions of isointensity within the lesion. On T2-weighted sequences the tumors show marked hyperintensity similar to or greater than that of CSF, with significant heterogeneity of the signal intensity. The low-intensity signals within the tumor hyperintense pattern are probably the result of the cellular debris and solid cholesterol crystals within the cysts . A high-intensity rim may surround the portion of the cyst on T2-weighted sequences that probably represents a CSF cleft.

21---d

Poor prognostic factors include patient age younger than 2 years, a short history of symptoms prior to presentation, presence of brainstem and cranial nerve deficits, lateral location of tumor, and high Ki-67 immunolabeling index.
The tumor arises within the fourth ventricle, extending into and through the outlets and the foramina of Luschka and the foramen Magendie, and giving impression of a plastic tumor mass. Extension of tumor through the outlets of the fourth ventricle into the cerebellopontine angle, in front of the brainstem, or down along the dorsal aspect of the cervical spinal cord may be visible on CT but is better seen on MRI

22.---e

Calcification in either the cyst wall or the solid component is highly indicative of this tumor

23.---c
Closure of the neural tube begins in the hindbrain

24.---a
Fungi that grow in infected tissues as yeast cells (Cryptococcus, Histoplasma) are spread hematogenously and, due to their small size, reach the meningeal microcirculation, penetrate the vessel walls, and result in acute or chronic leptomeningitis. Less frequently, parenchymal lesions such as granulomas and/or abscesses are encountered. Fungi that grow in infected tissues as hyphae (Aspergillus, Mucor) or pseudohyphae (Candida) tend to involve the parenchyma rather than the meninges because their larger size limits access to meningeal microcirculation

C. neoformans is the most common fungus to involve the CNS, and cryptococcosis is the most common fungus infection in AIDS patients

Cryptococcosis primarily manifests as meningitis, most pronounced in the cranial base. Four patterns of cryptococcal CNS infection may be encountered: parenchymal mass lesions, also known as cryptococcomas; dilated Virchow-Robin spaces ("gelatinous pseudocysts"); parenchymal/leptomeningeal nodules; and a mixed pattern.Virchow-Robin spaces of perforating arteries become distended with fungus and mucoid material, primarily in the basal ganglia and midbrainGelatinous pseudocysts do not display significant enhancement. The lesions may have mild mass effect, but there is no surrounding edema.The gelatinous pseudocysts are isointense to CSF on MR imaging, although they can often be slightly hyperintense on T1-weighted images. Primarily located in the midbrain and basal ganglia, they can be bilateral and are often symmetric . These pseudocysts do not enhance with gadolinium because the blood–brain barrier is not disrupted, and they are rarely associated with edema.

When there is hematogenous spread, usually from a pulmonary focus, Aspergillus hyphae lodge in cerebral vessels, cause occlusion, and grow through the vessel walls, producing infectious vasculopathy. Thus, an acute hemorrhagic infarction occurs at the beginning of the processes. Later, this converts to a septic infarction with associated cerebritis and abscess formation, usually in the distribution of the anterior and middle cerebral arteries . The basal ganglia and the thalami are characteristically involved in aspergillosis, as well as the corpus callosum and the brain stem. Involvement of the perforating arteries illustrates the invasive character of Aspergillus within the walls of the main cerebral arteries.

MR spectroscopy reveals

decreased NAA and markedly elevated lactate levels and the presence of succinate and acetate in CNS mucormycosis.

25.----b

Alzheimer disease (AD) is the most common cause of dementia in the elderly.

AD is characterized clinically by a progressive dementia, which typically begins with an isolated memory impairment.

Increased educational attainment and higher job complexity may reduce risk for late-onset AD.

The rare early-onset cases of AD present in individuals younger than the age of 65 years, some as young as the 30s.

The majority of individuals with autosomal dominant transmitted AD have mutations in one of three genes---the amyloid precursor protein gene on chromosome 21, the presenilin-1 gene on chromosome 14, and the presenilin-2 gene on chromosome 1. These known autosomal dominant mutations are involved in metabolism of amyloid protein, which implicates disordered amyloid protein in the causal pathway leading to AD.

The ε4 allele of apolipoprotein E (APOE), however, increases the risk of developing AD and also lowers the mean age at onset of the disease. APOE is a component of lipoproteins. Three normally occurring alleles of APOE have been identified: ε2, ε3, and ε4.

APOE ε3 is the most prevalent allele in the general population, with a frequency of roughly 80%.

The APOE ε3/4 genotype confers a roughly threefold increase in risk of developing AD, whereas ε4/4 confers an eightfold-increased risk of developing AD compared to the risk associated with the ε3/3 genotype. The ε2 allele decreases the risk of developing AD; however, this protective effect is not as strong as the risk conferred to carriers of ε4 allele.

26.---a

Pantothenate Kinase–Associated neurodegeneration and neurodegeneration with brain Iron Accumulation Type 1 is reffered as Hallervorden-Spatz Syndrome.

HD is inherited in an autosomal dominant fashion with complete penetrance. The genetic defect that causes HD is an expanded segment of chromosome 4 with a repeating pattern of the three nucleotide bases CAG. This segment of chromosome 4 encodes the huntingtin protein. In normal controls this segment of chromosome 4 typically has 29 or fewer CAG repeats; in HD patients this segment of chromosome 4 has 36 or more CAG repeats.

The putaminal measurement, when corrected for head volume, allowed the investigators to distinguish affected and control individuals in 100% of cases. The striatum (i.e., the caudate and putamen) is the largest subcortical gray matter structure in the brain. The globus pallidus forms the smaller part of the

lentiform nucleus, lying medial to the putamen.
The subthalamic nucleus is a lens-shaped nucleus on the dorsomedial surface of the peduncular part of the internal capsule .
The substantia nigra is the largest nucleus in the mesencephalon . It can be divided into the pars compacta, a cell-rich region containing melanin pigment, and the pars reticulata, a cell-poor region . The former is implicated in parkinsonian syndromes.
Selective bilateral pallidal necrosis is considered an organic hallmark of hypoxic-hypotensive insults of various origins
Dystonia commonly occurs with putaminal lesions in Leigh disease and Wilson disease
27.---c
70% of the patients with ONGs have NF1.
Optic nerve gliomas, especially those that present in childhood, are an important and often diagnostic feature of NF1
28.---d
Angiomatous" enlargement of the ipsilateral choroid plexus, and calvarial hemihypertrophy (widened diploic spaces and asymmetric sinus enlargement ipsilateral to the cortical atrophy) are secondary changes seen in Sturge-Weber Syndrome
29-.----d
Neither perilesional edema nor contrast enhancement is seen.in heterotopias.
30.---e
In true callosal hypogenesis

,posterior genu and anterior body of the CC is present whill eposterior body and splenium is small or absent. If the anterior portion of the CC is small or absent and the posterior portion is present, then, with certain exceptions, there has most likely been secondary destructive injury to the CC rather than a defect in development.

In holoprosencephaly,the splenium and callosal body may be present and the genu absent, or, in the case of the middle interhemispheric fusion variant of holoprosencephaly, the splenium and genu may be present and the body absent. Other examples of callosal dysgenesis include schizencephaly and porencephaly in which the telencephalon is injured and cannot send axons across the midline
Axons forming the CC has an aberrant course into the bundles of Probst
Some of the more commonly associated anomalies are the Chiari II malformation, the Dandy-Walker malformation, interhemispheric cysts, malformations of cortical development, cephaloceles, and midline facial anomalies . In general, these anomalies are the cause of clinical symptoms.
Isolated agenesis of the corpus callosum is usually asymptomatic and can be detected only by sophisticated neurologic testing.
31.---b
Three specific features help to

make the diagnosis of the trigeminal artery. First is the presence of a vessel that arises from the cavernous (or precavernous) carotid artery and courses directly posteriorly into the posterior fossa, where an abrupt medial bend is noted, and communication with the basilar artery is established.

The second feature is that the basilar artery will typically be of small caliber caudal to the trigeminal artery, and the ipsilateral PComA will also be small.

A variant trigeminal artery arises medially and courses through the sella and directly through the dorsum to reach the basilar artery. Thus, the third diagnostic feature is the identification of a vessel that appears to penetrate the dorsum sellae.

32.---d
Vein of Galen malformations comprise a spectrum of lesions ranging from those with numerous arteriovenous connections with no venous obstruction (choroidal type) to those with one or several arteriovenous fistulae with venous obstruction (mural type).

33.---e
ganglioneuroma, ganglioneuroblastoma and neuroblastomas show relatively low intensity on T2-weighted images, owing to the marked hypercellularity and paucity of free water content.

As tumor extends through the neural foramina, plain films disclose erosion of the pedicle, widening of the foramina, scalloping of the vertebral body, thinning of the ribs, or widening of the spinal canal

34.---a
The spinal cord receives its blood supply from the longitudinal anterior spinal artery (ASA) and the paired posterior spinal arteries (PSAs).

Predictable variations in caliber of the ASA occur along the length of the cord reflecting variations in metabolic requirement of the various cord regions. The relatively large amounts of gray matter found within the cervical and lumbar enlargements require a larger blood supply than the white matter tracts of the cord. Consequently, the larger size of the ASA in the lower cervical and lumbosacral regions, often exceeding 1 mm in diameter, reflects this relatively large blood flow requirement. The ASA often narrows to less than 0.5 mm in diameter in the thoracic region between T2 and T9, where the cord is largely composed of white matter tracts and the metabolic demand is correspondingly low

35.---e
Polio attacks principally motor neurons of the spinal cord and brainstem.

36.—d
Meningocele doesnot communicate with the terminal ventricle

37.---d
High-resolution T1-weighted images are standard for pituitary

pathology, they are not artifact free. An unusual artifact in the sella manifesting as focal T1 hyperintensity has been described in 14% of patients . Its presence could potentially obscure a lesion or could be mistaken for substances resulting in T1 shortening such as hemorrhage or protein. The artifact is secondary to focal susceptibility differences among the air-filled sphenoid sinus, bone, and the pituitary fossa soft tissue and is consistently related to the junction between the sphenoidal septum and sellar floor.

38.----b
Papillary lesions are solid with no calcification . In distinction from their adamantinomatous counterpart, MR shows papillary craniopharyngiomas as solid lesions. they are often situated within the third ventricle. These lesions demonstrate a nonspecific signal intensity pattern, without the characteristic hyperintensity on T1-weighted images of the cystic component of adamantinomatous tumors. Like all craniopharyngiomas, papillary lesions typically enhance.
On pathologic examination, papillary lesions do not show the features characteristic of the adamantinomatous variant, that is, the cholesterol crystals in a cystic component, wet keratin nodules, fibroinflammatory tissue, keratin, calcification, and nuclear palisades. In papillary lesions, there is extensive squamous differentiation.

39.----b
Trilateral" retinoblastoma ---- bilateral retinoblastoma with associated pineal tumor

40.---d
High Cho/NAA ratio is a strong indicator of a higher-grade neoplasm, but a low Cho/NAA ratio could arise from a low-grade neoplasm, low neoplastic cellular density, or nonneoplastic processes such as multiple sclerosis.

41.----a
The middle cerebral artery is divided into four anatomical segments: the horizontal segment (M1), insular segment (M2), opercular segment (M3) and cortical branches (M4 segments). The characteristic loops formed by the upward and downward course of the insular and opercular segments form a straight line on the lateral projection, which represents the upper border of the 'Sylvian triangle', its inferior border being formed by main middle cerebral artery trunk. The 'Sylvian point' is the highest and most medial point where the angular artery turns inferolaterally to exit the Sylvian fissure. Displacement of these landmarks has been used in the past to locate cerebral mass lesions.

42.---c
 Oligodendroglioma are diffusely infiltrating neoplasms that are found almost exclusively in the cerebral hemispheres, most commonly in the frontal lobes,

and typically involve subcortical white matter and cortex.

43.---c
Most macroadenomas are isointense with brain parenchyma on unenhanced T1W images and hyperdense on CT
The primary treatment of prolactin-secreting microadenomas is medical and the role of imaging in cases of hyperprolactinaemia is therefore mainly to exclude a macroadenoma.

44.---a
CT is positive for SAH in 98 per cent within 12 h of onset but this falls to less than 75 per cent by the third day.
No underlying cause of SAH is found on angiography in 15% cases

45.---a

46.----c
MRI in the coronal plane is mandatory to detect hippocampal sclerosis
The signs of hippocampal sclerosis on MRI are (1) volume loss and (2) increased signal on T2-weighted images.

47.---c
At full term, T1-weighted images should show high signal in the dorsal medulla and brain stem, the cerebellar peduncles, a small part of the cerebral peduncles, about a third of the posterior limb of the internal capsule, the central corona radiata, and the deep white matter in the region of the pre- and post-central gyrus.

48.---a
NF1 is associated with some characteristic bone dysplasias, including lambdoid sutural dysplasia, thinning of long bone cortices and kyphoscoliosis with a high thoracic acute curve

49.---a
Most dysembryoplastic neuroepithelial tumour (DNT) tumours do not enhance and if present, enhancement is faint and patchy.

50.---b
Generally, a guiding catheter is used to ensure stable access and provide a route for injection of contrast for road-mapping. Microcathctcrs, either flow guided or over the wire. are usually used to reach the target.

Endovascular procedures can he broadly divided into two categories: those that aim to restore a narrowed or obliterated cndovascular lumen supplying normal tissues and those that aim to exclude abnormal blood vessels from the circulation.

51.---e
Where preservation of patency of the parent vessel cannot be assured (fusiform or serpentine aneurysms, wide-necked aneurysms,false aneurysms and arterial dissection), sacrifice of the parent vessel may be considered, usually preceded by test occlusion. This can be achieved with either coils or detachable balloons, depending on the vessel configuration and indication for treatment.

52.----b

53.---e
High HU of contracted clot is mainly due to tightly packed haemoglobin. A contracted clot has Hb value of 30 gram with an absorption value of approx. 80. Iron percentage contributes about 4 units and tightly packed haemoglobin rest of the increase.
54.----e
55.---e
Blooming occurs on T2W imaging .
56.---b
Majority of CPA tumours are extra-axial in adult.
57.—e
Prognosis is excellent of brainstem glioma
58. ---b
75% of craniopharyngioma --- combined suprasellar /intrasellar cystic mass with mural nodule
59.---a
Optic nerve ,deep cerebellar white matter ,corticospinal tracts and pre/postcentral gyri show normal myelination at one month.
60.---e
CID, congenital HIV,MELAS/MERRF,Cockyne syndrome NF,methemoglobinopathy,carbon monoxide,lead intoxication are other causes of bilateral basal ganglia calcification

TEST PAPER 5

1. All are true regarding pathophysiology of stroke except
a. Normal cerebral blood flow is in the range of 50 to 55 mL/100 g brain tissue/min
b. cerebral blood flow values below 10 mL/100 g/min may lead to infarction within a matter of minutes
c. Cell depolarization is not observed until blood flow drops below 10 mL/100 g/min
d. penumbra surround the zone around the central core
e. In acute period there is a swelling and softening of the tissue with evidence of mass effect

2. All are true regarding Diffusion-weighted imaging except
a. uses pulsed gradients to make in vitro diffusion measurements
b. the b value alters the sensitivity of the image to the diffusion
c. hyperintensity indicate either restricted diffusion or T2 change or both.
d. ADC maps demonstrate contrast based purely on diffusion differences
e. ADC maps alone have very high sensitivity and accuracy for acute infarction

3. All are true regarding lacunar infarction except
a. defined as small-vessel infarctions up to 1.5 cm in diameter
b. typically seen in the deep gray matter, brainstem, and deep white matter of the hemispheres
c. spin echo MR is far more sensitive than CT for detecting lacunar infarction
d. lacunar infarctions were often multiple
e. conventional MR can readily age lacunar infarctions

4. All are features of acute haematoma except
a. markedly hypointense on T2W images and on GRE imaging
b. isointense or minimally hypointense to brain on T1-weighted images
c. high-intensity perimeter around the hemorrhage on the T2-weighted image due to edema
d. T1 shortening is observed on T1-weighted images
e. the hypointensity on what is called a T1-weighted image is actually a T2 effect

5. The most common atraumatic cause of SAH in the adult is
a. ruptured aneurysm
b. Intracranial arteriovascular malformations
c. Superficial intraparenchymal hemorrhage
d. Bleeding diathesis
e. Iatrogenic coagulopathy

6. All are associated with AVMS except
a. venous varices
b. intervening brain parenchyma found within the vascular nidus
c. gliosis and demyelination and parenchymal atrophy
d. presence of ferritin, hemosiderin, and other iron-storage forms

e. Calcification in vessel walls and adjacent brain parenchyma

7. All are true regarding cavernous angioma except
a. the second-most-common cause of symptomatic vascular malformation
b. Seizures are the most common symptom
c. Seizures associated with cavernous angiomas are most often focal
d. the risk of hemorrhage is in the range of 0.1% to 1.1% per year for each lesion
e. Extension of hemorrhage into subarachnoid or intraventricular space is common

8. All are true regarding developmental venous anomalies except
a. no arterial component
b. intervening brain tissue is usually abnormal
c. may be the most common cerebrovascular malformation
d. clinically silent
e. may be associated with cortical dysplasias

9. The most important factor that affects lesion visibility in MRI of trauma case is
a. lesion size and location
b. presence and age of hemorrhage
c. presence of edema
d. MR acquisition parameters
e. the MR pulse sequence

10. The most useful MR sequence for evaluating the progression of myelination during the first 6 months of life is
a. T1W
b. T2W
c. FLAIR
d. SW images
e. MR tractography

11. Which MR technique may be used to discern otherwise occult Multiple sclerosis disease in normal-appearing brain parenchyma?
a. MR spectroscopy
b. MT techniques
c. Diffusion-weighted MR imaging
d. T2W
e. T1W

12. Dilated perivascular spaces in the corpus callosum is seen in
a. mucopolysaccharidoses
b. Gaucher Disease
c. Fabry Disease
d. Krabbe disease
e. MLD

13. All are features of adrenoleukodystrophy except
a. The cerebral cortex and gray matter are of normal thickness
b. Symmetric areas of white matter abnormality in periatrial region extending across the splenium of the corpus callosum
c. The frontal white matter is most commonly involved
d. The demyelination tends to have a caudorostral progression with relative sparing of the subcortical arcuate fibers
e. Contrast enhancement appears at the lateral margin of the zones of demyelination

14. Enhancement after contrast administration is seen in
a. Adrenoleukodystrophy, Alexander disease and Krabbe disease
b. Alexander disease and Krabbe

disease
c. Adrenoleukodystrophy and Krabbe disease
d. Adrenoleukodystrophy and Alexander disease
e. Adrenoleukodystrophy only

15. All are true regarding anatomy of brain except
a. tangential gray matter (alveus) converge to form the fimbria
b. Fimbria projects into the temporal horn ventricular cavity and continues as fornix
c. The amygdala is located superomedial to the tip of the temporal horn
d. the tip of the temporal horn of lateral ventricle is known as the uncal recess
e. the uncal recess separates amygdala from hippocampal head

16. all are causes of bilateral basal ganglia lucencies except
a. severe hypoglycemia
b. MELAS
c. toxoplasmosis
d. Alexander disease
e. Hemolytic uremic syndrome

17. Profound hypervascularity are associated with all intracranial tumour except
a. hemangioblastoma
b. glioblastoma
c. medulloblastoma
d. anaplastic oligodendroglioma
e. metastase from renal cell carcinoma

18. All are true regarding brain lesions except
a. Hemorrhage is highly unusual in hemangioblastoma
b. The large, often nonenhancing cyst and the posterior fossa location are key feature of hemangioblastoma
c. the capsule of an abscess shows thin high intensity on T1W and thin hypointensity on T2W images
d. pyogenic abscesses show central restricted diffusion
e. lymphoma is usually homogeneous and hyperintense on T2W images

19. The most common primary intraaxial neoplasm of the adult posterior fossa is
a. hemangioblastoma
b. Meningioma
c. Schawannoma
d. dermoid cyst
e. Lhermitte-Duclos disease

20. All are true regarding metastases except
a. nonhemorrhagic metastases from melanoma are hyperintense on T1W and isointense on T2W
b. colonic mucinous adenocarcinomas metastases shows hypointensity on T2W standing out from hyperintense edema.
c. essentially all intracerebral metastases demonstrate contrast enhancement on MR imaging
d. contrast-enhanced MR imaging may detects many lesions that otherwise go undetected even on high-quality CT with contrast
e. high doses of MR imaging contrast agents doesnot increase number of the detection of metastatic lesions

21. All are true regarding epidermoid cysts except
a. congenital lesions of ectodermal origin
b. soft and very pliable

c. referred to as "pearly tumors" because of their gross internal appearance
d. hypodense and do not enhance with contrast material
e. tend to engulf and surround vessels

22. All are true regarding atypical teratoid/rhabdoid tumor except
a. highly malignant tumor
b. at a older age than PNET
c. very poor prognosis
d. large areas of PNET within the ATRT tumor
e. a tendency to occur in the cerebellar pontine angle / medullary pontine angle

23. All are true pineal glands and lesions except
a. the pineal gland normally enhances
b. Calcification within the pineal on CT is normal before age 6 years
c. A cyst in the pineal gland is a frequent normal finding
d. the most common tumor of the pineal gland in second decade of life is the germinoma
e. Parinaud syndrome may be noted

24. All are imaging features of pyogenic abscess except
a. center of the cavity is slightly hyperintense to CSF on T1W
b. signal intensities of center are quite variable on T2W
c. The rim is isointense to slightly hyperintense to white matter on T1-weighted images
d. The rim is hyperintense on T2-weighted images
e. smooth ring enhancement of an abscess capsule on postgadolinium MR images

25. All are true regarding tuberculous abscess except
a. TB abscesses are larger than tuberculomas
b. hypodense with surrounding edema and mass effect.
c. usually thin and uniform ring enhancement
d. Central area –variable signal on T2W
e. the rim --- a hypointense signal

26. Hypointensity on T2-weighted images in the extrapyramidal nuclei, thalami, and deep white matter due to iron deposition is seen in
a. multiple sclerosis
B. Pelizaeus-Merzbacher disease
c. cerebral infarctions
d. aging
e. all

27. All are true regarding NPH except
a. enlargement of the ventricular system out of proportion to the subarachnoid space
b. a prominent periventricular halo
c. a prominent CSF flow void in the cerebral aqueduct
d. reduced aqueductal flow velocity
e. triad of cognitive decline, gait disturbance, and incontinence

28. All are true regarding optic nerve glioma (ONG) in NF1 except
a. The presence of bilateral ONGs is considered specific for NF1
b. ONGs(sporadic and in NF1) are almost invariably juvenile pilocytic astrocytomas in childhood.
c. 20% of the patients with ONGs have NF1

d. 50% of childhood juvenile pilocytic astrocytoma present in the optic chiasm and hypothalamus
e. 5% to 40% of patients with NF1 develop ONGs

29. All are true regarding intracranial involvement of Sturge-Weber Syndrome except
a. ipsilateral to the port-wine nevus of the face
b. preferential involvement of the occipital lobe followed by the temporal and parietal lobes
c. Involvement of the posterior fossa structures
d. prominent medullary veins draining the cortex in a centripetal fashion to the periventricular vein.
e. the characteristic "tram-track" or railroad track appearance

30. All are true regarding cortical dyplasia of Tylor(CDT) except
a. CDT-D has balloon cells within dysplastic areas
c. CDT resembles the cortical tubers of tuberous sclerosis
d. one of most common causes of epilepsy attributable to focal cerebral dysgenesis
e. blurring of the gray–white matter junction
e. High-resolution imaging useful

31. All are true regarding Chiari I Malformation except
a. inferior displacement of the cerebellar tonsils through the foramen magnum into the rostral cervical spinal canal
b. Mild cerebellar ectopia refers to the caudal tips of the tonsils less than 5 mm below a line from the basion to the opisthion
c. descent of tonsil up to 2 mm is not considered pathologic (5yrs to 15yrs)
d. tonsillar protrusion of more than 5 mm below the foramen magnum is associated with a dramatic rise in the incidence of clinical symptoms (outside 5 to 15 yrs)
e. The concurrence of Chiari I malformations and syringohydromyelia has been estimated at between 25% and 65%

32. All are true regarding ICA agenesis except
a. persistent fetal communications through the sella turcica
b. enlargement of the basilar artery and posterior communicating artery
c. hypoplastic carotid canal on CT
d. externalization of the common carotid waveforms on usg
e. rete mirabile

33. -All are features of persistent trigeminal artery except
a. vessel arising from the cavernous (or precavernous) carotid artery
b. an abrupt lateral bend in posterior foss to communicate with the basilar artery
c. small caliber of the basilar artery caudal to the trigeminal artery
d. small ipsilateral PComA
e. the identification of a vessel that appears to penetrate the dorsum sellae

34. All are true regarding Chordoma except
a. 50% arise in the sacrum

b. the lumber spine most common site among spine
c. vacuolated physaliferous cells
d. amorphous calcification in 50% to 70% of the cases
e. high signal on T2-weighted and usually prominent enhancement

35. All are true regarding spinal cord hemangioblastoma except
a. considerable edema, similar to cord metastases
b. serpiginous areas of signal void or enhancement anterior to chord
c. markedly enhancing tumor nidus
d. widening of the spinal cord
e. cyst formation

36. All are true regarding spinal tuberculosis except
a. usually starts in the anteroinferior portion of the vertebral body
b. Grade III bone destruction with relative disc preservation
c. Focal and heterogeneous contrast enhancement
d. Well defined Signal intensity in paraspinal areas
e. Discal abscess with rim enhancement

37. All are true regarding sacrococcygeal teratomas except
a. most probably derived from cells of Hensen's node
b. Calcification found in about 50% of benign teratomas
c. typically lie cephalic to the intergluteal cleft
d. Altman type I tumors have minimal presacral component
e. Mostly mixed solid and cystic lesions

38. All are true regading pituitary gland except

a. the hyperintensity is not visible in diabetes insipidus in posterior pituitary gland
b. the suprasellar cistern resembles a six-pointed star in in the axial plane
c. The pituitary stalk is the central landmark in the suprasellar cistern
d. The pituitary stalk is approximately 6 mm thick
e. When viewed from below, the chiasm resembles the letter "X

39. All are true regarding imaging of adamantinomatous craniopharyngioma except
a. cystic component and solid component
b. cystic component hypointense T1- and hyperintense on T2- weighted images
c. frequent encasing of nearby cerebral vasculature
d. solid portion is frequently partially calcified and heterogeneous
e. moderate degree of enhancement of the solid portion of the tumor

40. All are true regarding diabetes insipidus except
a. due to failure to synthesize vasopressin in the paraventricular nuclei of the hypothalamus
b. Eighty percent or more of the vasopressin-secreting cells must be affected before clinical diabetes insipidus develops
c. imaging is directed at excluding a neoplastic or infiltrative lesion of the suprasellar cistern or hypothalamus
d. disappearance of hyperintensity of posterior

pituitary on T1-weighted images in any cause
e. visualization of the posterior lobe high signal in nephrogenic diabetes insipidus

41. All are true regarding ^{1}H MRS Changes in Neoplasia except
a. the hallmark of neoplasia is an elevation of the Cho resonance
b. a reduction of NAA
c. little or minor changes in Cr
d. low Cho/NAA ratio is a strong indicator of a higher-grade neoplasm
e. A Cho/NAA ratio of greater than 1.3 has been reported to have a high accuracy for detection of neoplasm

42. All are true regarding angiography except
a. At the bifurcation, the internal carotid lies usually posterior and lateral to the external carotid artery.
b. The petrous segment of ICA is intraosseous
c. in fetal arrangement ,the posterior cerebral artery arise directly from the internal carotid artery
d. The recurrent artery of Huebner may arise from the A1 or A2 segment
e. fusion of the A1 segment in the midline give a single 'azygos' anterior cerebral artery

43. All are true regarding pleomorphic xanthoastrocytoma (PXA) except
a. arises near the surface of the cerebral hemispheres
b. frequently cystic
c. may enhance strongly

d. usually associated with little or no oedema
e.. T1 hyperintense and T2 hypointense due to fat content.

44. All are true regarding chemodectomas except
a. arise from paraganglion cells
b. The most common site is the jugular bulb
c. bone destruction with enlargement of formen ovale
d. enhance intensely with IV contrast medium
e. tend to show areas of flow void corresponding to dilated vessels

45. All are true except
a. NASCET method of measuring carotid artery stenosis ---------[1– (minimum residual lumen/distal internal carotid lumen)] × 100
b. patients with symptomatic 70–99 per cent stenosis of the internal carotid artery are benefited from surgery
c. Surgery reduces the risk of stroke in asymptomatic carotid stenosis of 70 per cent or more as measured by US.
d. Carotid intervention should not be considered for a stenosis of less than 60 per cent regardless of symptoms.
e. Symptomatic 50–69 per cent stenoses may be a suitable target for intervention but in both cases the benefits are smaller.

46. All are causes of focal parenchymal mass with enhancement in HIV-related CNS disease except
a. Toxoplasmosis
b. Lymphoma
c. Tuberculosis
d. Candida

e. Cryptococcomas

47. Reduced frontal perfusion is noted in all except
a. frontotemporal dementia
b. schizophrenia, depression
c. human immunodeficiency virus (HIV) encephalopathy
d., Creutzfeldt–Jacob disease (CJD)
e. all

48. All are true regarding myelination of brain except
a. the myelination pattern seen at birth at full term is primarily in the motor tract
b. the process of myelination is easiest to follow on T1W during the first 6 months of life.
c. T1-weighted images at full term should show high signal in the dorsal medulla and brain stem
d. T2-weighted images are used to assess the myelination from 6 months to 24 months of age
e. the first signs of mature subcortical white matter on T2W are found around the calcarine fissure

49. All are true regarding 'neurofibromatosis bright objects (NBOs)' except
a. in 60–80% of NF1 cases
b. number remains static
c. multiple T2 hyperintense lesions with minimal mass effect and no contrast enhancement
d. the pons, cerebellar white matter, internal capsules are typical sites
e. normal signal on T1-weighted images

50. All are true regarding choroid plexus tumour except
a. most common brain tumour in children under 1 year
b. hyperdense or isodense, lobulated 'frond-like' mass
c. avidly and homogeneously enhancing masses with punctate calcifications
d. typical site is the frontal horn
e. Haemorrhage and localized vasogenic oedema are suggestive of carcinoma with invasion

51. Irreversible neurological deficit from diagnostic neuroangiography is in the range of
a. 0.3 to 3 /1000
b. 0.1 to 0.2/1000
c. 4 to 5/1000
d. 6 to 7/1000
e. 8 to 9 /1000

52. All are true regarding spine lesions except
a. the most common neoplastic extradural mass is metastases
b. the nidus of an osteoid soteoma frequently exceed 1.5 to 2.0 cm in diameter
c. feathered appearance at level of obstruction is noted in extradural masses
d. meningiomas are usually intradural extramedullary masses
e. Polka dot noted noted in hemangioma

53. All are true regarding endovascular therapy of aneurysm except
a. preffered approach in aneurysms in the posterior fossa
b. advantageous in acute SAH with two aneurysm
c. comparable rates of immediate neurological complication to conventional surgery
d. recurrence of aneurysms

especially of MCA following endovascular therapy
e. the most widely used technique is coil embolisation

54. All are true regarding calcification in infection except
a. congenital toxoplasmosis consist of multiple scattered flecks in the cortex and linear streaks in the basal ganglia
b. widespread periventricular calcification is noted in congenital CMV
c. Oat –shaped calcification is noted in neurocysticercosis
d. calcification in basal ganglia in congenital toxoplasmosis is linear
e. Neurofibromatosis show Extensive calcification of the choroid plexuses of the third and lateral ventricle
Oat –shaped calcification is noted in muscle cysticercosis

55. All are true regarding velum except
a. cyst of the cavum Vergae is reactangular on axial CT
b. velum interpositum lies below the third ventricle
c. velum interpositum is .triangular on axial CT with apex anteriorly
d. velum interpositum contains internal cerebral vein
e. .velum interpositum is normal condition

56. All are true regarding PCA except
a. P1 segment refers to precommunicating /peduncular segment
b. posterior thalmoperforating arteries supply the diencephalon and midbrain
c. parietooccipital sulcus froms the boundary between the PCA and the ACA
d. fetat origin of the PCA refers to its origin from the ICA
e. fetal origin of the PCA is seen in 1 to 2%

57. All are true regarding AVM except
a. strong serpentine enhancement
b. calcification in 2 % to 3%
c. tightly packed honeycomb of flow voids
d. steal phenomenon
e. may be atrophy and gliosis

58. All are true regarding intraventricular masses except
a. Choloid cysts are the most common mass in anterior third ventricle
b. stenosis is the most common intrinsic aqueductal abnormality
c. cerebellar astrocytoma is the most common posterior fossa tumour in children
d. ependymoma extend through the foramina of Luschka
e. the most common fourth ventricular neoplasm in an adult is ependymoma

59. All are common causes of "holes in the skull" except
a. dermoid
b. eosinophilic granuloma
c. metastases
d. surgical
e. epidermod

60. Which dimention is not part of Elster's rule for maximum normal height (in mm) of the pituitary gland?
a. 6mm
b. 8mm
c. 10mm

d.12mm
e.14mm

TEST PAPER 5(ANSWER)

1.----e

An initial acute period lasts for the first 2 days after the infarction in which gross examination demonstrates what appears to be normal tissue. This is followed by a subacute period during which there is a swelling and softening of the tissue with evidence of mass effect. This subacute period (with reference to pathology) generally extends for 7 to 10 days after the infarction, with maximal edema occurring at approximately 3 to 5 days. The chronic period extends from weeks to months after the infarction. During this time the infarcted tissue evolves into an area of encephalomalacia or cystic change.

Functionally the ischemic tissue can be divided into three compartments. The infarct core representing the dead or dying tissue is at the center of the infarction. The zone around the central core may have lost electrical activity, but it has more moderate reductions in blood flow and is defined as the penumbra. With reperfusion this tissue may be salvageable, but without reperfusion it may go on to infarction . Surrounding the penumbra is tissue with mildly reduced blood flow, often called the oligemic region. This tissue is more likely to survive; however, this region too may go on to infarct if perfusion is further hemodynamically altered.

2.---e

The diffusion-weighted image and the ADC image are read together. Diffusion-weighted image shows hyperintensity in acute infarction .The ADC map confirms the restriction of diffusion, seen as low intensity.If no hyperintensity is seen on DWI, then there is no acute infarction and no need for ADC maps because ADC maps alone have very low sensitivity and accuracy for acute infarction . Nonacute infarctions show no hyperintensity on DWI in the vast majority of cases, despite prolongation of T2 in the infarcted region.

3.---e

Conventional MR cannot readily age lacunar infarctions Diffusion-weighted MR has been found to improve the diagnostic detection of the acute lesions responsible for a patient's clinical symptoms. diffusion-weighted MR identifies multiple small acute infarctions that may be clinically silent.

4.-----d

No T1 shortening is observed on T1-weighted images in case of intracellular deoxyhaemoglobin.

5.---a

6.—b

There is no intervening brain parenchyma found within the vascular nidus.

7.---e

Extension of hemorrhage into subarachnoid or intraventricular space is not common. Progressive neurologic deficit is an uncommon manifestation of supratentorial cavernous angiomas but occurs more often with those in the infratentorial space

8.—b

Developmental venous anomalies (DVAs) /venous angiomas / venous malformations is an incidental malformations of venous drainage patterns. There is no arterial component in this entity. Intervening brain tissue is present between the veins comprising the lesion, and this brain tissue is usually normal without evidence of hemosiderin staining or gliosis .**9.—e**

10.---a

During the first 6 months of life, T1-weighted images are most useful for evaluating the progression of myelination. Inversion recovery images also provide improved T1-weighted contrast differences between tissues. After 6 months of age, most cerebral white matter appears high in signal intensity on the T1-weighted images, and beyond this time the T2-weighted images are generally relied on to further evaluate myelin progression. By 24 months of age, the process of myelination is essentially complete except for the terminal zones of myelination found in the occipital-parietal periventricular white matter

11.----b

MT techniques have been applied to brain MR in an attempt to characterize MS lesions and to discern otherwise occult disease in normal-appearing brain parenchyma. This pulse sequence technique exploits differences in relaxation between immobilized water transiently bound to macromolecules and water protons not associated with macromolecules. The hypothesis underlying these investigations is that demyelination results in more free water (i.e., a reduction in the "bound" fraction of water) compared with myelinated white matter or intact but edematous tissue. Selective suppression of immobilized water is accomplished by the application of an off-resonance saturation pulse, which saturates the broad resonance of protons bound to macromolecules. Transiently bound protons exchange with free water protons by diffusion

Using experimental design, it has been shown in some studies that MT ratios are higher (i.e., there is more signal reduction due to the saturation pulse) in normal mature (myelinated) white matter than in gray matter. A slight decrease of the magnetization transfer ratio was noted in early inflammatory lesions without demyelination in models of experimental allergic encephalomyelitis. More pronounced reductions in MT ratios have been described in demyelinating lesions in experimental models (proportional to the degree of demyelination) and in patients with MS

12.----a

13.---c

The parietal and occipital white matter is most commonly involved

14.---a

15----a

The hippocampus lies superior to subiculum and parahippocampal gyrus, forming a 4- to 4.5-cm-long curved elevation in the floor of the temporal horn of lateral ventricle .The convex ventricular surface is covered with ependyma, underneath which tangential white-matter tracts, called alveus, pass medially to converge to form the fimbria, which projects into the ventricular cavity and continues as fornix.

16.---b

17.---c

18.----e

Lymphoma most commonly is homogeneous and low intensity on T2-weighted images, a characteristic seen less commonly in glioblastoma

19.---a

20.---e

High doses of MR imaging contrast agents appear to allow the detection of more metastatic lesions

21.---c

The epidermoid cysts are frequently referred to as "pearly tumors" because of their gross external appearance(lobulated appearance)

On CT the lesions are hypodense and do not enhance with contrast material . They are difficult to differentiate from arachnoid cysts based on their density; however, their external surface is usually lobulated in configuration compared with the smooth surface of an arachnoid cyst. There may occasionally be focal calcifications in their walls. In contrast to arachnoid cysts, epidermoids tend to engulf and surround vessels and cranial nerves, whereas arachnoid cysts displace such structures.

22.---b

Atypical teratoid/rhabdoid tumor occurs at a younger age than PNET and is categorized as a WHO grade IV tumor

In fact, histologically there often are large areas of PNET within the ATRT tumor . However, in addition, there are areas of rhabdoid cells that appear quite different from the PNET component.

23.—b

Calcification within the pineal, seen on CT, is not normal before age 6 years (186). After age 6 years, and especially as a child approaches puberty, calcification becomes quite common and more prominent. The demonstration on CT of abnormally early calcification of the pineal, that is, before the age of 6years, especially if there is any soft tissue component surrounding it, should raise the concern that a pineal tumor is present . The bilaterality of congenital retinoblastoma raises the possibility of trilateral retinoblastoma with a pineoblastoma of the pineal gland, which is histologically identical to retinoblastoma in the eye

In the pediatric age group, the most common pineal tumor is the primitive neuroectodermal tumor (PNET), which usually occurs in younger children in the first decade of life and with an equal gender predilection. In the second decade of life, the most common tumor of the pineal gland is the germinoma.

Parinaud syndrome consist of vertical gaze paralysis and pupillary dilation if the mass exerts pressure on the tectum of the midbrain

24.----d

In a typical abscess with central liquefactive necrosis, the center of the cavity is slightly hyperintense to CSF, whereas the surrounding edematous brain is slightly hypointense to normal brain parenchyma on T1-weighted images. The rim is isointense to slightly hyperintense to white matter on T1-weighted images and is hypointense on T2-weighted images.

The rim may be a better indicator of response to treatment than residual enhancement, which can persist on contrast studies for months after completion of therapy . Other lesions that may have a hypointense rim on T2-weighted images include evolving hematomas, infrequent metastases, and high-grade gliomas with cystic necrosis

25.—d

The abscess is formed by semiliquid pus teeming with tubercle bacilli.The wall of a tuberculous abscess lacks the giant cell epithelioid granulomatous reaction of a TB granuloma.

On CT, the tuberculous abscess is hypodense with surrounding edema and mass effect. Postcontrast images demonstrate ring enhancement that is usually thin and uniform, but less often may be somewhat irregular and thick. The appearance is related to the central zone of liquefactive necrosis with pus and surrounding inflammation. This central area is thus of increased signal on T2-weighted images, and the rim can present a hypointense signal . The enhancement pattern on MR is similar to that on CT.

Infarction, meningeal enhancement, and parenchymal disease seem to be more common in patients with TB who are also HIV infected.

26.---e

27.---d

The prominent flow void in the cerebral aqueduct has been attributed to excessively rapid pulsatile CSF flow . The putative result of loss of brain elasticity in this condition produces excessively forceful transmission of the arterial pressure pulse during cardiac systole to the incompressible CSF in the ventricular system. This forceful pressure wave is transmitted from the CSF in the lateral ventricles through the third ventricle to the CSF in the aqueduct, resulting in pulsatile flow in the aqueduct that is more prominent than normal.

This in turn results in a loss of coherent signal in aqueductal CSF, which is more prominent than normal. MRI markers of this hyperdynamic aqueductal CSF flow have been prominent signal loss, prominent anteroposterior extent of the aqueductal CSF signal void, and excessive aqueductal flow velocity using formal velocity measurements with cine phase contrast methods

28.---c
70% of the patients with ONGs have NF1.
Optic nerve gliomas, especially those that present in childhood, are an important and often diagnostic feature of NF1

29.---c
The posterior fossa (infratentorial) structures are not affected by pial angiomatosis, presumably because their embryologic development is different.
The density and extent of calcification increases over time and advances from posterior to anterior .Controlling or eliminating the aggravating effects of the seizures may prevent f progression of both the atrophy and the calcification. For this reason, partial hemispherectomy for seizure control may be more beneficial than harmful, especially in patients younger than the age of 5 years.

30.---a
The cortical dysplasias of Taylor (CDTs) are characterized by the presence of abnormal neurons and glia within localized regions of the cerebral cortex.
At least two types of CDT are recognized: CDT with dysplastic neurons only and no balloon cells (CDT-D), and CDT with giant so-called balloon cells (BC) that are found within the area of dysplasia (CDT-BC)
The most common features seen in CDT in the series by Lawson et al. were blurring of the gray–white matter junction (80%), thick cortex (70%), and elevated signal on T2-weighted images in the affected gray matter (70%).
In the study by Lawson et al. both CDT-D and CDT-B most often involved the frontal lobe . In a study by Yagishitia et al., however, 60% of CDT was found within the temporal lobes.

31.---c
Descent of tonsil up to 6 mm is not considered pathologic (during 5yrs to 15yrs).

32.—c
Absent carotid canal is noted in ICA agenesisi
The primitive internal carotid arteries (ICAs) develop primarily from the third aortic arches

33.------b
Three specific features help to make the diagnosis of the trigeminal artery. First is the presence of a vessel that arises from the cavernous (or precavernous) carotid artery and courses directly posteriorly into the posterior fossa, where an abrupt medial bend is noted, and communication with the basilar artery is established.
The second feature is that the

basilar artery will typically be of small caliber caudal to the trigeminal artery, and the ipsilateral PComA will also be small.

A variant trigeminal artery arises medially and courses through the sella and directly through the dorsum to reach the basilar artery . Thus, the third diagnostic feature is the identification of a vessel that appears to penetrate the dorsum sellae.

34.---b

They arise from remnants of the notochord. Because the notochord, which forms the early fetal skeleton, extends from the clivus to the sacrum, chordomas can occur anywhere along the skull base and spine: 50% arise in the sacrum, 35% in the clivus, and 15% in the vertebrae.

In the spine, the areas most commonly involved are the cervical, lumbar, and finally the thoracic spine, in descending order of frequency .

35.---b

Myelography frequently shows expansion of the spinal cord and serpiginous filling defects posterior to the cord representing meningeal varicosities.

Spinal angiography reveals prominent feeding arteries and draining veins and an intense blush of the tumor nidus

Adjacent serpiginous areas of signal void or enhancement may be seen on MRI and, when present, clinch the diagnosis because the main mimic of these lesions, metastases, do not have associated enlarged vessels . These can represent large feeding arteries or, more commonly, draining meningeal varicosities associated with the very vascular tumor nidus.

The differentiation of edematous cord from cyst is important because metastases of the cord rarely are associated with cysts, whereas the other intramedullary lesion to show dramatic focal enhancement amid a larger region of nonenhancing abnormality, the hemangioblastoma, is frequently associated with a large syrinx.

36.---e

The thoracolumbar junction is affected most commonly, and the disease is relatively infrequent in the cervical and sacral segments of the spine.

Intraosseous abscess with enhancement of the vertebral body is noted in spinal tuberculosis

Differential Diagnosis Between Tuberculous Spondylitis and Pyogenic Spondylitis

	Tuberculosis spondylitis	Pyogenic spondylitis
Bone destruction	Grade III with relative disc preservation	Grade III with some peridiscal bone destruction
Contrast enhancement	Focal and heterogeneous	Diffuse and homogeneous
Signal intensity	Well defined	Ill defined

| Abscess with contrast rim enhancement | Intraosseous abscess with enhancement | Discal abscess with rim enhancement of the vertebral body |

37.---c

sacrococcygeal teratomas is the most common newborn tumor, the most common tumor of the sacrococcygeal region in childhood, and the most common sacrococcygeal germ cell tumor Most sacrococcygeal teratomas are visible externally (80% to 90%) . Sacrococcygeal teratomas account for 25% of skin-covered lumbosacral masses and typically lie within or below the intergluteal cleft.

Conversely, spinal lipomas nearly always lie cephalic to the upper end of the intergluteal cleft. Grossly, sacrococcygeal teratomas are classified by their relationship to the skin surface and the pelvis . Altman type I tumors (47%) lie predominantly external to the normal body and have minimal presacral component.

Altman type II tumors (35%) are evident externally but have significant intrapelvic extension. Altman type III tumors (9%) can be detected externally but lie predominantly within the pelvis and abdomen. Altman type IV tumors (10%) are entirely presacral.

38.---d

The pituitary stalk is approximately 2 mm thick

39.---b

The most characteristic MR finding is a suprasellar mass that is itself heterogeneous but contains a cystic component that is well defined, internally uniform, and hyperintense on both T1- and T2-weighted images.

Cyst contents vary in color and viscosity, but the typical content of the cyst is a dark-brown "machine oil" that contains characteristic suspended cholesterol crystals.

40.----e

A high percentage of MRs demonstrate high signal intensity in the posterior lobe of normal individuals on routine sagittal T1-weighted views. This percentage has been reported to be as high as 98% to 100% and as low as 60% . Arguments have been made, therefore,
particularly by the "high-percentage" reporters, that nonvisualization of the posterior lobe high signal should be interpreted as a sign of neurohypophyseal dysfunction. Nonvisualization has been reported in nephrogenic diabetes insipidus , a disorder in which the neurohypophysis is functionally intact. This seems to be a paradox, in that there should be abundance of neurosecretory activity to compensate for the insensitivity of the end organ, but Moses et al.proposed that in nephrogenic diabetes insipidus there is continuous stimulation

and release of hormones, thus depleting the posterior lobe of neurosecretory vesicles and hence the lack of signal.

41.---d
High Cho/NAA ratio is a strong indicator of a higher-grade neoplasm, but a low Cho/NAA ratio could arise from a low-grade neoplasm, low neoplastic cellular density, or nonneoplastic processes such as multiple sclerosis.

42.---e
The anterior cerebral artery is divided into three anatomical segments: the horizontal or precommunicating segment (A1), vertical or postcommunicating segment (A2), and distal ACA including cortical branches (A3). The recurrent artery of Huebner is the largest of the perforating branches and may arise from the A1 or A2 segment. It derives its name from the fact that it doubles back on its parent artery at an acute angle to join the lenticulostriate vessels.
A fusion of the A2 segment in the midline give a single 'azygos' anterior cerebral artery, which then supplies both hemispheres.

43.---e
Despite its fat content, it is T1 hypointense and T2 hyperintense on MRI.

44.----c
The most common site of chemodectomas is the jugular bulb and their presentation is with pulsatile tinnitus, deafness, vertigo and lower cranial nerve palsies. The tumour causes bone destruction with enlargement of the pars vasorum of the jugular foramen, well demonstrated on CT.

45.---d
Carotid intervention should not be considered for a stenosis of less than 50 per cent regardless of symptoms
Different ways of measuring percentage of carotid artery stenosis (adapted from): 1) NASCET method = $[1-(A/B)] \times 100$
2) ESCT method = $[1-(A/C)] \times 100$
3) common carotid method = $[1-(A/D)] \times 100$.
Where
A-- minimum residual lumen
B. distal internal carotid lumen
C. original internal carotid lumen
D. common carotid lumen

46.---e
47.----e
48.----a
The newborn has limited motor function but a well-developed sensory system. Thus the myelination pattern seen at birth at full term is primarily in the sensory tracts.

49.----b
They are few in number before the age of 4 years, increase in number and volume between 4 and 10 years and then decrease in the second decade, being rare over the age of 20. Therefore, they are rarely seen in the adult NF1 population.
The pons, cerebellar white matter, internal capsules, basal ganglia, thalami and hippocampi are typical sites

50.---d

The typical site is the trigone of the lateral ventricle, while in older children the cerebellopontine angle or fourth ventricle may be involved.

51.—a

52.---b

The nidus of an osteoid soteoma rarely exceed 1.5 to 2.0 cm in diameter

53.----d

Follow-up catheter or MR angiography has demonstrated recurrence of aneurysms, especially at the basilar and carotid terminations following endovascular therapy.

54.---c

Oat –shaped calcification is noted in muscle cysticercosis

55.---b

Velum interpositum lies above the third ventricle

56.---e

Fetal origin of the PCA is seen in 15 to 20 % cases

57.---b

Calcification is noted in 20 to 30% of AVM.

58.---e

The most common fourth ventricular neoplasm in an adult is metastases

59.----e

60.---e

6mm (infants and children),8mm (men and postmenopausal women),10mm(women of child bearing age),12 mm(women in late pregnancy or postpartum women) are maximum normal height (in mm) of the pituitary gland according to Elster's rule.

TEST PAPER 6

1. All are true regarding holoprosencephaly (HPE) except
a. Alobar holoprosencephaly is the most severe form of HPE
b. The alobar form is most common (46% to 54%)
c. The most common chromosomal association is with trisomy 13
d. mutation of the sonic hedgehog gene (SHH) is implicated
e. The olfactory bulbs and tracts are almost always present

2. All are true regarding Diffusion-weighted imaging except
a. poor sensitivity to otherwise occult infarction
b. high specificity for infarction
c. a routine imaging sequence in all stroke patients
d. reflect the microvascular water environment
e. sensitive to translational movement/ diffusion of water over short distances

3. All are true regarding Diffusion-weighted imaging except
a. uses pulsed gradients to make in vitro diffusion measurements
b. the b value alters the sensitivity of the image to the diffusion
c. hyperintensity indicate either restricted diffusion or T2 change or both.
d. ADC maps demonstrate contrast based purely on diffusion differences
e. ADC maps alone have very high sensitivity and accuracy for acute infarction

4. All are true regarding watershed infarctions except
a. the pattern of perfusion deficit useful in identifying underlying the etiologies
b. located at boundaries of vascular territories
c. often precipitated by an episode of systemic arterial hypotension
d. more commonly non-hemorrhagic
e. commonly enhance earlier than thromboembolic infarctions.

5. All are causes of spinal stenosis except
a. Morquio syndrome
b. Achondroplasia
c. spondylosis
d. OPLL
e. Hurler syndrome

6. All are true regarding aneurysm except
a. narrow neck means –neck of fewer than 4mm
b. the average packing density of coils with GDC coil within the aneurysm is approx.75%
c. Polymer –Enhanced coils is designed to iniate stronger healing response in aneurysm
d. platinum coils coated with a volume-expanding hydrogel is designed to increase the packing density in time dependent fashion
e. advantage of liquid polymer embolisation is its use in irregularly shaped aneurysm

7. Hypointense signal on T2 W image is produced by
a. Deoxyhemoglobin in patent veins

b. Mucinous material
c. Rapid or turbulent flow
d. Ferromagnetic artifact
e. all

8. All are true regarding AVMs except
a. wedge-shaped clusters of vessels with the apex directed toward the cortical surface
b. no Intervening brain parenchyma found within the vascular nidus
c. usually no mass effect on adjacent structures
d. Approx. 10% of AVMs associated with arterial aneurysms
e. feeding and draining vessels in AVMs separated by parenchyma

9. All are true regarding cavernous angioma except
a. familial pattern in 10% to 15% of patients
b. the peak incidence of symptom onset is between the first and second decades of life
c. frequently multiple (approximately 20% to 30% of cases),
d. superficial location with proximity to the subarachnoid space /ventricle is common.
e. The pons is the most common brainstem location.

10. A young patient undergoes MRI of brain which show no abnormality on unenhanced SE images. The pons reveals lacelike region of stippled contrast enhancement on contrast study .The patient is asymptomatic. The most likely diagnosis is
a. lymphoma
b. cavernous angioma
c. capillary telangiectasia
d. venous angioma
e. developmental venous anomaly

11. The diagnostic study of choice for initial evaluation of head injury patients is
a. MRI
b. CT
c. USG
d. PET
e. X-ray

12. All are myelination milestones after birth (months) except
a. 3 month, cerebellar white matter on T1W
b. 4 month, corpus callosum (splenium) on T1W
c. 6 month, corpus callosum (genu) on T2W
d. 11 month, anterior limb of internal capsule T2W
e. 14 month, frontal white matter T2W

13. Which spectroscopic finding has been shown to be significantly lower in patients with relapsing-remitting MS.
a. whole-brain NAA
b. whole-brain choline
c. whole- brain myo-inositol
d. whole- brain lactate
e. whole-brain gulatmine

14. Which is not involved in Krabbe disease /globoid cell leukodystrophy (GLD)
a. the parietal periventricular white matter
b. splenium of the corpus callosum
c. corticospinal tracts
d. auditory pathway involvement
e. cerebellar white matter and deep gray nuclei

15. Dilated perivascular spaces is

seen in
a. Mucopolysaccharidoses
b. Zellweger syndrome
c. Alexander disease
d. MELAS
e. Krabbe disease

16. All are true regarding hippocampus except
a. lies inferior to subiculum and parahippocampal gyrus
b. form a 4- to 4.5-cm-long curved elevation in the floor of the temporal horn
c. the hippocampal head has three to four digitations on its superior surface
d. the hippocampal body extends posteriorly around the midbrain
e. the tail of hippocampus lies behind the brainstem

17. The most frequent cause of seizures beyond 50 yrs is
a. stroke
b. tumor
c. hippocampal sclerosis
d. trauma
e. phakomatoses

18. Pigmented neoplasm are all except
a. medulloblastoma
b. melanotic neuroectodermal tumor of infancy
c. schwannoma
d. melanoma
e. choroid plexus papilloma

19. All are true regarding enhancement pattern in glioblastoma multiforme except
a. ringlike enhancement (thick and irregular)
b. contrast enhancement correlate with the degree of hypervascularity demonstrated on angiography
c. enhancing region of tumour correlate with areas of tumor tissue on pathology
d. enhancement is helpful in guiding surgical biopsy
e. useful in identifying postoperative residual or recurrent tumor

20. All are true regarding subependyma except
a. the fourth ventricle is the most common site (75%)
b. the only glial tumors that can be truly considered benign
c. sharply demarcated and lobulated
d. typically does not enhance
e. hypointense to gray matter on T2-weighted images

21. All are true regarding edema of brain metastases except
a. On MR, metastatic foci are often separable from edema on T2-weighted images
b. Intravenous contrast clearly shows the tumor focus separate from the surrounding edema
c. Peritumoral edema follows white matter boundaries
d. The edema accompanying metastases usually cross the corpus callosum
e. Edema is not a significant component of cortical metastases.

22. All are true regarding arachnoid cyst except
a. Intensity usually follows almost exactly that of CSF
b. low intensity on T1-weighted images
c. isointensity on long-TR/short-TE images
d. hyperintensity on T2-weighted images

e. no suppression of signal on FLAIR

23. All are true regarding medulloblastoma except
a. Dissemination may occur in subarachnoid space
b. Low-risk tumors are up to 3 cm in greatest dimension
c. the brain imaging enough in the initial work-up of medulloblastoma
d. No need to get immediate postoperative study to exclude any residual tumor
e. The recommended interval between imaging studies is every 3 to 4 months during the first year of surgery

24. Supratentorial ependymomas differs from infratentorial ependymomas in respect of
a. origin
b. presence of cyst lesion
c. presence of a mural nodule
d. evidence of calcification
e. contrast-enhancement

25. All are true regarding Rasmussen encephalitis except
a. an abrupt onset of severe and intractable epilepsy
b. usually begins in childhood, between 6 and 8 years of age
c. tends to affect hemisphere bilaterally
d. Serial scans show focal or hemispheric atrophy
e. earliest change on MRI--- cortical swelling with hyperintensity on T2-weighted image

26. All are imaging features of pyogenic abscess except
a. center of the cavity is slightly hyperintense to CSF on T1W
b. signal intensities of center are quite variable on T2W
c. The rim is isointense to slightly hyperintense to white matter on T1W
d. The rim is hyperintense on T2W
e. smooth ring enhancement of an abscess capsule on postgadolinium MR images

27. All are true regarding tuberculoma except
a. "Target sign" on CT
b. noncaseating granulomata ---- hypointense on T1-W and hyperintense on T2-W
c. caseating granuloma ---- hypo to isointense to gray matter on T1-W
d. caseous tuberculomas ----- consistently hyperintense signals on T2W
e. intense nodular and ringlike enhancement

28. All are true regarding signal changes with aging except
a. the extrapyramidal nuclei ----- are isointense to cortical gray matter during the first 10 years of life
b. the globus pallidus become hypointense relative to cortical gray matter and to white matter in the most patients by age 25yrs
c. the dentate nucleus decreases in signal intensity more slowly and inconsistently
d. hypointensity in the caudate and putamen may equal that in the globus pallidus in individuals in their eighth decade
e. Low-intensity changes in the cortical ribbon, particularly in the motor cortex, ---is always pathological

29. The tau-positive pathology are all except
a. Pick disease
b. progressive supranuclear palsy
c. CBD
d. FTLD syndromes associated with FTDP-17-MAP
e. FTLD-MND

30. All are true regarding FASI in NF-1 except
a. bright foci on T2-weighted MR
b. absence of significant mass effect
c. absence of contrast enhancement or hemorrhage
d. Globus pallidus FASI shows abnormally high signal intensity on T1W
e. FASI in the the hippocampi most commonly resolve spontaneously during the teen years

31. All are true regarding Sturge-Weber Syndrome except
a. cortical calcification
b. delayed myelin maturation on T2W
c. enlargement of the choroid plexus glomerula
d. Cerebellar developmental venous anomalies
e. unilateral cerebral atrophy

32. All are true regarding cobblestone complex except
a. related to the overmigration of neuroblasts and glia through the external glial limitans
b. related to merosin overactivity
c. diffuse cobblestone cortex is noted in the Walker-Warburg phenotype
d. Absence of the septum pellucidum noted in muscle-eye-brain disease
e. reverse of the normal pattern of myelin maturation noted in Fukuyama congenital muscular dystrophy

33. All are true reagading cephaloceles except
a. In general, the herniated brain contents --dysplastic and nonfunctioning in occipital cephaloceles
b. The pituitary gland and optic chiasm are often located within transsphenoidal cephalocele
c. agenesis or hypogenesis of the corpus callosum noted in transsphenoidal cephalocele
d. hypotelorism on an axial series is noted in transsphenoidal cephalocele
e. Transalar sphenoidal cephaloceles occur through defects in the lateral wall of the sphenoid sinus

34. All are true regarding rhombencephalosynapsis except
a. undifferentiated midline cerebellum
b. Aqueductal stenosis
c. better preserved rostral vermis than rostarl vermis
d. fused middle cerebellar peduncles
e. The dentate nuclei in shape of horseshoe-shaped arch

35. All are true regarding sacrococcygeal teratoma except
a. arise from multipotential cells of Hensen's node
b. Type 2 tumors are almost always completely external
c. a pelvic soft tissue mass with calcification and fat
d. solid portions of the tumor enhance

e. Mostly benign

36. All are true regarding hemangioblastoma of spinal cord except
a. associated with meningeal varicosities and usually are located on the dorsal surface of the cord.
c. Approximately 30% of the patients have von Hippel-Lindau syndrome
c. the spinal cord tend to be single (79%)
d. the cervical cord --most often involved (51%)
e. 43% cases associated with cysts

37. All the features favour brucellosis over tuberculosis except
a. predilection for the lower lumbar spine
b. height of the vertebral bodies usually preserved
c. tends to involve the posterior elements
d. rarely extends into the epidural space
e. paraspinous soft tissues rarely affected

\38. All are true regarding lipoma of filum terminale except
a. no association with tight filum terminale syndrome
b. Intradural lipomas tend to be fusiform in shape
c. extradural lipoma tend to be far more diffuse, tend to be larger
d. extradural lipoma commonly elevate and distort the distal thecal sac
e. round midline appearance in axial MRI is classic of intradural lipoma

39. All are true regarding imaging of pituitary gland except
a. the anterior lobe is similar in signal intensity to cerebral gray matter on all pulse sequences
b. the posterior lobe is hyperintense on T1-weighted images
c. the anterior lobe, the posterior lobe, and the pituitary stalk all enhance intensely
d. increased signal intensity on T1W in the neonate and in pregnancy
e. pituitary gland acquire adult signal by about 4 to 6 months of age

40. All are true regarding adamantinomatous craniopharyngioma except
a. suprasellar masses during the first two decades of life
b. The presence of increased T2 signal along the optic nerves
c. the presence of clumps of "wet keratin" often with dystrophic calcification.
d. dark-brown "machine oil" like content with suspended cholesterol crystals
e. has the inflammatory and fibrotic nature

41. All are true regarding retinoblastoma except
a. the most common intraocular malignancy of childhood
b. trilateral" retinoblastoma ---- bilateral retinoblastoma with associated pontine tumor
c. bilateral tumors occur in up to one third of patients
d. The majority of tumors contain calcification
e. MR is a more sensitive

evaluation for extraocular tumor along the optic nerve

42. All are true regarding MR spectroscopy except
a. Lipid ---0.8 to 1.4 ppm
b. Lactate ---1.32 ppm
c. NAA—3.0ppm
d. creatinine ---3.0ppm
e. choline---3.2ppm

43. All are true regarding catheter angiography except
a. The transfemoral route is now almost exclusively used for catheterization of the cerebral vessels
b. femoral sheath is mandatory for interventional procedures.
c. The most frequently used catheters are 4F or 5F with a tapered J-shaped tip
d. The use of hydrophilic guidewires greatly facilitates catheterization of the cerebral vessels
e. The right vertebral artery is the first-line approach to angiography of the posterior circulation

44. All are true regarding pleomorphic xanthoastrocytoma (PXA) except
a. arises near the surface of the cerebral hemispheres
b. frequently cystic
c. may enhance strongly
d. usually associated with little or no oedema
e.. T1 hyperintense and T2 hypointense due to fat content.

45. All are true regarding Chordomas except
a. most frequent location in the skull base ---- the spheno-occipital synchrondrosis of the clivus
b. cause bone destruction and contain calcification
c. Fat-suppressed T1W spin-echo sequences particularly useful
d. may have a 'soap-bubble' appearance
e. poor contrast enhancement

46. All are true regarding perfusion-weighted imaging in infarction except
a. TTP provides a qualitative overview of brain perfusion
b. A threshold of 8 s delay in TTP correlates with a CBF of under 20 ml 100 g^{-1} min
c. a CBV deficit seems to be the best predictor of initial infarct
d. a CBV deficit seems to be the best predictor of final size in successful reperfusion
e.. The MTT and CBF indicate tissue at risk (the final infarct volume)

47. All are true regarding imaging of herpes encephalitis except
a. low attenuation in the antero-medial temporal lobe on CT
b. CT appears normal in the first 3–5 days after onset
c. Haemorrhage is seen as a early and prominent feature
d. The abnormal signal is mainly cortical on MRI
e. MRI is more sensitive than CT to haemorrhagic foci

48. All are true regarding dementia except
a. symmetrical posterior temporal and parietal perfusion defects on regional cerebral blood flow (rCBF) SPECT in AD
b. deficit of central benzodiazepine receptors on receptor imaging in AD

c. markedly symmetric atrophy in the anterior and medial parts of the temporal lobe in Picks disease
d. Lewy body dementia is recognized as the second most common degenerative dementia after AD
e. AD incidence increases sharply over 70 years

49. All are true regarding imaging of normal myelination except
a. progressive reduction in water diffusion, fractional anisotropy and magnetization transfer
b. brain myelination is detected in grey matter earlier on T2-weighted fast spin-echo (FSE)
c. brain myelination is detected in the white matter tracts earlier on T1-weighted spin-echo (SE) or STIR
d. The brain should appear virtually fully myelinated on T2-weighted sequences by 2 years
e. The brain should have almost an adult appearance on T1-weighted sequences by 10 months

50. All are true regarding Sturge–Weber syndrome except
a. leptomeningeal angiomas with a primarily fronto –parietal distribution
b. abnormal venous drainage with chronic ischaemia
c. involved hemisphere progressively becomes atrophied
d. enlargement of the ipsilateral choroid plexus
e. 'tramline calcifications' on x ray of skull by the age of 2yrs

51. All are true regarding CNS germ cel tumour (GCT) except
a. more common in Europe
b. germinoma is the most common type of CNS GCT
c. most pineal region GCTs occur in boys and suprasellar GCTs in girls
d. germinoma --a hyperdense, solid mass and enhance avidly and homogeneously
e. germinoma --- T2 hypointensity relative to grey matter

52. Imaging indicators of intraventricular obstructive (noncommunicating) hydrocephalus are all except
a. dilatation of the temporal horns disproportionate to lateral ventricular dilatation
b. enlargement of the anterior and posterior recesses of the third ventricle
c. dilatation of the sulcal spaces, major fissures and basal cisterns
d. inferior convexity of the floor of the third ventricle
e. transependymal oedema and bulging of fontanelles

53. All are true regarding carotid and vertebral artery occlusion except
a. to assess the ability of the cerebral circulation to tolerate its permanent sacrifice
b. A temporary (non-detachable) occlusion balloon is inflated for approxi- 30 minutes at the site of anticipated permanent occlusion
c. an injection of the contralateral ICA during inflation of the test occlusion balloon is made to assess cross flow through the circle of Willis
d. A delay in cerebral vein oacification of 4 seconds or more indicates that occlusion is unlikely

to be tolerated
e. Routine use of heparin during the test occlusion limits the incidence and severity of complications.

54. Bracket sign is noted in
a. oligodendroglioma
b. craniopharyngioma
c. corpuas callosum lipoma
d. meningioma
e. medulloblastoma

55. All are true regarding pellucidum septum except
a. The double septum /fifth ventricle is due to the abnormal persistence of the fetal cavum septi pellucidi
b. cavum septi pellucid persists in 1-2% of adults
c. cyst of the cavum Vergae represents the so-called `sixth ventricle'
d. cyst of the cavum Vergae is backward expetion of the septal cyst
d. cyst of the cavum Vergae lies beneath the posterior part of corpus callosum with the velum interpositum above

56. All are true regarding MCA except
a. lateral lenticulostriate arteries arise from M2
b. lateral tenticulostriate arteries supply the lentiform nucleus and caudate nucleus
c. M2 refers to insular segment of MCA
d. much of cerebral cortex and white matter is supplied by MCA branches
e. fenetstration and duplication is very common variants

57. All leads to Early Draining veins on angiogram except
a. venous angioma
b. AVM
c. cerebral infarction with luxury perfusion
d. glioblastoma multiforme
e. mets from renal cell carcinoma

58. All are true regarding intraventricular masses except
a. astrocytoma is the most common neoplasm in body of ventricle in older children and adult
b. body of lateral ventricle is the most common location for supratentorial ependymomas
c. Choroid plexus papilloma is the most common trigone mass in young children
d. temporal horn choroid plexus may be calcified in NF 2
e. xanthogranuloma of choroid plexus are usually bilateral

59. All are true regarding glioblastoma multiforme except
a. most malignant of all glial neoplasm
b. necrosis is the hallmark
c. deep white matter of the frontal and temporal lobes—usual location
d. thick irregular regular ring enhancement
e. peripheral edema represent pure edema only

60. All are true regarding intracranial lesions except
a. dermoid enhances strongly
b. tubulonodular lipoma is associated with callosal dysgenesis
c. 50% to 60% arachnoid I middle cranial fossa
d. two-third colloid is hyperdense

e.Rathke cleft cyst show no calcification

TEST PAPER 6(ANSWER)

1----e
The olfactory bulbs and tracts are almost always absent.

2.---a
DWI has revolutionized the evaluation of early stroke patients due to its high sensitivity to otherwise occult infarction and its high specificity for infarction.

3.---e
The diffusion-weighted image and the ADC image are read together. Diffusion-weighted image shows hyperintensity in acute infarction .The ADC map confirms the restriction of diffusion, seen as low intensity.If no hyperintensity is seen on DWI, then there is no acute infarction and no need for ADC maps because ADC maps alone have very low sensitivity and accuracy for acute infarction . Nonacute infarctions show no hyperintensity on DWI in the vast majority of cases, despite prolongation of T2 in the infarcted region.

4.---d
DWI and PWI have been used to evaluate patients with border zone infarctions . Analysis of the pattern of perfusion deficit may be helpful in identifying the etiologies of the border zone infarction.

Three patterns have been identified .Most of patients seen with normal perfusion had a history of pre- or periinfarction hypotension as a presumed stroke mechanism.

A pattern in which the perfusion deficit was equivalent to the diffusion deficit suggested a cardiac or aortic embolic source. Patients with extensive perfusion deficit had severe stenosis or occlusion of a large artery, Higher rates of severe progression in volume appeared to occur in patients with perfusion-diffusion mismatch.

There are two types of hemispheric watershed or border zone infarction .One of these is a superficial border zone infarction seen in the cortical regions of the brain. These areas represent the boundary zone between leptomeningeal collaterals from adjacent arterial territories.Cortical infarctions may occur between the middle cerebral and anterior cerebral territory or between the middle cerebral and posterior cerebral artery territory .

Another group of border zone infarctions comprise the deep or medullary infarctions seen in the deep white matter of the hemisphere, in the corona radiata and centrum semiovale . These watershed areas occur between medullary arteries arising from the cortical branches of the middle cerebral artery and lenticulostriate arteries from the proximal portions of the middle cerebral artery.

5.---e

6.—b
The average packing density of coils with GDC coil within the

aneurysm is approx.20 to 40% ,there is relatively high long term recanalisation and there is little healing response.
Polyglycolic lactic acid copolymer-coated cells is an example of polymer –enhanced coils.Ethylene vinyl alcoholbcoplymer –Onyx is an example of liquid polymer.

7.---e
8.----a
Classically, AVMs appear as wedge-shaped clusters of vessels, with the apex of the wedge directed toward the ventricular surface and the base located at the cortical margin

9.—b
Cavernous angioma is believed to be congenital,but the peak incidence of symptom onset is between the third and fifth decades of life.

10.---c
The key to distinguishing the enhancement of capillary telangiectasia from other, similar enhancing lesions, notably lymphoma when periventricular, is the absence of any signal abnormality on the unenhanced images.

11.—b
12.---c
Myelination Milestones After Birth (Months)
T1-weighted image----3 mo, cerebellar white matter, 4 mo, corpus callosum (splenium), 6 mo, corpus callosum (genu)
T2-weighted image--6 mo, corpus callosum (splenium), 8 mo, corpus callosum (genu), 11 mo, anterior limb of internal capsule,14 mo, frontal white matter

13.----a
14.---d
Auditory pathway involvement is characteristic of adrenoleukodystrophy and is not seen in GLD

15.---a
16.---a
The hippocampus lies superior to subiculum and parahippocampal gyrus, forming a 4- to 4.5-cm-long curved elevation in the floor of the temporal horn of lateral ventricle.

17.---a
18.----e
19.----b
Contrast enhancement does not correlate with the degree of hypervascularity demonstrated on angiography

20.---e
The MR diagnosis of subependymoma hinges on its periventricular location, with the most common sites being the foramen of Monro and the fourth ventricle. The subependymoma typically does not enhance after intravenous contrast, which, along with its hyperintensity to gray matter on T2-weighted images, can help to distinguish it from many of the other lesions that can occur in similar locations, particularly when related to the lateral ventricle.

21.---d
The edema accompanying metastases usually does not cross the corpus callosum nor does it involve cortex, features that often

help to distinguish these lesions from primary infiltrative brain malignancy.

Peritumoral (metastases) edema is usually prominent and follows white matter boundaries which are readily identified as fingerlike projections with intervening unaffected cortex.

22.---e
FLAIR is particularly useful in arachnoid cysts because the signal should be completely suppressed if the contents represent CSF

23---d
In the follow-up of patients who have undergone surgery for posterior fossa PNET, the routine is to get immediate postoperative study to exclude any residual tumor.

The recommended interval between imaging studies is every 3 to 4 months during the first year and every 6 to 8 months in subsequent years, for a maximum of 7 to 8 years . Most medulloblastomas recur in close proximity to the primary tumor site with a mean time to recurrence of 13 to 15 months.

24.----a
Supratentorial ependymoma has an appearance that is similar to that seen in the posterior fossa with one important exception, that it most frequently arises in the white matter and not in the ventricle. In the posterior fossa it is always an intraventricular and/or cerebellar pontine angle mass. In the supratentorial brain, it is most frequently a hemispheric, cerebral white matter tumor and rarely an intraventricular tumor.

25.----c
The disease tends to affect one hemisphere. Classification and staging criteria have been proposed based on MR imaging findings on T2-weighted and FLAIR images: normal volume and signal (stage 0), swelling and hyperintense signal (stage 1), normal volume and hyperintense signal (stage 2), atrophy and hyperintense signal (stage 3), and progressive atrophy and normal signal (stage 4).

26.----d
In a typical abscess with central liquefactive necrosis, the center of the cavity is slightly hyperintense to CSF, whereas the surrounding edematous brain is slightly hypointense to normal brain parenchyma on T1-weighted images. The rim is isointense to slightly hyperintense to white matter on T1-weighted images and is hypointense on T2-weighted images.

The rim may be a better indicator of response to treatment than residual enhancement, which can persist on contrast studies for months after completion of therapy . Other lesions that may have a hypointense rim on T2-weighted images include evolving hematomas, infrequent metastases, and high-grade gliomas with cystic necrosis

27.----d
In patients with parenchymal tuberculomas, 10% to 34% have multiple lesions.

A caseating granuloma is hypointense to isointense to gray matter on T1-weighted images and may have a slightly hyperintense rim (possibly secondary to the presence of paramagnetic species that shorten the T1 relaxation time) . On T2-weighted images, caseous tuberculomas exhibit variable signals. They are often isointense or hypointense to brain parenchyma, and it is postulated that this relative hypointensity is related to T2 shortening by paramagnetic free radicals produced by macrophages heterogeneously distributed throughout the caseous granuloma . Alternatively, the diminished signal on T2-weighted images may be attributed to the mature tuberculoma's being of greater cellular density than the brain. Granulomas may also be hyperintense to brain on T2-weighted images, and this is likely due to a greater degree of central liquefactive necrosis in these lesions. There is usually an associated mass effect. Surrounding edema may be minimal in small lesions, and there is generally less edema than that surrounding a pyogenic abscess of comparable size, based on CT studies.

28.----e
Low-intensity changes in the cortical ribbon, particularly in the motor cortex, presumably from iron deposition also have been correlated with usual aging as well as certain neurodegenerative disorders such as amyotrophic lateral sclerosis .
In most patients by age 25 years, the globus pallidus, followed by the red nucleus and pars reticulata of the substantia nigra, become hypointense relative to cortical gray matter and to white matter on the long–repetition time (TR)/echo time (TE) sequence.

29.---e
Tau-negative pathologies are associated with the recently discovered dysfunctional protein TAR-DNA binding protein (TDP-43). In the tau-negative category is FTLD-U, which comprises about 60% of all FTLD cases. It is characterized by ubiquitin-positive inclusions. Also under the tau-negative category are autosomal dominant mutations associated with the progranulin gene (FTD-17 PGRN). Finally, FTLD-MND falls under the tau-negative category.

30.---e
Foci of abnormal signal intensity (FASI) refers to multifocal signal changes (bright foci on T2-weighted MR) in the brainstem, cerebellar white matter, dentate nucleus, basal ganglia, periventricular white matter, optic nerve, and optic pathways . The radiologic criteria for distinguishing these lesions as hamartomas (rather than more ominous neoplasms) are absence of significant mass effect, absence of a spreading (vasogenic) pattern of edema, and absence of

contrast enhancement or hemorrhage.
Lesions peak in late childhood and those in the basal ganglia, cerebellum, and brainstem most commonly resolve spontaneously during the teen years; they are uncommon in adults with NF1. Lesions in the hippocampi, however, are seen in approximately 80% of patients without any change in prevalence over time..With large numbers of FASI or extensive lesions at an atypical
age should be followed due to the increased risk of proliferative change.

31.---b
Pseudo–accelerated myelin maturation on T2-weighted images is noted due to transient hyperperfusion.

32.---b
Merosin is absent or deficient in most cases of the cobblestone complex. These disorders are characterized by ocular abnormalities, brain anomalies (cobblestone cortex), and congenital muscular dystrophy of varying severity
Walker-Warburg syndrome ,also known as HARD +/- E, in which patients may have hydrocephalus (H), agyria (A) (cobblestone complex), retinal dysplasia (RD), and encephalocele (E).

33.----d
Hypertelorism on an axial series is noted in transsphenoidal cephalocele

34---c
The caudal vermis usually appears better preserved (e.g., the flocculonodulus is formed), whereas the rostral vermis is more severely hypoplastic. This pattern contrasts with that of DWM, in which the rostral vermis is better preserved.
The dentate nuclei are fused and classically describe a horseshoe-shaped arch crossing the midline draped along the fourth ventricle
The fourth ventricle is characteristically diamond or keyhole shaped on axial images , resulting from dorsal and rostral fusion of the dentate nuclei, the cerebellar peduncles, and the inferior colliculi.
The inferior olivary nuclei are usually absent

35.---b
Type 1 tumors are almost always completely external and distort the buttocks. Type 2 tumors have an intrapelvic portion, but most of the tumor is external. Type 3 tumors are predominantly intrapelvic with significant displacement of invasion of surrounding structures. Type 4 tumors have no external portion, and almost all of the tumor is intrapelvic

36.-----d
Hemangioblastomas involving the spinal cord tend to be single (79%).In spinal hemangioblastomas, the thoracic cord is most often involved (51%), followed by the cervical cord (41%)

37.---c
Brucellosis has a predilection for the lower lumbar spine , whereas

tuberculosis tends to favor the lower thoracic spine. In brucellosis the height of the vertebral bodies is usually preserved even though signal abnormalities consistent with osteomyelitis are noted. In tuberculosis the vertebral bodies are severely damaged, with marked gibbous deformity. Brucellosis tends to spare the posterior elements that may be affected by tuberculosis. The disc tends to be preserved in brucellosis and in tuberculosis, although it may also be affected in both conditions. Brucellosis rarely extends into the epidural space, whereas tuberculosis often extends to form epidural abscesses and involve the meninges. The paraspinous soft tissues are rarely affected by brucellosis and are commonly affected by tuberculosis, which causes cold abscesses. Spinal deformities are rare with brucellosis and common in tuberculosis.

\38.—a

Filar lipomas are commonly associated with the tight filum terminale syndrome and may require sectioning for untethering of the cord.

The filum terminale is thickened by high-signal fat. It is closely applied to the dorsal surface of the canal but may be distinguished from normal dorsal epidural fat by its continuous extension over multiple segments, its slight line of separation from the segmented dorsal epidural fat, and its classic round midline appearance in axial MRI.

Lipomas of the extradural portion of the filum are far more diffuse, tend to be larger, and tend to merge with adjacent extradural fat. They commonly elevate and distort the distal thecal sac.

39.---a

With the exception of the neonate and in pregnancy, the anterior lobe is similar in signal intensity to cerebral white matter on all pulse sequences, whereas the posterior lobe is distinctly hyperintense on T1-weighted images

In neonates the anterior lobe has higher signal intensity on T1 weighting than in the adult . At about 2 months of age, the intensity begins to diminish. By about 4 to 6 months of age, it resembles that of the adult . In both pregnancy and in the neonate, lactotroph hypertrophy and increased protein synthesis in the pituitary gland have been proposed as explanations for the high signal

40.----b

The presence of increased T2 signal along the optic tracts, rather than along the optic nerves, may suggest a craniopharyngioma over other parasellar lesions

Adamantinomatous tumors are almost always grossly cystic and usually have both solid and cystic components.

Calcification is seen in the vast majority of these tumors

Extensive fibrosis and signs of inflammation are often found with these lesions, particularly when they are recurrent, so that they adhere to adjacent structures, including the vasculature at the base of the brain. Moreover, adamantinomatous craniopharyngiomas are often invasive into adjacent brain, which evokes a dense gliosis that may be difficult to distinguish from a primary glial neoplasm. The inflammatory and fibrotic nature of the lesions makes recurrence a not-uncommon event, typically occurring within the first 5 years after surgery.

41.----b
Trilateral" retinoblastoma ---- bilateral retinoblastoma with associated pineal tumor

42.----c

Lipids	0.8–1.4	Breakdown of tissue, contamination from subcutaneous fat from skull
Lactate	1.32	Marker of anaerobic glycolysis (inverted at 135–144 ms)
NAA	2.0	Marker of neuronal health
Glutamine and glutamate	2.1–2.6	Neurotransmitter
Creatine	3.0, 3.9^a	Marker of cellular energetics
Choline	3.2	Membrane marker, marker of cell proliferation
Myo-inositol	3.5	Osmolytic marker, proposed glial marker

43.—e
The left vertebral artery is larger or of equal size than the right vertebral artery in approximately 75 per cent and therefore represents the first-line approach to angiography of the posterior circulation
Mani catheter and Sidewinder catheter are other catheters used.

44.---e
Despite its fat content, it is T1 hypointense and T2 hyperintense on MRI.

45.---c
Fat-suppressed T1W spin-echo sequences are particularly helpful for demonstrating the extent of the tumour and distinguishing pathological enhancement from the high signal of adjacent clival fat. The differential diagnosis includes chondrosarcoma, metastasis and nasopharyngeal carcinoma.
Most frequent location in the skull base ---- the spheno-occipital synchrondrosis of the clivus, followed by the basiocciput and petrous apex.
Often marked contrast enhancement is noted

46.----b
TTP provides a qualitative overview of brain perfusion. A threshold of 4 s delay seems to indicate tissue at risk and correlates with a CBF of under 20 ml 100 g^{-1} min^{-1} [30]. However proximal vessel stenosis can delay TTP even if CBF via collaterals is normal and tissue viability not

threatened. As outlined earlier, within an area of prolonged MTT (or TTP), moderate ischaemia may cause increased CBV, however reduced CBV indicates inadequate collateral supply and high risk of infarction.

47.---c
Haemorrhage is seen as a late feature and not usually prominent feature.
MRI is more sensitive than CT ,T2W and FLAIR sequences show high signal within 2 d of onset DWI shows cortical hyperintensity with greater sensitivity than conventional MR. Cerebral blood flow, measured by perfusion CT or SPECT, is increased in the acute phase.

48.---c
MRI and even CT in Pick disease show atrophy in the anterior and medial parts of the temporal lobe, which usually is markedly asymmetric (right or left) , and diminishes posteriorly.
Asymmetric frontal lobe atrophy may also be present.

49.---a
Advanced MRI techniques show progressive reduction in water diffusion, increased fractional anisotropy (assessed by diffusion tensor imaging), and increased magnetization transfer in normal maturation process.

50.---a
Sturge–Weber syndrome is a congenital syndrome characterized by a port-wine naevus on the face and ipsilateral leptomeningeal angiomas with a primarily parieto-occipital distribution

51.----a
CNS germa cel tumour (GCT) is more common in Asia.

52.---c
The sulcal spaces, major fissures and basal cisterns are small or obliterated in intraventricular obstructive (noncommunicating) hydrocephalus.
Other features, such as changes in the configuration of the frontal horns of the lateral ventricles, specifically widening of the radius of the frontal horn, and a decrease in the angle it makes with the midline plane, are less useful. Further features classically described in chronic hydrocephalus, such as erosion of the dorsum sellae and copper beaten skull, are even less reliable.

53.---d
A delay in cerebral vein oacification of 2 seconds or more indicates that occlusion is unlikely to be tolerated

54.---c

55.----d
Cyst of the cavum Vergae lies beneath the posterior part of corpus callosum with the velum interpositum below

56.---a
MCA has three segments --- M1(horizontal segment),M2(insular),M3(opercular).Lateral lenticulostriate arteries arise from M1

57.---a

58.----b
Supratentorial ependymomas are

mostly extraventricular
59.---e
GBM show thick irregular ring enhancement .It is a highly vascular mass and hemorrhage and edema are common. Peripheral edema actually represent tumour plus edema
60.----a
Dermoid doenot enhances

TEST PAPER 7

1. **Clinical Indications for Performing Susceptibility-Weighted Gradient Echo Scan is/are**
a. Hemorrhagic infarction
b. cavernous hemangioma
c. Seizure history
d. Metastases from melanoma
e. all

2. **All are true regarding FLAIR imaging except**
a. null CSF signal and produce a strongly T2-weighted image
b. more sensitive than T2W imaging for the detection of infarction in periventricular and cortical regions
c. generally not able to detect infarctions in hyperacute time period (less than 6 hours after the onset of symptoms)
d. occluded vessels or vessels with reduced blood flow appear as hyperintense
e. acute hemorrhage appear hyperintense

3. **All are features of hyperacute hematoma except**
a. slightly hypointense or isointense to brain on T1W images
b. slightly hyperintense to brain on T2W images
c. a thin, irregular rim of marked hypointensity at the periphery of the lesion on T1W images
d. no enhancement
e. restricted diffusion

4. **Hypointense signal on T2 W image is produced by**
a. Iron without hemorrhage
b. Calcification or bone
c. Air
d. Very high nonparamagnetic protein content
e. all

5. **All are true regarding intracranial AVMs except**
a. supratentorial location in approximately 40% to 53% of cases
b. most often solitary lesions
c. enlarges the deep venous system in case of deep seated AVMs
d. enlargement of the vein of Galen in children
e. multiple in Rendu-Osler-Weber disease and Wyburn-Mason syndrome

6. **All are true regarding MRA except**
a. turbulent / in-plane, or extremely slow flowing blood may manifest as low intensity
b. flowing blood can be differentiated from subacute-chronic intravascular clot by TOF
c. major advantage of PC MRA is its specificity for flow
d. conventional arteriography is superior to MRA in depicting overall angioarchitecture
e. MRA has poorer spatial and temporal resolution in comparison to catheter cerebral angiography

7. **MR features of cavernous angioma is /are**

a. focal central heterogeneity containing areas corresponding to subacute-chronic hemorrhage (methemoglobin)
b. circumferential complete rings of markedly hyperintense iron-storage forms around low - intensity central areas
c. no mass effect or edema
d. no demonstrable feeding arteries or draining veins associated with developmental venous anomalies
e. contrast enhancement

8. All are true regarding Capillary telangiectasias (capillary angiomas) except
a. usually small, solitary lesions
b. most common location --the medulla
c. a collection of pathologically dilated capillaries
d. Intervening brain parenchyma present
e. most of lesions clinically silent

9. All are measures to to reduce the problem of insensitivity of intracranial MRA (particularly 3D TOF) to slow flow as in large aneurysms except
a. The use of an off-resonance saturation pulse
b. use of PC MRA
c. reducing the thickness of the slab in 3D acquisitions and combining multiple thin slabs for anatomic coverage
d. using a spatially varying excitation pulse
e. all

10. All are true regarding myelination except

a. T1- and T2-weighted images remain the standard sequences for evaluating myelination
b. white matter myelination appears hyperintense on T1 and hypointense on T2 relative to gray matter
c. the occipital white matter myelinate before the frontotemporal white matter
d. the genu myelinates before the splenium of the corpus callosum
e. Optic nerve, chiasm, tract remain myelinated at the time of birth or shortly after birth

11. Which is true regarding multiple sclerosis
a. Tumefactive MS exert significant mass effect
b. decreased perfusion within the tumefactive lesion in comparison with contralateral, normal-appearing brain parenchyma
c. enhancing along with nonenhancing lesions is quite common in MS
d. "black holes" does not show correlation with demyelination and axonal loss
e. MS lesions may display clearly defined rings within or surrounding plaques of demyelination

12. The most characteristic MR finding in both the infantile and late-onset forms of Krabbe disease/globoid cell leukodystrophy (GLD) is
a. the corticospinal tracts involvement
b. cerebellar white matter and deep gray nuclei involvement
c. involvement of the posterior portion of the corpus callosum

d. early involvement of the subcortical U fibers
e. auditory pathway involvement

13. Cortical dysgenesis is seen in
a. Zellweger syndrome
b. Alexander disease
c. MELAS
d. Pelizaeus-Merzbacher disease
e. Krabbe disease

14. All are true regarding hippocampus except
a. curved structure
b. on medial aspect of temporal lobe
c. consisting of the dentate gyrus and cornu ammonis
d. The cornu ammonis segmented into four portions, CA1 through CA4.
e. CA1(the end-folium) is completely enveloped by the dentate gyrus.

15. Late-onset or delayed posttraumatic seizures are defined as
a. seizures occurring 1 week after initial trauma
b. seizures occurring 2 week after initial trauma
c. seizures occurring 3 week after initial trauma
d. seizures occurring 4 week after initial trauma
e. seizures occurring 5 week after initial trauma

16. All are true regarding intracranial tumour except
a. Fat-containing neoplasms are teratoma and dermoid
b. chemical shift artifact is big hurdle in detecting presence of fat in tumour
c. Fat-selective suppression methods –useful n the distinction of etiologies of hyperintense tumors on T1W
d. Melanin in tumors is seen as high intensity on T1-weighted and intermediate intensity on T2-weighted images
e. fat is hyperintense on T1-weighted and intermediate intensity on conventional T2-weighted images

17. All are true regarding glioblastoma multiforme except
a. typically demonstrate central necrosis, hemorrhages of varying ages, and hypervascularity
b. marked intratumoral heterogeneity on MRI
c. significant mass effect mainly due to fairly extensive white matter edema
d. Nearly all glioblastomas at least partially enhance with intravenous contrast
e. Multicentric malignant gliomas easily differentiated from metastases on MRI

18. All are true intaventricular lesions except
a. central neurocytoma typically show attachment to the septum pellucidum
b. Subependymomas in the lateral ventricles typically show intense contrast enhancement
c. Heterotopic gray matter doesnot r enhance and have no calcifications
d. Intraventricular meningiomas and choroid plexus are usually situated within the atrium of the lateral ventricle
e. ependymoma, subependymoma, and oligodendroglioma are most often

hyperintense to gray matter

19. All are true regarding brain metastases except
a. renal cell carcinoma metastases has tendency to involve the infratentorial brain
b. Early metastatic foci are commonly found in gray matter
c. Metastases are notoriously surrounded by massive amounts of edema
d. The extent of associated edema bears no direct relationship to the size of the metastasis
e. MR imaging with intravenous contrast is more sensitive than CT for diagnosis of metastases

20. All are true regarding arachnoid cysts except
a. about one half to two thirds occur in the middle cranial fossa
b. frequently associated primary hypogenesis of the temporal lobe
c. frequently cause erosion and expansion of the overlying portion of the calvarium
d. develop calcifications in their walls
e. demonstrate no contrast enhancement

21. All are true regarding imaging of medulloblastoma except
a. isodense or slightly increased at the site of the solid portion of the tumor on CT
b. Contrast enhancement occurs in 95% of cases on CT
c. restricted diffusion in 95% on MRI
d. low signal of the solid portion on T2
e. decreased Taurine

22. All are true of primitive neuroectodermal tumors of the supratentorial brain except
a. higher incidence of calcification in compartison to PNET of the posterior fossa
b. a lower frequency of large cysts and necrosis in compartison to PNET of the posterior fossa
c. markedly elevated choline and depressed NAA
d. decreased diffusion with decrease in ADC values;
e. MRI is the method of choice for localization

23. All are imaging features of ADEM except
a. Asymmetric patchy areas of hyperintensity on T2WI
b. Mild mass effect
c. Variable enhancement
d. hemorrhage constant feature
e. DTI: no ↓ FA values on normal-appearing white matter perilesional area

24. All are true regarding tuberculosis of CNS except
a. the isodense to slightly hyperdense exudate in the basal cistern in TBM
b. Hydrocephalus is related to poor prognosis
c. The most common parenchymal form of CNS TB is the tuberculous granuloma (tuberculoma)
d. Tuberculoma is mostly infratentorial in adult and supratentorial in children
e. tuberculoma is associated with meningitis in about 10% of cases

25. All favour diagnosis of dilated perivascular spaces over lacunar infarction except
a. usually are isointense to CSF on all pulse sequences
b. bilaterally symmetric

c. less than 5 mm in diameter
d. located in the inferior one third of the putamen
e. restricted diffusion

26. All are true regarding frontotemporal lobar dementia except
a. predominant frontal lobe atrophy seen in behavioral variant
b. behavioral variant ---- associated with bilaterally symmetric frontal atrophy
c. Semantic dementia ---- predominant atrophy involving the anterior temporal lobes.
d. Nonfluent aphasia is characterized by left frontal and insular atrophy.
e. Pick bodies are seen in most of FTLD cases

27. All are true regarding neurofibromatosis type 1 except
a. the most common of the neurocutaneous syndromes
b. autosomal dominant disorder without racial or sexual predilection
c. estimated incidence 1 in 3,000 to 1 in 4,000 persons
d. high rate of spontaneous mutation
e. the gene locus for NF1 is at 17 p11.2

28. Diagnostic criteria for neurofibromatosis type 1 includes all except
a. Café-au-lait spots ≥5(5 mm child, 15 mm adult)
b. Neurofibromas: ≥2
c. Plexiform neurofibroma: 1
d. Lisch nodules (iris hamartomas): ≥2
e. sphenoid wing dysplasia

29. All are true regarding Sturge-Weber Syndrome except
a. clinical triad ------seizures, mental handicap, and a "port-wine" nevus of the face
b. Somatic hemiatrophy (ipsilateral to malformation)
c. Leptomeningeal capillary/venous malformation
d. Cerebral hemiatrophy (ipsilateral to malformation)
e. Facial hemihypertrophy (ipsilateral to malformation)

30-. All are true regarding hemimegalencephaly except
a. enlargement of the affected cerebral hemisphere due to cortex overgrowth
b. ipsilateral ventricular enlargement
c. frontal horn straight and pointing anteriorly and superiorly
d. malformations of cortical development
e. Hemimegalencephaly most often involves only one the cerebral hemisphere

31. All are true regarding atretic cephalocele except
a. small, skin- covered, subscalp lesions
b. contain meninges and neural and glial rests
c. generally occur near the nasion
d. associated with persistent falcine sinus
e. also known as meningocele manqué

32. All are true regarding rhombencephalosynapsis except
a. undifferentiated midline cerebellum
b. Aqueductal stenosis
c. rostral vermis preserved better than rostarl vermis

d. fused middle cerebellar peduncles
e. The dentate nuclei in shape of horseshoe-shaped arch

33. All are true regarding spinal tumour except
a. osteoid osteoma may regress spontaneously
b. the most common location of osteoblastoma in spine is the lumber spine
c. ABC never cross the intervertebral disc space
d. ABC of the spine is an expansile lytic lesion usually involving the posterior elements
e. Multiple small fluid/fluid levels and internal septations may be present in ABC

34. All are true regarding myxopapillary ependymoma except
a. large, soft, expansile masses
b. always found in the region of the filum terminale
c. presence of fat spaces
d. generally hyperintense
e. may be found in brain

35. All are true regarding spinal lesions in ADEM except
a. monophasic course
b. spinal cord lesion is typically large and swollen
C. always shows intense enhancement
d. myelopathy is often complete in ADEM
e. predominantly affects the thoracic region

36. All are true regarding tight filum terminale syndrome except
a. Due to failure of complete involution of the distal cord
b. the filum greater than 2 mm in diameter
c. the tip of the conus medullaris lies below L-2
d. normal x ray of L/S spine
e. filar fibrolopoma present in 29% of cases

37. All are true regading pituitary stalk except
a. Prolactin and growth hormone-secreting cells predominate in lateral aspect of anterior pituitary
b. oxytocin and vasopressin are synthesisized in posterior gland
c. posterior lobe occupies only 10% to 20% of the volume of the sella turcica
d. the differential rates of enhancement of the pituitary gland on dynamic scans
e. posterior lobe lies in almost always in the midline and directly applied to the dorsum sella

.38. All are true regarding craniopharyngioma except
a. epithelially derived neoplasms
b. the suprasellar cistern as the epicenter in most cases
c. more than half cases in childhood or adolescence,
d. a second, smaller peak in the sixth decade
e. the most frequent form --- squamous or papillary type

39. All are true regarding diabetes insipidus except
a. due to failure to synthesize vasopressin in the paraventricular nuclei of the hypothalamus
b. Eighty percent or more of the vasopressin-secreting cells must be affected before clinical diabetes insipidus develops
c. imaging is directed at excluding a neoplastic or infiltrative lesion

of the suprasellar cistern or hypothalamus
d. disappearance of hyperintensity of posterior pituitary on T1-weighted images in any cause
e. visualization of the posterior lobe high signal in nephrogenic diabetes insipidus

40. All are true regarding NAA except
a. the most prominent spectral peak in normal brain
b. 2.02 ppm
c. serves as a marker of neuronal density and viability
d. NAA levels may reflect neuronal dysfunction rather than just neuronal loss
e. decreased NAA levels have been observed with Canavan disease

41. All are true regarding Hemorrhagic Infarction except
a. more commonly seen in cardioembolic stroke than in atherothrombotic stroke
b. revascularization therapy does increase the rate of hemorrhagic transformation
c. High levels of MMPs may be predictive of the risk of hemorrhagic transformation
d. T2*-sensitive gradient echo technique is the most sensitive method of detecting acute hemorrhage
e. MR is less sensitive to hemorrhage in infarction than CT

42. All are true regarding functional MRI except
a. used to study cortical activation
b. measure tiny increase in signal intensity on T2* WI in the relevant cortex during neuronal activation.
c. use of the magnetic susceptibility effects of oxyhaemoglobin
d. a net decrease in oxyhaemoglobin concentration in the venules and veins in the vicinity of the activated brain
e. The magnitude of MR signal change is field dependent, being greater at higher field strengths

43. All are true regarding astrocyoma except
a. diffuse astrocytomas WHO grade II are infiltrating low-grade tumours
b. contrast enhancement is usually absent in diffuse astrocytomas WHO grade II
c. Anaplastic astrocytomas (WHO grade III) usually show contrast enhancement
d. Pleomorphic xanthoastrocytoma (PXA) is usually associated intense oedema
e. GBM is the commonest primary intracranial neoplasm in adults

44. Imging features suggestive of a haemangiopericytoma rather than meningioma are all except
a. a lobulated dural-based mass
b. absence of calcification
c. hyperostosis
d. multiple areas of flow void on MRI
e. extensive edema

45. All are true regarding venous infarcts except
a. do not conform to arterial territories

b. often haemorrhagic and multifocal
c. The superior sagittal sinus is most commonly involved
d. 'delta sign'
e. DSA is frequently needed to confirm the diagnosis of venous thrombosis

46. CT criteria of abnormal basal meningeal enhancement is /are
a. linear enhancement of the middle cerebral artery cisterns
b. obliteration by contrast of the CSF spaces around normal vascular enhancement
c. Y-shaped enhancement at the junction of the suprasellar and middle cerebral artery cisterns
d. asymmetry of enhancement
e. all

47. All are true regarding hydrocephalus except
a. The American neurosurgeon Walter Dandy coined the term 'communicating hydrocephalus'
b. The most common cause in children of hydrocephalus is aqueduct stenosis
c. In young children the occipital horns are often most affected in communicating hydrocephalus
d. the cerebral sulci are characteristically enlarged in communicating hydrocephalus
e. in 'normal pressure hydrocephalus' lumbar CSF can be normal

48. All are true regarding brain maturation except
a. myelination is virtually complete by the age of 2 years
b. Gyral and sulcal development mainly occurs in utero
c. progressive T1 and T2 shortening of the white matter is noted with maturation
d. myelination maturation follows a centripetal posterior-to-anterior and inferior-to-superior pattern
e. Most myelination occurs post-term in the first 8 months

49. All are true regarding Hemimegalencephaly except
a. hamartomatous overgrowth of all or part of one hemisphere
b. may be in association with tuberous sclerosis
c. diffuse cortical thickening
d. the contralateral ventricle is enlarged
e. the frontal horn --- straight and pointed

50. All are true regarding craniopharyngioma except
a. the most common suprasellar tumour in children
b. calcified, mixed cystic and solid tumour
c. enhancement of the solid component and the cyst wall
d. high lipid peaks
e. T1 lenthening due to proteinacaeous components

51. Congenital causes of hydrocephalus
a. aqueductal stenosis/gliosis
b. Chiari II malformation
c the Dandy–Walker malformation
d. vein of Galen malformation
e. all

52. All are true regarding ONYX except
a. non-adhesive liquid embolic agent
b cosists of ethyl-vinyl alcohol polymer (EVOH)
c. dimethyl sulfoxide (DMSO)

used as solvent
d. tantalum used to make it radiopaque
e. it solidifies more rapidly than NBCA

53. All are true regarding following syndromes except
a. unilateral AVMs of visual pathways and midbrain seen in Wyburn –Mason syndrome
b. Progressive cerebellar hypertrophy is seen in Louis-Bar synsrome
c. Multiple AVMs are found in Rendu-Osler-Weber Disease
d. soft issue or bone hypertrophy is seen in Klippel-Trenaunay-Weber Syndrome
e. Gorlin syndrome shows medulloblastoma

54. All are true regarding calcification in brain tumour except
a. oligodendroglioma calcify in 50% cases
b. craniopharyngioma show calcification in over 75% of cases
c. calcification in craniopharyngioma is in midline and above the sella
d. calcification in meningioma is characteristically ball-like and amorphous
e. medulloblastoma calcify.frequently

55. All are causes of large head in infancy except
a. Pelizeazius –merzbacker disease
b. Lipidoses
b. Spongy degeneration
c. Alexander's disease
d. Tuberous sclerosis

56. All are true regarding azygous ACA except
a. solitary unpaired vessel
b. arise as single trunk
c. arise from the confluence of the A1 segment of the right and leftACAs
d. very common anomaly
e. often associated with other intracranial anomalies

57. All the factors increase the hemorrhagic risk of AVM except
a. smaller size
b. central/deep venous drainage pattern
c. peri-or intraventricular location
d. presence of an intranidal aneurysm
e. presence of angiomatous changes

58. All are true regarding lateral ventricles except
a. septum is absent in corpus callosum dysgenesis
b. septum pellucidum thicker than 3mm is suspicious for neoplasm
c. the most common primary septal tumour is astrocytoma
d. dysplastic thickening of septum is seen in NF1
e. subependymoma show strong predilection for frontal horn

59. All are true regarding anaplastic astrocytoma except
a. absent necrosis
b. presence of at least 20% gemistocytes in a glial neoplasm is a poor prognostic sign
c. protopplasmic astrocytoma is located superficially in the cerebral cortex
d. spread through the extracelluar space and along compact white matter tracts
e. uniform strong enhancement

60. All are true regarding

epidermoid tumour except
a.mother pf pearl appearance
b.lobulated cauliflower like mass
c.40 % to 45 % in middle fossa
d.insinuates in CSF spaces
e.TIW and T2W image like CSF

TEST PAPER 7(ANSWER)

1.---e

2.---e
FLAIR has been particularly helpful in the evaluation of brain parenchyma immediately adjacent to CSF-filled spaces such as the ventricular compartment and cortical sulci. A specific limitation of FLAIR is the lack of specificity of hypointensity for acute hemorrhage, which on FLAIR alone can look identical to water-containing cystic regions.

3.----C
A thin, irregular rim of marked hypointensity at the periphery of the lesion on T2-weighted images is paramount to recognize hyperacute hematoma . This has been attributed to very rapid deoxygenation of blood within the hematoma at the blood–tissue interface. The hypointensity may be more evident in 3-T than lower-field systems and more obvious on GRE images regardless of field strength; regardless of scanner field strength. So, T2*-weighted GRE should be part of all routine stroke MR protocols.

4.-----e

5.----a
Intracranial AVMs are located in the supratentorial compartment in approximately 80% to 93% of cases. Supratentorial AVMs usually arise over the convexities and involve the distribution of the middle cerebral artery (MCA).

6.---b
A subacute-chronic intravascular clot is often difficult or impossible to distinguish from intravascular flowing blood on the GRE images that comprise TOF MRA. Two-dimensional and 3D PC MRA techniques differentiate flowing blood from clot.

7.----b
Cavernous angioma shows circumferential complete rings of markedly hypointense iron-storage forms around high-intensity central areas

8.----b
The most common location is the pons. Intervening brain parenchyma is identifiable within the lesion (in distinction from cavernous hemangiomas) In most cases, the intervening and adjacent brain tissue is normal on pathologic examination, without gliosis or residua of prior hemorrhage

9.---e

10.---d
The splenium myelinates before the genu of the corpus callosum.

11.----d
Increasing hypointensity of MS plaques on T1-weighted images has been correlated with increased demyelination and axonal loss on pathology . These lesions may approach the signal intensity of CSF, referred to as "black holes," and have been shown to be correlated more

closely with clinical disability and outcome.

MS lesions may display clearly defined rings within or surrounding plaques of demyelination . Peripheral lesional high signal intensity on T1-weighted images is frequently encountered, suggesting the presence of paramagnetic material and likely corresponds to the presence of free radicals in the macrophage layer forming the margin of an acute plaque . Atrophy is common with progression of disease, usually manifested by ventricular enlargement and thinning of the corpus callosum , and increased iron deposition is concomitantly found in the basal ganglia, thalami, cortex, and subcortical white matter.

12.---a

The most characteristic MR finding in both the infantile and late-onset forms of GLD is high signal intensity on the T2-weighted images found along the lengths of the corticospinal tracts.

13.---a

14.----e

The hippocampus is a curved structure on the medial aspect of temporal lobe consisting of complex U-shaped layers of the dentate gyrus and cornu ammonis, which are interlocked together.The cornu ammonis is segmented into four portions, CA1 through CA4. CA4 is completely enveloped by the dentate gyrus and is known as the end-folium. The cornu ammonis blends into the subiculum, which forms the transition to the neocortex of parahippocampal gyrus.

15.---a

16.---b

Chemical shift artifact provides clue to the presence of fat in tumour. This artifact is displayed as a region of signal void at fat–water interfaces and hyperintensity at water–fat interfaces along the frequency-encoding axis . Fat-selective suppression methods can play a role in the distinction of etiologies of hyperintense tumors on T1-weighted images.

17.---e

Vascular endothelial proliferation within and adjacent to the tumor and intratumoral necrosis are highly characteristic of glioblastoma and are of great prognostic significance . (Exuberant neovascularization is also a characteristic of the pilocytic astrocytoma, so by itself it cannot be used as a pathognomonic sign for glioblastoma.)

MR imaging demonstrates marked intratumoral heterogeneity, reflecting sites of hemorrhage, necrosis, and varying degrees of hypercellularity. These changes are best seen on T2-weighted images, often showing foci of cystic necrosis and hemorrhage with debris–fluid levels and lower-intensity regions in areas of hypercellularity.

Linear or serpentine regions of signal void within the tumor mass on spin echo MR imaging indicate the often prominent angiogenesis that characterizes glioblastomas . Calcification is usually rare . Glioblastomas, along with oligodendroglioma and ependymoma, have a tendency to bleed.

Enhancement patterns are usually very heterogeneous , often with ringlike enhancement depicted as being thick, irregular, and nodular and surrounding necrotic areas, findings virtually indistinguishable from those seen in metastases and radiation necrosis

18.---b
Subependymomas in the lateral ventricles typically lack contrast enhancement. Intraventricular meningiomas and choroid plexus are usually situated within the atrium of the lateral ventricle and typically enhance diffusely

19.---b
Early metastatic foci are commonly found at gray matter–white matter interfaces, a feature shared by all hematogenously disseminated embolic disease. This distribution has been ascribed to the dramatic narrowing of the diameter of arterioles supplying the cortex as these vessels enter the white matter . As noted by Henson and Urich, tumor emboli measuring 100 to 200 μm in diameter are often found lodged in the 50- to 150-μm lumina of arterioles.

20.---d
Arachnoid cyst do not develop calcifications in their walls and demonstrate no contrast enhancement

21.---e
Proton spectroscopy shows evidence of malignant neoplasm by demonstrating a significant increase of choline relative to NAA, often a ratio of 3 or 4 to 1 .
 Taurine, an amino sulfonic acid, is elevated in PNETs.Taurine concentration is another marker for the differential diagnosis of PNET from other tumors
The tumors that showed restricted diffusion (hyperintense on diffusion sequence,dark and decreased in signal intensity on the ADC map)
 Measurements of ADC values for solid components of PNETs (range 0.67 to 0.99, mean 0.83×10^{-3} mm^2/s) are consistently lower than those for ependymomas (range 1.0 to 1.3, mean 1.23×10^{-3} mm^2/s) and can be useful for differential diagnosis.
Measurements of ADC values for solid components of PNETs (range 0.67 to 0.99, mean 0.83×10^{-3} mm^2/s) are consistently lower than those for ependymomas (range 1.0 to 1.3, mean 1.23×10^{-3} mm^2/s) and can be useful for differential diagnosis .

22.-----b
The appearance of supratentorial PNET on CT is similar to that seen with the primitive neuroectodermal tumor (medulloblastoma) of the posterior fossa, with the exception of a higher incidence of calcification (which approaches 50% to 70%) and also a higher frequency of large cysts and

necrosis.

23.---d

No hemorrhage seen in ADEM. The presence of hemorrhage in a more severe clinical form characterizes acute hemorrhagic encephalomyelitis .MR reveals moderate to large, usually asymmetric, patchy areas of increased signal intensity on T2-weighted images in the deep and subcortical white matter of the cerebral hemispheres, cerebellar white matter, and brainstem . The spinal cord may be involved. Clinical correlation is absolutely essential to narrow the differential diagnosis. The differential diagnosis for this MR appearance includes astrocytoma, vasculitis (which may also involve both gray and white matter), acute hemorrhagic leukoencephalopathy (which would reveal evidence of hemorrhage), tumefactive MS, PML in immunocompromised patients, and posterior reversible leukoencephalopathy particularly (e.g., hypertensive encephalopathy or chemotherapy related) in cases involving brainstem and relatively symmetric white matter patterns. MS and ADEM are indistinguishable by MR, regardless of lesion location or enhancement . The clinical course of the disease, or the clear relationship of the usually monophasic ADEM to previous viral illness or immunization, will suggest the correct diagnosis. Diffusion-weighted images may differentiate acute from subacute lesions because the acute lesions may have some restricted diffusion, but the value of DWI in demyelinating diseases is generally low. Even though acute demyelination can show restricted diffusion, it must be understood that significant restricted diffusion, particularly in gray matter lesions, should prompt consideration of acute vasculitic infarction and not acute demyelination.

24.---d

Tuberculoma is mostly infratentorial when in children, and it is supratentorial in adults. On CT, the most common finding of tuberculous meningitis is the isodense to slightly hyperdense exudate in the basal cistern, with basal homogeneous enhancement of the meninges. Cisternal enhancement is often quite striking and is far better demonstrated by postgadolinium MR than by
One third of tuberculomas may be multiple and are associated with meningitis in about 10% of cases . Parenchymal disease can occur with or without coexistent meningitis .Parenchymal disease can occur with or without coexistent meningitis .

25.---e

Small VR spaces (less than 2 mm) are found in all age groups and probably represent a normal anatomic finding . With advancing age, VR spaces are found with increasing frequency and larger apparent size .

In one report, lenticulostriate VR spaces had a mild correlation with age, whereas high-convexity VR spaces, although more rare, had a much stronger correlation with age .
Age, hypertension, dementia, and incidental subcortical white matter lesions were significantly associated with large (greater than 2 mm) VR spaces.
Migraine patients have been reported to show prominent perivascular spaces.
Distinction between dilated perivascular spaces and lacunar infarction is a common problem on clinical MR images. Three criteria must be assessed by the radiologist in these cases: location, morphology, and signal intensity.
Generally useful guidelines are that lacunar infarctions often are larger than 5 mm, are not symmetric, are located in the upper two thirds of the putamen, and are not isointense to CSF on all imaging sequences
. Conversely, dilated perivascular spaces usually are isointense to CSF on all pulse sequences, bilaterally symmetric, less than 5 mm in diameter, and located in the inferior one third of the putamen .Size is certainly the weakest discriminator of those mentioned.

26.---e

Pick bodies are intraneuronal inclusions, which are seen in minority of FTLD cases
Whereas AD and DLB account for the majority of neurodegenerative dementias in individuals older than age 65 years, FTLD is as common as AD in individuals under the age of 60 years
Frontotemporal lobar dementia (FTLD) describes a family of neurodegenerative disorders characterized by focal lobar degeneration of the frontal and/or temporal lobes. The umbrella term frontotemporal lobar dementia was divided into three clinical syndromes or subtypes at a consensus conference in 1998 . These are frontotemporal dementia----the frontal variant of FTLD or the behavioral variant of FTLD.
 Semantic dementia (SD) is also known as the temporal variant of FTLD
 Nonfluent aphasia---the nonfluent aphagia subtype of FTLD
FTLD is commonly associated with three other neurodegenerative syndromes with motor findings. These are cortical basal degeneration, progressive supranuclear palsy, and amyotrophic lateral sclerosis (labeled FTD-MND, or motor neuron disease).
The behavioral FTD subtype is the most common of the three FTLD subtypes to be associated with ALS, whereas the nonfluent aphasia subtype is the most common to be associated with cortical basal degeneration and progressive supernuclear palsy.

27.---e

Genetic linkage analyses have

shown that the gene locus for NF1 is at 17q11. Less than half of the patients with NF1 have a positive family history, a fact that suggests a high rate of spontaneous origin

28.---a
Two or more must be present for diagnosis of neurofibromatosis type1
Café-au-lait spots ≥6(5 mm child, 15 mm adult)
Neurofibromas: ≥2
Plexiform neurofibroma: 1
Axillary (intertriginous) freckling
Optic nerve glioma
Lisch nodules (iris hamartomas): ≥2
"Distinctive bone lesions": sphenoid wing dysplasia or long bone dysplasia
First-degree relative with neurofibromatosis 1

29.---b
Somatic hemiatrophy (contralateral malformation)

30----a
Enlargement of the affected cerebral hemisphere in hemimegalencephaly is due to white matter overgrowth

31.---c
Atretic cephalocele generally occur near the obelion

32.---c
The caudal vermis usually appears better preserved (e.g., the flocculonodulus is formed), whereas the rostral vermis is more severely hypoplastic. This pattern contrasts with that of DWM, in which the rostral vermis is better preserved.
The dentate nuclei are fused and classically describe a horseshoe-shaped arch crossing the midline draped along the fourth ventricle
The fourth ventricle is characteristically diamond or keyhole shaped on axial images, resulting from dorsal and rostral fusion of the dentate nuclei, the cerebellar peduncles, and the inferior colliculi.
The inferior olivary nuclei are usually absent

33.--c
ABC can cross the intervertebral disc space and involve an adjacent vertebral body
In osteoblastoma, the lumbar spine is most often involved, followed by the thoracic and cervical spine. Osteoblastomas occur most often in the posterior element.

34.---c
Mucin accumulation around vessels and between cells surrounding vessels is characteristic of myxopapillary ependymoma.

35.----c
The typical spinal cord lesion in ADEM is large and swollen, showing variable enhancement, and predominantly affects the thoracic region. Most frequently, ADEM is clinically differentiated from MS by its clinically monophasic course, in contrast to MS, which classically has periods of exacerbation and remission. Myelopathy in MS is frequently partial, but in ADEM it is often complete and associated with areflexia. Most ADEM patients recover completely, without further neurologic deficit.

A study using magnetization transfer and diffusion tensor MRI in patients with ADEM, patients with MS, and normal controls showed that, in contrast to what happens in MS, the normal-appearing brain and cervical tissues in ADEM are spared in the pathologic process.

36.----d
In a large series, 100% of cases had midline defects in the arches of the lumbosacral spine, usually at L-4, L-5, and/or S-1, leading Hendrick et al. to suggest that normal spine radiographs almost exclude this diagnosis.

37.---b
Oxytocin and vasopressin (antidiuretic hormone). The posterior lobe does not synthesize hormones,oxytocin and vasopressin They are synthesized in the hypothalamus and transported to the neurohypophysis down the axons of the pituitary stalk..
The pituitary gland receives its blood supply principally from the hypophyseal portal venous system.
combination of arterial and portal venous blood supply explains the differential rates of enhancement of the pituitary gland on dynamic scans after bolus administration of intravenous (i.v.) contrast agents

38.----e
The most frequent form is the classic adamantinomatous type, but a distinct squamous or papillary type is becoming recognized with increasing frequency.

39.----e
A high percentage of MRs demonstrate high signal intensity in the posterior lobe of normal individuals on routine sagittal T1-weighted views. This percentage has been reported to be as high as 98% to 100% and as low as 60% . Arguments have been made, therefore, particularly by the "high-percentage" reporters, that nonvisualization of the posterior lobe high signal should be interpreted as a sign of neurohypophyseal dysfunction. Nonvisualization has been reported in nephrogenic diabetes insipidus , a disorder in which the neurohypophysis is functionally intact. This seems to be a paradox, in that there should be abundance of neurosecretory activity to compensate for the insensitivity of the end organ, but Moses et al.proposed that in nephrogenic diabetes insipidus there is continuous stimulation and release of hormones, thus depleting the posterior lobe of neurosecretory vesicles and hence the lack of signal.

40.---e
Increased NAA levels have been observed with Canavan disease, an inherited disorder in which the enzyme aspartoacylase, which is involved in the process of degrading NAA to aspartate and acetate, is not being produced, resulting in the accumulation of NAA to toxic levels

41.----e

When hemorrhage is suspected within the first few hours to days after an infarction, it is essential that MR is performed with a T2*-sensitive gradient echo technique, the most sensitive method of detecting acute hemorrhage. When echo planar imaging is used in conjunction with DWI studies, the T2-weighted "b = 0" image is also very useful to depict acute hemorrhage as areas of hypointensity or signal loss. MR is more sensitive to hemorrhage in infarction than CT. MR may also detect more scattered "petechial" hemorrhage than CT.

42----d

Functional MRI techniques can be used to study cortical activation. During cortical activation there is an increase in rCBF and thus an increase in oxygen delivery to the activated brain, which exceeds the local oxygen metabolic requirement. There is, therefore, a net increase in oxyhaemoglobin concentration in the venules and veins in the vicinity of the activated brain, which results in a tiny increase in MR signal, the so called *blood oxygenation level dependent* or, BOLD effect. Although fMRI is being increasingly used for brain mapping, the technique has limited clinical applications and is used primarily for the identification of eloquent cortex, particularly the motor strip, prior to surgery in patients with structural lesions and arteriovenous malformations

43.----d

Pleomorphic xanthoastrocytoma (PXA) is usually associated with little or no oedema

44.----e

45.----e

The superior sagittal sinus is most commonly involved, which can lead to bilateral parasagittal infarcts
Using a combination of structural images, MR and CT venography, there is very little need to resort to DSA to confirm the diagnosis of venous thrombosis.

46.----e

47.----d

The cerebral sulci are characteristically not enlarged in communicating hydrocephalus

48.----d

Myelination maturation follows a centrifugal posterior-to-anterior and inferior-to-superior pattern

49.----d

The ipsilateral ventricle is enlarged and there is a very characteristic configuration of the frontal horn which is straight and pointed. Occasionally this may be the only imaging clue to an underlying malformation. Hemimegalencephaly may occur in isolation or in association with syndromes such as proteus, epidermal naevus and Klippel–Trenaunay–Weber, syndromes neurofibromatosis type 1 (NF1) and tuberous sclerosis.

50.----e

On T1-weighted sequences the cyst may demonstrate T1 shortening due to proteinacaeous components, which have been described macroscopically as

appearing like 'machine oil'. The cystic components are of increased signal on T2-weighted FSE.
51.---e
52.---e
Onyx is a new non-adhesive liquid embolic agent which consists of a mixture of ethyl-vinyl alcohol polymer (EVOH), dimethyl sul-occlufoxide (DMSO) as a solvent and tantalum to render it radiopaque. In contrast to NBCA, it solidifies slowly, minimises the danger of insitu gluing of a microcatheter. Onyx has been used for cerebral arteriovenous malformations (AVMS) and giant cerebral aneurysms in which other forms of endovascular or surgical treatment are difficult
53.---b
Progressive cerebellar atrophy is seen in Louis-Bar synsrome
54.----e
Medulloblastoma is a tumour that is unlikely to calcify.
55.-----a
Causes of large head in infancy
Hydrocephalus
Subdural effusions
Normal (sometimes familial)
Migrational abnormalities
Lipidoses
Spongy degeneration
Alexander's disease
Tuberous sclerosis
56.---d
Azygous ACA is rare anomaly
57.---e
The presence of peripheral or mixed venous drainage pattern and the presence of angiomatous change (the tresence of dilated cortical vessels derived from arteries not usually expected to supply the territory occupied by an AVM .
The cumulative risk of hemorrhage from a parenchymal AVM is estimated at 25 to 4% per year.
58.---c
The most common primary septal tumour is central neurocytoma
59.---e
Anaplastic astrocytoma enhance strongly but nonuniformly
60.---c
40 % to 45 % in CP angle

TEST PAPER 8

1. **Susceptibility –weighted imaging is an important sequence for**
a. venous vasculature
b. hemorrhage
c. iron-containing structures in the brain
d. useful in imaging of trauma and occult vascular diseases
e. All

2. **Which MR imaging is used to detect longitudinal changes due to Wallerian degeneration?**
a. Spin –echo imaging
b. Gradient-echo imaging
c. Diffuion-tensor imaging
d. FLAIR
e. Inversion recovery imaging

3. **All are true regarding infarction except**
a. both both microabscesses and large-vessel infarction in case of septic emboli
b. infarction in more than one vascular distribution in case of emboli
c. Vasculitis can produce a pattern similar to that of embolic disease
d. Infarctions with vasculitis can involve the deep gray and deep white matter structures in concert or alone
e. MR angiography is a valuable diagnostic tool in the search for vasculitis

4. **Which is diamagnetic?**
a. oxyhemoglobin
b. deoxyhemoglobin
c. methemoglobin
d. transferrin
e. lactoferrin

5. **Hypertintense signal on T1 W image is produced by**
a. Mucinous material, Hypermyelination
b. Intratumoral melanin
c. Ferromagnetic artifact
d. Slow flow
e. all

6. **All are true regarding intracranial hemorrhage in AVMs except**
a. rate of hemorrhage is 2% to 4% per year
b. Each occurrence of hemorrhage from an AVM is associated with a mortality of 10% to 15%
c. permanent neurologic deficit associated with hemorrhage is estimated to be approx. 20% to 30% per episode of hemorrhage
d. The risk of rebleeding after the initial hemorrhage from cerebral AVM is estimated to be 6% during the first year
e. smaller AVMs (less than 2.5 cm) present less frequently with hemorrhage than larger one

7. **The size of circle of Willis aneurysms that can be detected in most of cases by intracranial MRA by state-of-the-art acquisition and postprocessing methodology**
a. >2mm
b. >3mm
c. >4mm
d. >5mm
e. >6mm

8. All are CT features of cavernous angioma except
a. focal high-attenuation lesion
b. variably present calcification
c. no edema or mass effect
d. strong enhancement
e. less sensitivity than MR for its the detection

9. All are at higher Risk for Intracranial Aneurysms except
a. Polycystic kidney disease
b. Coarctation of the aorta
c. Fibromuscular dysplasia
d. Marfan syndrome
e. Moya moya disease

10. Myelinated Regions at Birth (or Shortly After Birth) are all except
a. Dorsal brainstem
b. Inferior, superior cerebellar peduncles
c. Perirolandic region
d. Corticospinal tract
e. peripheral portion of centrum semiovale

11. All are true regarding multiple sclerosis except
a. the MR appearance of corpus callosal lesions is specific for MS
b. lesions at callosal–septal interface is noted in up to 93% of MS patients
c. MS lesions typically decrease in size over time
d. MS plaques may enhance after the administration of intravenous contrast
e. steroids treatment may be associated with a marked reduction in lesion enhancement

12. All are MR finding in Metachromatic Leukodystrophy except
a. symmetric confluent areas of high signal intensity within the periventricular
b. predominant involvement of the frontal white matter in juvenile and adult forms
c. absence of contrast enhancement,
d. cerebellar white matter rarely involved
e. lack of involvement of deep gray matter.

13. Cystic white matter changes is seen in
a. Megalencephalic leukoencephalopathy with subcortical cysts
b. Cytomegalovirus infection and Megalencephalic leukoencephalopathy with subcortical cysts
c. Vanishing white matter disease and Cytomegalovirus infection
d. Megalencephalic leukoencephalopathy with subcortical cysts and Cytomegalovirus infection
e. Vanishing white matter disease ,Megalencephalic leukoencephalopathy with subcortical cysts and Cytomegalovirus infection

14. All are true regarding hippocampus except
a. located on the medial aspect of the temporal lobe
b. situated below the parahippocampal gyrus
c. located posterior to the amygdala
d. has head, body and tail
e. connection with the mammillary body via the fornix and fimbria

15. All are true regarding imaging

of cortical malformations except
a. Inversion recovery sequences are well suited for detection of subtle gray matter thickening and indistinctness of gray and white matter junction
b. High spatial resolution can be achieved through the use of thin-section three-dimensional volume imaging
c. High spatial resolution can be achieved through the use of smaller in-plane resolution imaging,

d. phased-array surface coils or high–field strength magnets are used to achieve high spatial resolution
e. a spoiled gradient recalled echo sequence yield very poor spatial resolution

16. All are features of intratumoral hemorrhage except
a. Markedly heterogeneous signal intensities
b. identification of nonhemorrhagic tumor component
c. early evolution of blood-breakdown products
d. Absent/diminished/irregular ferritin/hemosiderin rim
e. Persistent surrounding high intensity on long–repetition time images

17. ---All are true regarding glioblastoma multiforme except
a. most commonly involved lobe frontal lobe followed by the temporal lobe
b. bihemispheric involvement with corpus callosum infiltration (butterfly) distribution characteristic
c. tendency to invade leptomeninges and dura
d. dissemination via the subarachnoid space.
e. metastasize outside the CNS very common

18. All are true regarding central neurocytoma except
a. specifically within the lateral ventricle
b. typically show attachment to the septum pellucidum
c. No calcification
d. nearly isointense to gray matter
e. Contrast enhancement common

19. All are true regarding brain metastastes except
a. roughly 80% to 85% of metastases are located in the supratentorial compartment
b. Clinically silent lesions are most frequently seen in patients with adenocarcinoma and oat cell carcinoma of lung and melanoma
c. the optimal screening examination is intravenous-enhanced MR imaging
d. Most common cause of brain metastases is lung cancer
e. incidence of solitary metastasis is estimated to range from 5% to 10%

20. All are true regarding MR cisternogram except
a. thin-section
b. heavily T1-weighted images
c. allow for excellent depiction of the contents of the cerebellopontine angle
d. allow for excellent visualization of the seventh and eighth nerve complexes

e. high resolution

21. All are true regarding medulloblastoma except
a. associated in Gorlin syndrome and Turcot syndrome
b. Eighty percent of the PNETs involve the vermian tissue to some extent
c. cysts more typical of medulloblastoma than the cerebellar astrocytoma
d. brainstem involvement seen in up to 38% of patients
e. very high incidence of hydrocephalus

22. All are true regarding subependymal giant cell tumors except
a. most often in association with tuberous sclerosis
b. arise from subependymal nodules
c. typically near the foramen of Monro
d. No contrast enhancement of the mass
e. calcification and iron deposition

23. All are true regarding ADEM except
a. multiphasic
b. 5 days to 2weeks of preceding viral infection
c. inflammatory reaction around the vessels and multifocal perivenous demyelination
d. white matter involved more than gray matter
e. The location of lesions on MR often correlates with the clinical signs and symptoms

24. The most common radiographic findings associated with CNS TB are all except
a. enhancement of the basal cisterns
b. granulomata and calcifications
c. hydrocephalus
d. meningeal enhancement
e. infarction, usually of cerebellum

25. All are true regarding space of Virchow-Robin (VRS) except
a. isointense to CSF on all pulse sequences
b. type 2 lacunae
c. lack mass effect
d. round, oval, or curvilinear with well-defined, smooth margins
e. common in relation to anterior commissure

26. All are true regarding Dementia with Lewy bodies(DLB) except
a. the second-most-common neurodegenerative cause of dementia in the elderly,
b. aggregation of α-synuclein protein in neurites form Lewy bodies
e. occipital hyperperfusion in functional imaging
f. decreased dopamine transporter activity in the basal ganglia with SPECT/PET radioligands
g. decreased uptake of metaiodobenzylguanidine on cardiac scintigraphy.

.27. All are true regarding spinocerebellar Ataxias except
a. SCA2 shows with the "hot cross bun" sign
b. Friedreich ataxia is the commonest hereditary ataxia
c. spinal cord atrophy with preservation of the basis pontis and the cerebellum is noted in Friedrich ataxia

d. Ataxia Telangiectasia is characterized by atrophy of the cerebellar vermis and cerebellar hemispheres
e. Vit E causes ataxia

28. All are true regarding Motor neurone disease except
a. neurodegenerative disorders of the upper and/or lower motor neurons
b. Amyotrophic lateral sclerosis (ALS) is the most frequent type of motor neuron disease
c. hyperintense signal coursing along the corticospinal tract from precentral gyrus to the level of the cord on FLAIR
d. Hypointense signal on the T2-weighted and FLAIR sequences in the motor cortex
e. an increase in mean diffusivity and a increase in fractional anisotropy of the corticospinal tract

29. All are seen in Tuberous sclerosis except
a. lymphangiomyomatosis.
b. "honeycomb" lung
c. spontaneous pneumothorax
d. simple cysts and/or angiomyolipomas
e. contracted lung

30. Hemimegalencephaly may be associated with all except
a. Klippel-Trenaunay syndrome
b. epidermal nevus syndrome
c. Proteus syndrome
d. neurofibromatosis type II
e. tuberous sclerosis

31. All are true regarding cephalocoeles except
a. cerebral MR venography may be useful in the assessment of frontal cephaloceles
b. the ventricles or subarachnoid space that subtends the cephalocele to "point" toward the defect
c. the ventricle often appear to be elongated
d. generalized widening of the subarachnoid space may be seen.
e. most of cephaloceles occur in the midline

32. All are true regarding Joubert Malformation except
a. Vermian hypogenesis
b. separation of the cerebellar hemispheres
c. deepening of the interpeduncular fossa and elongation and thinning of the isthmus
d. thick and horizontally oriented superior cerebellar peduncle to the dorsum of the pons
e. bat shaped fourth ventricle

33. All are true regarding osteoid osteoma of vertebral spine except
a. The most common locations in the spine -- the lumbar region (59%)
b. Osteoid osteomas involve the posterior elements in 75% of cases.
c. presence of the nidus (less than 2.5 cm)
d. focally "hot" on bone scan
e. enhancement of nidus

34. All are true regarding spinal cord hemangioblastoma except
a. considerable edema
b. serpiginous areas of enhancement anterior to chord
c. markedly enhancing tumor nidus

d. widening of the spinal cord
e. cyst formation

35. All are true regarding neuromyelitis optica except
a. interval usually of days or weeks between optic neuritis and transverse myelitis
b. longitudinally confluent lesions
c. hyperintense on T2W
d. extend five or more vertebral segments
e. only monophasic course

36. All are true regarding spine except
a. The tip of the normal dural sac begins to rise from S-5 after 14 weeks' gestation
b. the tip of the dural sac terminates between the S1-2 /S2-3nterspace in adult.
c. a conus that lies at or below L-3 is regarded as abnormal
d. the tip of the conus and the tip of the dural sac both end "high" or "low" concordantly
e. fila thicker than 1mm are abnormal.

37. All are true regarding size of pituitary gland except
a. weighs about 0.5 g in the adult
b. average size is 12 mm in width, 8 mm in anteroposterior diameter, and 3 to 8 mm in height
c. greatest size noted in adolescent girls and pregnant women
d. the increased T1 signal intensity in the anterior gland during pregnancy is abnormal
e. signal on T1 of anterior gland progressively normalizes in the first 12 months after delivery

38. the most reliable indicator of cavernous sinus invasion by pituitary macroadenoma is
a. Lateral extension and interposition of abnormal tissue between the lateral wall of the cavernous sinus and the artery
b. normal pituitary between the adenoma and cavernous sinus
c. intact medial venous compartment
d. less than 25% ICA encasement
e. marked constriction or occlusion of the cavernous portion of the internal carotid artery

39. All are true regarding cranial pathology except
a. Carotid cavernous fistulas are mostly due to trauma
b. The ipsilateral cavernous sinus, orbital veins, and petrosal sinus fill slowly and lately in Carotid cavernous fistulas
c. The fistulous communication in Carotid cavernous fistulas is most often occult on MR
d. pituitary enlargement noted in cavernous sinus dural arteriovenous malformations
e. contrast-enhanced MRA is useful at detecting fistulas

40. All are true regarding BOLD contrast except
a. used in Functional MRI
b. BOLD signal response arises from localized hemodynamic changes
c. BOLD contrast is a negative contrast effect
d. surrogate marker of increased neuronal activity.
e. Cognitively more difficult tasks produce a larger BOLD contrast

41. All are regading PET imaging except

a. cerebral glucose uptake use fluorodeoxyglucose (FDG)
b. oxygen metabolism study use $^{15}O_2$ or ^{11}CO
c. rCBF study use $H_2{}^{15}O$.
d. ^{11}C methionine and Fα-methyl tyrosine are used for tumour imaging.
e. ^{99m}Tc hexamethylpropylene amine oxide (HMPAO) is used for rCBF study

42. All are true regarding pilocytic astrocytomas except
a. WHO grade I1
b. predilection for the posterior fossa
c. primarily seen in children
d. usually a significant cystic component and show enhancement
e. frequently mistaken for haemangioblastomas in adult

43. All are true regarding imaging of meningioma except
a. atypical meningiomas have lower ADC values than the typical meningioma
b. an choline peak on MRS – characteristic of meningioma
c. Meningiomas have usually a markedly elevated rCBV on PWI
d. supplied from meningeal vessels
e. a dense, homogeneous, persistent blush on angiography

44. All are true regarding stroke except
a. A matched defect of core and penumbra ----a completed infarct without areas of reversibility.
b. core shows restricted diffusion and CBV deficit
c. penumbra --- salvageable ischaemic tissue
d. IV thrombolysis is given within 3 h of symptom onset
e. quantifying the ADC does not increases specificity for infarcts in patients with strokes or TIAs

45. All are true regarding tuberculosis of CNS except
a. Involvement of the central nervous system occurs in 5 per cent of cases of tuberculosis
b. Tuberculous meningitis is the most frequent manifestation and tends to involve the basal leptomeninges
c. Infarctions of the basal ganglia and internal capsules can occur
d. The 'target sign' of central high attenuation with rim enhancement is not pathognomonic for tuberculoma.
e. Tuberculous abscesses are common

46. All are true regarding diseases of skull except
a. 'ground-glass' pattern in fibrous dysplasia
b. a spotty 'cotton-wool pledget' – early feature of Paget in skull
c. typical 'spoke wheel' appearance noted in haemangioma of skull
d. 'Tam O'Shanter' deformity inPaget is due to foraminal narrowing
e. osteo- or fibro-sarcomas arise in about 1% of patients with cranial Paget's disease

47. All are true regarding spinal lesion except
a. polka dot appearance noted in vertebral lymphoma hemangioma
b. axial skeleton is one of the commonest sites of involvement in Paget disease

c. The lateral and dorsal spinal cord columns are affected in Subacute combined degeneration of the spinal cord
d. Cobb's syndrome is associated with vascular malformations
e. iophendylate (Myodil) may cause arachnoiditis

48. All are true regarding transmantle cortical dysplasia except
a. abnormal cells extend all the way from the wall of the ventricle to the cortex
b. blurring of the junction between the cortex and the white matter
c. hypointensity (compared to the white matter on T2) extending from the lateral ventricular wall to the blurred cortex
d. correlation between abnormal venous drainage and dysplastic cortex
e. may be calcified

49. All are DD of posterior fossa tumour with CT hypersedsity and T2 hypointensity except
a. Medulloblastoma
b. Choroid plexus carcinoma
c. Ewings' sarcoma
d. ependymoma
e. Chordoma

50. All are true regarding Nonaccidental head injury except
a. retinal haemorrhages
b. subdural haemorrhages
c. extradural haemorrhage
d. diffuse cerebral oedema
e. cerebral contusions

51. All are true regarding N-butyl-cyanoacrylate (NBCA) except
a. acrylate glue
b. liquid embolic agent cause transient vascular occlusion
c. used for embolisation of cerebral AVMs and dural fistula
d. diluted in Lipiodiol
e. made radiopaque with Tantalum powder

52. The cardinal sign of raised intracranial pressure is
a. suture diastasis
b. thick skull vaults
c. sellar erosion
d. craniolacunae
e. cupper beaten appearance

53. All the features distinguish acquired fusion from failure of segmentation of vertebra except
a. fused segment taller than adjacent unfused bodies
b. reduced AP diameter
c. wasp waist at the level of fusion
d. usually associated arch fused
e. angulation

54. Anterior inferior cerebellar artery supply all except
a. supply nerve VII and VIII
b. inferolateral pons
c. middle cerebellar peduncle
d. flocculus
e. posterolareal surface of cerebellar hemisphere

55. All are true regarding parenchymal AVM except
a. solitary in 90% cases
b. 85% in cerebral hemishphere
d. prominent capillary bed
d. shaped like cone with base on the cortex
e. flow related aneurysm in 10 to 12 %

56. All are true regarding lateral ventricles except
a. septum pellucidum is a triangular membrane

b.septum pellucidum is absent in holoprosencephaly
c.80% of normal fetus hace cavum septum pelllucidi (CSP)
d.a persistent CSP is present in 2 % to 5% of normal adults
e.Cavum vergae (CV) can occur without CSP

57.All are true regarding low-grade astrocytoma except
a.hypointense on T1W
b.5% to 10% calcify
c.no necrosis
d.edema and hemorrhage rare
e.enhancement absent/mild inhomogenous

58.All are true regarding Schwannoma except
a.encapsulated ,round and focal
b.undergoe malignant degeneration
c.cyst heamorrhage and necrosis common
d.enhances strongly
e.,hyoointense on T1W

59.All are true regarding CNS infection except
a.medulla is the most common affected part in cryptococcosis
b.thr posterior centrum semiovale is the most common site for PML
c.lesions inADEM is typically bilateral and asymmetric
d.atrophy is seen in Rasmussen's encephalitis
e.CMV does not cause periventricular calcification in AIDS

60.All are true regarding amino-acid disorders except
a.marked,generalized diffuse edema is seen in Maple syrup urine disease
b.saggital sinus thrombosis may be seen in homocystinuria
c.batwing dilatation of sylvian fissure and frontotemporal atrophy is seen in Glutaric aciduria type 1
d.corpuas callosum appears abnormally thick in non-ketotic hyperglycinemia
e.bilateral low density lesions in the globus pallidus is seen in Methylmalonic academia

TEST PAPER 8(ANSWER)

1.—e
2.---c
3.---e
That MR angiography is not a valuable diagnostic tool in the search for vasculitis but the recent development of CT angiography has shown promise in this diagnosis.
4.---a
Oxyhemoglobin is diamagnetic ,while deoxyhemoglobin,methemoglobin, transferring, lactoferrin, ferritin, hemosiderin are paramagnetic.
5..—e
Larger AVMs (less than 2.5 cm) present less frequently with hemorrhage than larger one.Hypertension and cocaine abuse is positively associated with hemorrhage in patients harboring intracranial AVMs.
6.----e
7.---b
8.---d
Enhancement cavernous angima is typically mild on CT but may not be identifiable.
9.------e
10.----e
11.----a
The MR appearance of MS lesions is highly variable and certainly not specific. The corpus callosum is a region that is especially vulnerable to demyelination in MS, possibly due to its intimate neuroanatomic relationship to the lateral ventricular roofs and to small penetrating vessels. Studies have shown focal areas of high signal intensity on T2-weighted images in the inferior aspect of the corpus callosum (callosal–septal interface) in up to 93% of MS patients . Sagittal T1-weighted images nicely depict these lesions as focal areas of thinning of the inferior aspect of the corpus callosum .

It has been advocated that the MR appearance of these corpus callosal lesions may be specific for MS , there is no question that ischemic lesions can have a virtually identical appearance MS plaques may enhance after the administration of intravenous contrast , reflecting transient abnormality of the blood–brain barrier. The enhancement patterns are extremely variable and may appear homogeneous, ringlike, or nodular. Treatment with steroids may also be associated with a marked reduction in lesion enhancement and morphology

Contrast enhancement may be used to add specificity to the finding of multiple hyperintensities on T2-weighted images because the finding of enhancing along with nonenhancing lesions is quite common in MS but makes many other diagnoses unlikely. Similarly, the temporal changes in enhancing and nonenhancing lesions common in MS are very different from those in other entities. The enhancement of the demyelinating lesions depends on the amount of contrast administered, with increased conspicuity of lesions with triple-dose studies

12.---d

Distinguishing features of MLD include absence of contrast enhancement, frequent involvement of cerebellar white matter, and lack of involvement of deep gray matter.

In the late-infantile form of MLD , there is a posterior (occipital) predominance of signal abnormality with dorsofrontal progression of disease .

Involvement of the corticospinal tracts (typically ascribed to X-linked adrenoleukodystrophy) may also be seen in the late-infantile form of MLD. The corpus callosum is invariably affected, and hypointensity within the thalami on T2-weighted images may be seen. The so-called tigroid and "leopard skin" pattern of demyelination (alternating areas of normal white matter within areas of demyelination, suggestive of perivascular white matter sparing) in the periventricular white matter and centrum semiovale has been typically described in Pelizaeus-Merzbacher disease but has also been noted in the late-infantile form of MLD.

13.---e

14.---b

Broca intralimbic gyrus is composed primarily of the hippocampus (hippocampal formation or HF) and the vestigial supracallosal and paraterminal gyri. The hippocampus is located on the medial aspect of the temporal lobe situated above the parahippocampal gyrus and posterior to the amygdala . The hippocampus is composed of the bulbous digitated hippocampal head , body , and tail . The hippocampus connects with the mammillary body and in turn the thalamus via the fornix and fimbria .

15.----e

Dedicated pulse sequences are needed to detect subtle cortical malformations—sequences that emphasize high contrast between gray and white matter or high spatial resolution. Inversion recovery sequences are well suited for allowing detection of subtle gray matter thickening and indistinctness of gray and white matter junction.

High spatial resolution can be achieved through the use of thin-section three-dimensional volume imaging, such as a spoiled gradient recalled echo sequence, or smaller in-plane resolution imaging, such as with phased-array surface coils or high–field strength magnets . Multiplanar reconstruction of volume-acquired data or photographic image reversal of inversion recovery or T2-weighted sequences may also be helpful.

16.----c

There is delayed evolution of

blood-breakdown products.

Intratumoral Hemorrhage Versus Benign Intracranial Hematomas

Intratumoral hemorrhage	Benign hemorrhage

Markedly heterogeneous, related to:
  Mixed stages of blood
  Debris–fluid (intracellular–extracellular blood) levels
  Edema + tumor + necrosis with blood
	Shows expected signal intensities of acute, subacute, or chronic blood, depending on stage of hematoma

Identification of nonhemorrhagic tumor component	No abnormal nonhemorrhagic mass
Delayed evolution of blood-breakdown products	Follows expected orderly progression
Absent, diminished, or irregular ferritin/hemosiderin	Regular complete ferritin/hemosiderin rim
Persistent surrounding high intensity on long–repetition time images (i.e., tumor/edema) and mass effect, even in late stages	Complete resolution of edema and mass effect in chronic stages

17.----e

There is a distinct tendency for malignant gliomas, especially those that are located superficially, to invade leptomeninges and dura with subsequent dissemination via the subarachnoid space. It is quite rare for these lesions to metastasize outside the CNS.

18.---c

Calcification is considered characteristic feature of central neurocytoma.

Central neurocytoma (WHO grade II) is a relatively benign intraventricular neoplasm that occurs mainly in young to middle-aged adults. On microscopy, the tumor is made up of small, well-differentiated cells with features reminiscent of oligodendroglioma.

19.—e

Intraparenchymal metastases are the most common type of metastatic disease to affect the intracranial space. Most common, in decreasing incidence, are lung cancer, breast cancer, melanoma, gastrointestinal cancers, renal cell carcinoma, and tumors of unknown primary. Furthermore, the brain is often the only site of metastases among patients with extracranial malignancy, a situation particularly common in those with bronchogenic carcinoma and melanoma. It is generally accepted that most intracerebral metastases are multiple, regardless of the site of origin; however, there is a high incidence of solitary metastasis, estimated to range from 30% to 50% and especially common in melanoma, lung, and breast carcinoma.

20.----b
High-spatial-resolution, thin-section, heavily T2-weighted images used to acquire an "MR cisternogram" allow for excellent depiction of the contents of the cerebellopontine angle and visualization of the seventh and eighth nerve complexes. Acquisition can be performed either with three-dimensional half-Fourier rapid acquisition with relaxation enhancement or three-dimensional constructive interference in the steady-state techniques

21.---c

22.---d
Contrast enhancement of the mass is the rule, but enhancement alone does not prove the presence of SGCT. Hypointensity on T2 is nonspecific because calcification and iron deposition are present in both subependymal nodules and tumors.

23.---a
Classically ADEM has monophasic clinical course. A multiphase variant also has been described, called "multiphasic disseminated encephalomyelitis" or "relapsing disseminated encephalomyelitis."

24.----e
The most common radiographic findings associated with CNS TB include enhancement of the basal cisterns, granulomata, calcifications, hydrocephalus, meningeal enhancement, and infarction, usually of the basal ganglia.
Central nervous system TB is represented by different and possibly concomitant forms; the most common are tuberculous meningitis and parenchymal involvement, including focal cerebritis and tuberculoma, followed by tuberculous abscesses and miliary tuberculosis. The most frequent complications are parenchymal infarction, hydrocephalus, and mycotic aneurysms.
Arteritis is present in approximately 28% to 41% of cases with basilar meningitis. Infarctions are even more common in children. The middle cerebral artery and its branches are most often affected, especially the small perforating branches supplying the basal ganglia.

25.---b
Type I lacunae are small infarcts, type II are small hemorrhages, and type III are dilated VRS Perivascular space of Virchow-Robin (VRS) is an extension of the subarachnoid space that accompanies penetrating vessels into the brain to the level of the capillaries. The VRS at the base of the brain follow the lenticulostriate arteries as they enter the basal ganglia through the anterior perforated substance. On axial images they are typically adjacent to the anterior or posterior surface of the lateral portion of the anterior commissure. In the coronal or sagittal plane they are adjacent to the superior surface of the commissure or just lateral to the putamen.

Those in the high convexity follow the course of the penetrating cortical arteries and arterioles from the high-convexity gray matter into the centrum semiovale.

High signal intensity (i.e., higher intensity than CSF, most notably on proton density–weighted or FLAIR images) foci in the midbrain can be seen from enlarged perivascular spaces(along branches of the collicular and accessory collicular arteries)

26.---e

Occipital hypoperfusion noted functional imaging of dementia with Lewy bodies(DLB) cases. Dementia with Lewy bodies (DLB) is considered to be the second-most-common neurodegenerative cause of dementia in the elderly, The defining neuropathology of dementia with Lewy bodies is pathologic aggregation of α-synuclein protein in neurites to form Lewy bodies.

A pattern of focal atrophy confined to the dorsal pontomesencephalic junction, peri third ventricular gray matter, and substantia innominata had been identified on a voxel-based morphometry study in DLB.

REM sleep behavior disorder is a sentinel sign of Lewy body disorders.

α-synuclein pathology first appears in brainstem nuclei such as the locus ceruleus and reticular activating system,

27.---a

SCA3 (Machado-Joseph disease) shows abnormal signal of the transverse pontine fibers (with the "hot cross bun" sign) together with atrophy of the pons, middle cerebellar peduncles, and cerebellum, similar to MSA-C. Differences exist, however. SCA3 shows neuropathologic and MRI findings not seen in MSA-C, including atrophy of the superior cerebellar peduncles, frontal and temporal lobes, and globus pallidi and abnormal linear hyperintense signal along the medial margins of the internal segments of the globus pallidi bilaterally on long-TR and FLAIR images . The latter imaging finding correlates pathologically with degeneration of the lenticular fasciculus, a major outflow of the internal segment of the globus pallidus.

Gross pathology and MRI of Friedreich Ataxia reveal atrophy of the spinal cord . Spinal cord atrophy has been variably reported to affect the cervical spinal cord and/or along the length of the entire cord, from the cervicomedullary junction through the conus medullaris. These atrophic changes are due to degeneration with myelin loss and gliosis of the posterior columns and roots and spinocerebellar and corticospinal tracts .

The absence or milder nature of the cerebellar atrophy in Friedreich ataxia serves as a useful differential diagnostic feature on MRI and contrasts with the imaging findings in primary cerebellar degenerative processes.

28.---e
Advanced MR techniques, particularly DTI and MRS, are more sensitive than conventional MRI in detecting upper motor neuron degeneration, particularly early in the disease. When compared with normal controls, ALS patients show an increase in mean diffusivity and a decrease in fractional anisotropy of the corticospinal tract . Mean diffusivity correlated with disease duration, whereas fractional anisotropy correlated with disease severity.

29---e
The lung volume in tuberous sclerosis is expanded rather than contracted, and these patients may suffer multiple episodes of spontaneous pneumothorax

30.---d
Hemimegalencephaly may be associated with Neurofibromatosis type I .

31.---a
In general, MR is the most sensitive and accurate imaging modality for both the detection and characterization of cephaloceles. Cerebral MR venography may be useful in the assessment of parietal and occipital cephaloceles because the superior sagittal sinus and torcular herophili are commonly found within the cephalocele sac. Contrast-enhanced MR sequences may also be helpful in delineating transsphenoidal and postsurgical temporal cephaloceles.
Associated anomalies, such as agenesis or hypogenesis of the corpus callosum, the Dandy-Walker malformation, and subependymal heterotopic gray matter, are common.

32.---d
There is deepening of the interpeduncular fossa and elongation and thinning of the isthmus defined as the region between the inferior colliculi and the pontomesencephalic junction. The interpeduncular fossa (cistern) is elongated.
The superior cerebellar peduncles are thick and are abnormally oriented perpendicular to the dorsum of the pons. The appearance of the mesencephalon and the superior cerebellar peduncles has been described as the "molar tooth sign" . The molar tooth sign may be seen in other posterior fossa malformations such as pontine tegmental cap dysplasia.

33.---c
Plain films demonstrate the classic findings in 66% to 75% of the cases, show a lucent nidus in classic cases . The size of the nidus is less than 1.5 cm (if greater than 1.5 cm, the lesion would be classified as an osteoblastoma),. The nidus is surrounded by sclerotic bony reaction
The administration of gadolinium, like that of iodinated contrast material, causes intense enhancement within the very vascular nidus. This enhancement may help not only to localize the nidus, but also to differentiate it from a nonenhancing lytic lesion such as Brodie's abscess .

34.---b
Myelography frequently shows expansion of the spinal cord and serpiginous filling defects posterior to the cord representing meningeal varicosities.
Spinal angiography reveals prominent feeding arteries and draining veins and an intense blush of the tumor nidus
Adjacent serpiginous areas of signal void or enhancement may be seen on MRI and, when present, clinch the diagnosis because the main mimic of these lesions, metastases, do not have associated enlarged vessels . These can represent large feeding arteries or, more commonly, draining meningeal varicosities associated with the very vascular tumor nidus.
The differentiation of edematous cord from cyst is important because metastases of the cord rarely are associated with cysts, whereas the other intramedullary lesion to show dramatic focal enhancement amid a larger region of nonenhancing abnormality, the hemangioblastoma, is frequently associated with a large syrinx.

35.—e
The course of NMO is unpredictable, and it may have a mono- or multiphasic course . The relapsing form of NMO primarily affects women, and most patients experience clusters of attacks months or years apart followed by partial recovery during periods of remission. The monophasic form of NMO is characterized by a single, severe attack extending over 1 to 2 months and affects men and women with equal frequency.

36.---e
Gryspeerdt measured the thickness of the normal filum terminale at myelography and concluded that fila thicker than 2 mm were abnormal. Yundt et al. confirmed that observation by direct measurement of the filum terminale in the operating room . In their series, the normal filum measured 1.2 ± 0.2 mm.

37.---d
Pituitary gland achieves its greatest size in adolescent girls and pregnant women.
The gland height progressively decreases during the first 8 months after delivery, and the increased T1 signal intensity in the anterior gland normally seen in pregnancy progressively normalizes in the first 12 months after delivery. Termination of lactation has no effect on these changes.

38.---a
Lateral extension and interposition of abnormal tissue between the lateral wall of the cavernous sinus and the artery is the most reliable indicator of cavernous sinus invasion
Vieira et al. recently performed a logistic regression analysis with correlation with surgical findings . MR signs studied included (1) presence of normal pituitary between the adenoma and cavernous sinus, (2) status of cavernous sinus venous compartments, (3) cavernous

sinus size, (4) cavernous sinus lateral wall bulging, (5) displacement of the intracavernous internal carotid artery (ICA), (6) Knosp-Steiner grade of parasellar extension, and (7) percentage ICA encasement. They found that accurate criteria for noninvasion included (1) normal pituitary between the adenoma and cavernous sinus (positive predictive value 100%), (2) intact medial venous compartment (positive predictive value 100%), and (3) less than 25% ICA encasement (negative predictive value 100%). Cavernous sinus invasion was certain with greater than 45% ICA encasement and three or more cavernous sinus venous compartments not depicted. The most valuable criterion of invasion was ICA encasement of 30% or more, a value considerably different from Cottier's 67%. Significant asymmetry between cavernous sinuses, very high serum prolactin levels (greater than 1,000 ng/mL), and markedly elevated growth hormone levels in the GH-secreting adenomas correlate well with invasion.

One should note that despite the fact that cavernous sinus involvement by pituitary adenomas is not uncommon, marked constriction or occlusion of the cavernous portion of the internal carotid artery is very rare. This is of some differential diagnostic significance in distinguishing adenomas from meningiomas.

39.----b
The ipsilateral cavernous sinus, orbital veins, and petrosal sinus fill prematurely because of arteriovenous shunting and are dilated

40.----c
the $T2^*$-weighted MR signal intensity increases with BOLD contrast so BOLD contrast is a positive contrast effect and is a surrogate marker of increased neuronal activity.

The BOLD effect depends not only on the nuclear transverse relaxation rate of blood and the oxygenation state of hemoglobin, but also on the compartmentation of hemoglobin within erythrocytes. The effect is also magnified due to the magnetic susceptibility differences between the vascular compartment of the capillaries and the surrounding tissues.

The other feature of BOLD contrast is that the magnitude of the response depends on task difficulty. Cognitively more difficult tasks produce a larger BOLD contrast.

Because magnetic susceptibility effects are field strength dependent, higher-field magnets offer increased BOLD sensitivity. This property suggests that 3-T scanners have an advantage over 1.5-T scanners

41.---e
^{99m}Tc hexamethylpropylene amine oxide (HMPAO) is used for rCBF study in SPECT

42---a

43.---b

MRS may show an alanin peak, which is characteristic for a meningioma but this is seen in less than 50 per cent of cases. Meningiomas have usually a markedly elevated rCBV on PWI, which can be used to differentiate from dural metastases, which tend to have a lower rCBV.

44.---e
Quantifying the ADC increases specificity for infarcts in patients with strokes or TIAs
Management strategies of stroke vary but frequently IV thrombolysis is given within 3 h of symptom onset as soon as haemorrhage or an obvious large infarct has been excluded. Because early DWI lesions may reverse, some thrombolysis centres treat patients presenting within 3 h, even if perfusion imaging shows a matched defect
Intra-arterial thrombolysis or mechanical disruption may be attempted if the patient does not rapidly improve and a proximal vessel occlusion is shown angiographically or as a dense artery on CT. Beyond 3 h restricted diffusion is less likely to be reversible so thrombolysis is usually only appropriate if there is mismatch and many centres opt for primary intra-arterial treatment if there is also a proximal vessel occlusion.

45.---e
Tuberculous abscesses are uncommon; they may resemble tuberculomas but are usually larger with a thinner enhancing rim

46.---d
Basilar invagination, due to softening of bone; occurs in about a third of cases of cranial Paget and can lead to a 'Tam O'Shanter' deformity.

47.---a
Polka dot appearance noted in vertebral hemangioma

48.----c
Typical features of transmantle cortical dysplasia include blurring of the junction between the cortex and the white matter, and hyperintensity (compared to the white matter on T2) extending from the lateral ventricular wall to the blurred cortex.

49.---d
DIFFERENTIAL DIAGNOSIS OF POSTERIOR FOSSA TUMOUR WITH CT HYPERDENSITY AND T2 HYPOINTENSITY
Medulloblastoma/primitive neuroectodermal tumour/atypical teratoid/rhabdoid tumour
Choroid plexus carcinoma
Chondrosarcoma
Chordoma
Lymphoma
Langerhans' cell histiocytosis

50---c

51.---b
Prior to injection, NBCA are diluted in a lipophylic contrast agent (Lipiodol) or made radiopaque with Tantalum powder. On contact with an ionic solution, such as blood, NBCA solidifies rapidly, causing permanent vascular occlusion. The microcatheter through which it has been delivered has to be swiftly withdrawn to avoid the

risk of gluing the catheter in-situ. It is a very effective but dangerous embolic agent,

52.---c

53.---e

Angulation is common in postinflammatory fusion as there is no bone destruction.Association with spina bifida is common.

54—e

AICA supply anterolateral surface (petrosal)of the cerebellar hemisphere

55.---d

There is no intervening capillary bed in AVMs .AVMs consist of arterial feeders ,arterial collaterals ,the AVM nidus and enlarged venous outflow channels

56.---e

A CV appears as a posterior extention of a CSP ,so CV never occur without a CSP

57.---b

15% to 20% of low –grade astrocytoma calcify.Most low grade astrocytomas eventually undergo malignant degeneration .

58.---b

Schwannoma doesnot undergo malignant degeneration

59.---a

The meninges,basal ganglia and midbrain are most commonly affected site in cryptococcosis.

60.---d

Corpus callosum appears abnormally thin in non-ketotic hyperglycinemia

TEST PAPER 9

1. Structures that can be distinguished from the background using susceptibility-weighted imaging is/are
a. deoxyhemoglobin in veins
b. hemorrhage
c. iron-laden tissue (caudate nucleus, red nucleus, substantia nigra,)
d. calcium depositions in pathologic tissue
e. all

2. All are true regarding contrast infarction except
a. Gyral parenchymal enhancement typically begins toward the end of the first week
b. Gyral parenchymal enhancement persists for approximately 6 to 8 months
c. early cortical enhancement suggested a more favorable clinical outcome
d. No contrast enhancement during chronic infarction
e. early arterial enhancement without significant early parenchymal enhancement seen in most patients with a completed stroke

3. All are true regarding arterial supply except
a. The posterior inferior cerebellar artery (PICA) is the major lateral branch of the vertebral artery
b. the anterior inferior cerebellar artery (AICA) and the superior cerebellar artery are branch of basilar artery
c. PICA supply a portion of medulla, the inferior vermis and the posterior and inferior cerebellar hemispheres
d. The superior cerebellar artery generally supplies the superior vermis and the upper surface of the cerebellar hemispheres
e. The AICA in general has the largest area of supply to the cerebellum and feeds the anterior portions

4. All are true regarding MR except
a. Spin echo imaging minimizes the effects of static magnetic field variations (field inhomogeneities)
b. gradient echo imaging is extremely sensitive to field inhomogeneities
c. air–tissue interfaces produce signal loss in GRE
d. higher magnetic field strengths enhance susceptibility effects and the related signal loss
e. Number of unpaired electrons in Oxyhemoglobin is 4

5. All are correctly matched except
a. Oxyhemoglobin in RBCs (hypeacute)---isointense on T1W and increased signal on T2W image
b. Deoxyhemoglobin in RBCs(acute ,Hours to days)---iso to decreased on T1W ,decreased signal on T2W image
c. Methemoglobin in RBCs(First several days)---increased signal on T1 and decreased signal on T2W
d. Extracellular methemoglobin (Subacute to chronic ,Days to months)—decreased signal on T1

and T2W images
e. Ferritin and hemosiderin(remote Days to indefinitely)----iso to decreased signal on T1W and decreased signal on T2W images

6. Hypertintense signal on T1 W image is produced by
a. Fat
b. Very high nonparamagnetic protein content
c. Paramagnetic or iodinated contrast agents
d. Calcification
e. all

7. Factors associated with increased hemorrhage from an AVM are all except
a. peripheral venous drainage
b. periventricular/intraventricular / basal ganglia AVM
c. arterial supply from perforating vessels /from the vertebrobasilar system
d. intranidal aneurysms
e. high intranidal pressure

8. All are indication of MRA in case of AVMs except
a. The search for dural vessels involved in AVMs
b. the assessment of AVM nidus size
c. Quantification of intravascular flow in AVMs
d. the search for associated aneurysms
e. The presence of major venous sinus occlusion

9. Angiographically "occult cerebrovascular malformations" refers to
a. AVMs
b. cavernous angioma
c. capillary telangiectasia
d. venous angioma
e. developmental venous anomaly

10. Morbidity and mortality on operation of an unruptured aneurysm is
a. morbidity (4%) and mortality (approaching 0%)
b. morbidity (8%) and mortality (approaching 5%)
c. morbidity (12%) and mortality (approaching1 0%)
d. morbidity (16%) and mortality (approaching15 %)
e. morbidity (20%) and mortality (approaching 20%)

11. Myelination starts in the second trimester of gestation and continues into adulthood. Myelination begins with
a. the peripheral nervous system
b. the spinal cord
c. the brainstem
d. the supratentorial brain
e. all at the same time

12. All are true regarding lesions of multiple sclerosis except
a. high signal intensity on T2-weighted images
b. conventional MR is specific in determining the age of lesions
c. frequently situated in the periventricular white matter, internal capsule, corpus callosum
d. proton density– weighted images / FLAIR images usually better define periventricular lesions
e. Dawson fingers refers to linear or ovoid lesions oriented perpendicular to the lateral ventricle

13. All are true regarding most of metabolic disorder of brain except

a. One of the most common nonspecific MR findings is a delay in the normal myelination in the infant
b. H-MR spectroscopy may be more sensitive to early changes in the brain than conventional MR imaging
c. The most common findings on ^{1}H-MR spectroscopy is a nonspecific pattern of decreased NAA with or without a lactate peak
d. Canavan disease is the only metabolic disorder characterized by an increase in the choline peak
e. In Pelizaeus-Merzbacher disease, the NAA peak may be normal

14. Occipital white matter predominance is seen in
a. X-linked ALD and Krabbe disease
b. MELAS and Krabbe disease
c. X-linked ALD and MELAS
d. MELAS , Krabbe disease and X-linked ALD
e. MELAS

15. All are component of limbic lobe except
a. the uncus
b. parahippocampal gyrus
c. hippocampus
d. cingulate gyrus
e. subcallosal area

16. All are true regarding cortical organization defect except
a. polymicrogyria, schizencephaly, and non–balloon cell cortical dysplasia are examples
b. congenital bilateral perisylvian syndrome is characterised by polymicrogyria
c. cortical thickening and indistinctness of the gray–white matter junction
d. Schizencephaly is usually lined by polymicrogyric cortex
e. non - the balloon cell type of cortical dysplasia usually presents as hyperintense signal on long TR with radial bands.

17. All the following intracranial neoplasms has tendency to haemorrhage except
a. glioblastoma/anaplastic astrocytoma
b. anaplastic oligodendroglioma/oligodendroglioma
c. Ependymoma
d. medulloblastoma
e. metastatic melanoma

18. All are true regarding glioblastoma multiforme
a. approximately 15% to 20% of all intracranial tumors
b. the most common primary brain neoplasm in adults
c. most glioblastomas arise de novo
d. its peak incidence in the sixth decade
e. a male predominance of approximately 3:2

19. All are true regarding Lhermitte-Duclos disease except
a. masslike thickening of cerebellar folia
b. usually discovered in adults.
c. irregular stripes of alternating low and high intensity
d. intense contrast enhancement
e. may be associated with Cowden syndrome

20. MRI of brain of AIDS-patient shows single deep mass having

relatively homogeneous intensity similar to that of gray matter, dense contrast enhancement, and minimal edema.The findings which favour lymphoma over toxoplasmosis are all except
a. the presence of subependymal spread
b. marked choline peak elevation
c. substantially elevated rCBV
d. Hemorrhage
e. enhancement along the perivascular spaces

21. All are true regarding imaging of acoustic schwannoma except
a. thin-section (3 mm) axial T1-weighted images reveal most tumors
b. mild hypointensity noted on T1W
c. significant heterogeneity with cystic and/or hemorrhagic regions on MR
d. The widening of the internal auditory canal usually appreciated best on coronal images
e. erosion of the posterior wall of the canal best appreciated in the axial view

22. The most common malignant pediatric brain tumor is
a. Medulloblastoma
b. pineoblastoma
c. haemangioblastoma
d. central neuroblastoma
e. retinoblastoma

23. All are true regarding gliomatosis cerebri except
a. involve at least two cortical lobes
b. preservation of anatomic architecture and sparing of neurons
c. focal mass effect in type 1
d. increased signal intensity within the affected structures on T2 and FLAIR
e. elevation of choline relative to NAA with preserved creatine

24. All are true regarding variant CJD except
a. acquired by eating infected beef
b. low intensity in the pulvinar of the thalami on T2W
c. bilaterall involvement of thalamus
d. periaqueductal gray matter abnormality
e. the absence of significant atrophy

25. All are true regarding neurosyphilis except
a. Vascular neurosyphilis usually appears around 5 to 10 years after primary infection
b. Heubner endarteritis is the most common form of syphilitic arteritis, affecting small arteries
c. Syphilitic gummas occur 3 to 10 years after infection
d. General paresis usually presents 10 to 20 years after the initial infection
e. MR imaging shows hyperintense signal on T2-weighted images and contrast enhancement in the posterior spinal cord and dorsal nerve roots.

26. All the parts of brain shows hyperintense signal normally on T2W except
a. the parietopontine tracts of the posterior limb of the internal capsule
b. Triangular-shaped regions

posterior and superior to the trigones
c. anterior and lateral to the frontal horns
d. ependymitis granularis
e. periaqueductal areas

27. All are true regarding dementia except
a. Braak and Braak staging is related to neurofibrillary or amyloid pathology
b. Lobar hemorrhages in amyloid angiopathy have a tendency to affect the occipital lobe more frequently
c. severe confluent white matter ischemic disease is noted in Biswanger disease
d. CADASIL is due to due to a mutation in the notch three gene.
e. white matter hyperintensities in the frontal lobe is noted in CADASIL

28. All are true regarding atrophy except
a. pronounced vermian atrophy is noted in cerebellar cortical atrophy
b. the basis pontis is preserved in cerebellar cortical atrophy
c. Dilantin, diphenylhydantoin cause cerebellar atrophy
d. involvement of the inferior olivary nuclei in FXTAS
e. the atrophic basis pontis in FXTAS maintains its oval shape

29. All are true regarding tuberous sclerosis except
a. The signal intensity patterns of SEN can change over time
b. the enhancement in SENs always indicate neoplastic transformation
c. The SGCA is a benign and slowly growing tumor
d. the SGCA show a predilection for arising near the foramen of Monro
e. The spinal cord and peripheral nerves are not affected in TS.

30. All are true regarding the Chiari II malformation except
a. cervicomedullary kink
b. beaked shaped medulla
c. stenogyria
d. wrapping of cerebellum around the brainstem
e. trapped fourth ventricle

31. All are true regarding the Chiari II malformation except
a. nearly always hypoplastic or absent splenium
b. frequently enlarged caudate heads and massa intermedia
c. colpocephaly due to obstruction
d. interdigitatation of gyri across the interhemispheric fissure
e. herniation of cerebellar vermis

32. All are true regarding arachnoid cyst except
a. Mostly in the temporosylvian region
b. extraaxial lesions
c. signal characteristics of CSF
d. restricted diffusion
e. may exert mass effect on adjacent bone

33. All are true regarding Persistent Blake's Pouch except
a. cystic malformation of the posterior fossa
b. Blake's pouch normally regresses during 5 to 8 weeks of gestation
c. widening of the valleculum
d. malformation of the cerebellar hemispheres

e. a constant association with hydrocephalus

34. All are true regarding osteochondroma of vertebral column except
a. has predilection for the spinous processes
b. Mostly in the cervical region
c. Three fourth occur in younger than 20 years
d. cortex in direct contiguity with the cortex of the adjacent bone
e. malignant degeneration 5% to 25% in multiple hereditary exostosis

35. All are true regarding hemangioblastoma of spinal cord except
a. usually are located on the dorsal surface of the cord.
c. Approx. 30% of the patients have von Hippel-Lindau syndrome
c. single in spinal cord (79%)
d. the cervical cord --most often involved (51%)
e. 43% cases associated with cysts

36. All are true regarding Multiple sclerosis lesions in spinal cord except
a. isolated involvement of the spinal cord occur in 5% to 24% of cases
b. Approx.60% of spinal cord lesions in the cervical region on MRI
c. tend to be elongated in the direction of the long axis of the cord
d. tend not to involve the entire cross-sectional area of cord
e. peripherally located and generally respect boundaries between white and gray matter

37. All are true regarding development of spinal cord except
a. The distal spinal cord forms by the process of primary neurulation
b. caudal cell mass give rise to the neural tissue and the vertebrae caudal to S-2
c. common concurrence of distal vertebral, neural, anorectal, renal, and genital anomalies
d. "ascent" of the cord results from disproportionately greater longitudinal growth of the vertebrae
e. a conus that lies at or below L-3 is regarded as abnormal

38. All are true regading The Klippel-Feil syndrome except
a. failure in the segmentation of two or more cervical vertebrae
b. Type II shows massive fusion of most of the cervical and upper thoracic spine
c. heritable disorder, a defect of the segment polarity genes
d. classic triad of short neck, low posterior hairline, and limited cervical motion
e. Sprengel deformity in 15% cases

39. All are true regarding pituitary macoadenoma except
a. Intratumoral hemorrhage occurs in 20% to 30% of pituitary adenomas
b. bleeding much higher in patients receiving bromocriptine
c. Larger pituitary adenomas may be accompanied by cystic degeneration with or without hemorrhage
d. The presence of T1

hyperintensity in the optic nerves correlates with degree of chiasm compression
e. interposition of abnormal tissue between the lateral wall of the cavernous sinus and the artery is the most reliable indicator of cavernous sinus invasion

40. All are the radiopharmaceuticals used to produce images of a rCBF (SPECT) except
a. ^{133}Xe
b. ^{123}I isopropyl iodoamphetamine (IMP)
c. ^{99m}Tc ethyl cysteinate dimer (ECD)
d. ^{123}I α-methyl tyrosine
d. ^{99m}Tc hexamethylpropylene amine oxide (HMPAO)

41. All are true regarding gliomas except
a. gliomas are the commonest neuroepithelial tumours
b. astrocytomas account for approx. 75%of glial tumours.
c. haemangioblastomas is the commonest primary intra-axial tumour below the tentorium cerebelli in adults
d. anaplastic astrocytomas usually occurs after 40 years
e. About 20 % of haemangioblastomas occur in association with von Hippel–Lindau disease.

42. All are true regarding imaging features of meningioma except
a. Hyperostosis indicates the site of the tumour attachment to the meninges.
b. frequently isointense to cerebral cortex on both T1W and T2W i

c. signal intensity of capping cyst similar to CSF
d. 'dural tail sign'
e. The extent of the vasogenic oedema correlate with the size of the meningioma

43. All are true regarding imaging strategies in acute stroke except
a. CT is usually the first-line investigation
b. early infarcts are much easier to detect on DWI
c. DWI better for the demonstration of a new infarct on a background of chronic ischaemia
d. the correct diagnosis of a transient ischaemic attack on DWI
e. Cervical angiography is often not important after stroke

44. All are true regarding follow-up of brain abscess except
a. recommended at biweekly intervals or when new symptoms arise.
b. Sufficient treatment is indicated by resolution of rim enhancement
c. Sufficient treatment is indicated by disappearance of the low signal rim on T2W images
d. Treatment response may be better assessed with PWI than conventional MRI
e. low signal on DWI correlates with a good clinical response

45. All are true regarding fibrous dysplasia of skull except
a. involves the base and/or facial skeleton
b. bones appear expanded and dense
c. Lower density areas within the sclerotic bone

d. the most common cause of 'leontiasis ossea'
e. extension of lesion from the sphenoid bones into the facial skeleton much less common than meningioma

46..All are true regarding spine diseases except
a. spine involvement usually up to about 15 per cent of rheumatoid arthritis
b. The commonest causes of arachnoiditis is iatrogenic
c. MRI changes in scute myelitis commonly extends over multiple segments
d. arteriovenous fistulas located in the spinal dura mater responsible for over 80% of spinal AVM
e. venous congestion may cause the Foix–Alajouanine syndrome

47..All the following points favour subependymal hamartomas (tuberous sclerosis) over subependymal heterotopias except
a. irregular
c.parallel to the ventricular wall
c.more heterogeneous due to calcification, gliois
d.do not have signal characteristics of grey matter
e.may enhance

48..All are true regarding posterior fossa tumour in children except
a. lateral location of medulloblastoma is a poor prognostic feature
b. the cerebellar low-grade astrocytoma (CLGA) is in most cases (85%) a pilocytic tumour
c. the posterior fossa is the most common site for ependymomas in children
d. ependymoma disseminate throughout the neuro-axis by leptomeningeal spread
e. most brainstem tumours in children are astrocytomas

49..All are true regarding paediatric spinal trauma except
a. The distance between the anterior arch of C1 and the dens can be up to 5 mm in normal children
b. The prevertebral soft tissues should not exceed one -thirds of the width of the C2 vertebral body
c. significant injury to the spinal cord may be seen in the absence of detectable bony injury
d. rotation between C1 and C2 remains constant throughout all positions in Atlanto-axial rotatory fixation
e. Atlanto-axial rotatory fixation should be suspected if the symptoms of torticollis persist for more than 2 weeks

50.All are true regarding dehydrated alcohol (98%) except
a.liquid embolic agent
b.potent
c.sclerosing effect
d.cause dehydration and desaturation of fats
e.used in percutaneous treatment of haemangiomatous malformation in head and neck

.51.All are features of raised intracranial pressure in infants and children except
a. suture diastasis
b. thick skull vaults
c. sellar erosion

d. craniolacunae
e. cupper beaten appearance

52. indication of spinal angiography except
a. pre-embolisation elucidation of arteriovenous fistula
b. confirmation of haemangioblastoma
c. pre-operative investigation of hypervascular lesions of vertebrae
d. showing the anatomy of reticulomedullary arteries
e. all

53. All are true regarding carotid-vertebrobasilar anastomosis except
a. the most common is primitive trigeminal artery
b. primitive trigeminal artery arises from ICA at its exit from the carotid canal
c. primitive hypoglossal artery connects the cervical ICA with vertebral artery
d. persistent otic artery originate from petrous ICA
e. proatlantal intersegmental artery connects the ECA or cervical ICA and vertebral artery

54. All are true regarding frequency of glioma except
a. two-thirds of all brain tumours are primary neoplasm
b. almost half of all primary brain tumours are gliomas
c. three quarters of all gliomas are astrocytomas
d. 45 % to 50 % of all glioma is glioblastoma multiforme
e. 4 % to 10% of all gliomas is anaplastic astrocytoma

55. -All are true regarding medulloblastoma except
a. 75%---in vermis
b. 75% ---under 15 yrs of age
c. hypodense on NECT
d. associated with Gorlin syndrome
e. Zuckerguss phenomenon

56.. All are true regarding Toxoplasmosis Gondi infection except
a. solitary or multiple ring enhancing lesios
b. vasogenic edema
c. target appearance
d. basal ganglia common site of involvement
e. capsulated

57. All are peroxisomal disorder except
a. Zellweger syndrome
b. adrenoleukodystrophy
c. infantile Refsum disease
d. acatalasia
e. PML

58.. All are split notochord syndrome except
a. dorsal enteric fistula/sinus
b. caudal regression syndrome
c. dorsal enteric diverticulae
d. diastematomyelia
e. neuroenteric cyst

59. All are true regarding Joubert's syndrome except
a. split or segmented vermis
b. the inferior and superior cerebellar peduncle are often small
c. hydrocephalus
d. conenital retinal dystrophy
e. callosal dysgenesis

60. All are true regarding neurocutaneous syndrome except
a. the commonest CNS tumour in NF I is optic nerve glioma
b. 90% of the white matter lesion

in NFI show mass effect and contrast enhancement
c. subependymal nodules is seen in 95% in Tuberous sclerosis
d. Subependymal giant cell astrocytoma is seen in 15% of Tuberous sclerosis patients
e. calcification in Sturge-Weber syndrome is most commonly found in parietal and occipital lobe

TEST PAPER 9(ANSWER)

1.---e
2.----b
Contrast enhancement on conventional MR images play an important role in the diagnosis of subacute infarction . Gyral parenchymal enhancement in the subacute infarction typically begins toward the end of the first week, when mass effect has resolved, and persists for approximately 6 to 8 weeks. This discordance between enhancement and mass effect is an extremely useful radiologic sign because enhancing lesions with significant mass effect are unlikely to represent cerebral infarction . Subacute infarction represents one of the lesions that demonstrate significant enhancement and no mass effect .(Chapter 15,,Atlas)
3.---e
AICA in general has the smallest area of supply to the cerebellum and feeds the anterior portions. The AICA can be variable in size, often having a shared or balanced relationship with the PICA. It generally courses laterally to the cerebellopontine angle. (Chapter 15,,Atlas)
4.---e
Number of unpaired electrons in Oxyhemoglobin is 0.
5.---d
Extracellular methemoglobin (Subacute to chronic Days to months)—decreased signal on T1 and T2W images.
6.---e.

7.—a
Central venous drainage is associated with increased hemorrhage from an AVM.
8.—c
Quantification of intravascular flow in AVMs may be a future indication for MRA as an adjunct to the multifaceted treatment plan and follow-up of patients harboring these lesions by using PC MRA techniques .
9.----b
10.—a
11.---a
12.---b
Conventional MR is sensitive in detecting MS plaques but is nonspecific in determining the age of lesions and distinguishing the underlying histopathologic substrates (demyelination, transient inflammation, edema, or even remyelination).
13.----d
Canavan disease is the only metabolic disorder characterized by an increase in the NAA peak
14.---d
15.---c
The limbic system is composed of a series of arches: the limbic lobe , the callosal and hippocampal sulci , the intralimbic gyrus , and the fornix . The limbic lobe is composed of the uncus , parahippocampal gyrus , isthmus of the cingulate gyrus , cingulate gyrus, and subcallosal area . Broca intralimbic gyrus is composed primarily of the hippocampus (hippocampal formation or HF)

and the vestigial supracallosal and paraterminal gyri.

16.---e
Regarding differentiation between balloon cell and non–balloon cell focal cortical dysplasia, the balloon cell type usually presents as hyperintense signal on long–repetition time (TR) acquisitions with radial bands, whereas the non–balloon cell type usually does not.

17.---d
Hemorrhagic Tumours
Primary brain tumors
  Glioblastoma/anaplastic astrocytoma
  Anaplastic oligodendroglioma/oligodendroglioma
  Ependymoma
  teratoma
Metastatic disease
  Melanoma
  Renal cell carcinoma
  Choriocarcinoma
  Lung carcinoma
  Breast carcinoma
  Thyroid carcinoma

18.----c
Most glioblastomas arise from an existent astrocytoma or anaplastic astrocytoma, some arise de novo

19.---d
It demonstrates minimal if any contrast enhancement. Cowden syndrome is an autosomal dominant tumor-suppressor-gene syndrome characterized by ductal carcinoma of the breast, thyroid cancer, and multiple hamartomas.

20.---d
Hemorrhage is very common in cerebral toxoplasmosis, particularly after treatment, and, if present, argues against lymphoma.
Glioblastoma, like lymphoma, can cross the corpus callosum and enhance.
Densely enhancing dural-based lesions could implicate lymphoma, sarcoidosis, metastases (especially breast carcinoma), and meningioma (which would be the only tumor to calcify among these).
In both children and adults, Posttransplant lymphoproliferative disorder (PTLD) is the most common cause of cancer-related mortality after solid organ transplantation.

21.---d
The widening of the internal auditory canal is usually be appreciated best on axial images, which demonstrate the entire length of the canal on a single slice, in contrast to the coronal image, which generally does not reveal the entire length of the canal on a single section.

22.—a

23.---c
The WHO classifies these tumors into two types. Type 1 exhibits the diffuse infiltrating enlargement of affected structures with no focal mass effect. In type 2 there is a diffuse lesion with a focal mass effect, which is a malignant glioma.

24.---b
The most characteristic abnormality is high intensity on

T2-weighted images in the pulvinar of the thalami. This has been termed the "pulvinar sign" of vCJD. The bilaterally abnormal pulvinar on MR had a sensitivity of 78% and a specificity of 100% in the large series of vCJD cases. Although thalamic abnormality can be seen in non-vCJD cases, it is more characteristic in the anterior and median thalamus.

25.---b

Two types of vascular involvement have been described in neurosyphilis—Heubner endarteritis and Nissl-Alzheimer endarteritis.

The Heubner type is the most common form of syphilitic arteritis, affecting large and medium-sized arteries. Pathophysiologically, there is fibroblastic proliferation of the intima, thinning of the media, and adventitial fibrous and inflammatory changes, resulting in an irregular luminal narrowing and ectasia

. Less frequently, the Nissl-Alzheimer type of arteritis is present, primarily involving small vessels in which a luminal narrowing occurs as a consequence of intense proliferation of endothelial and adventitial cells. Both types of arteritis may lead to vascular occlusion. Moreover, syphilis can be associated with a venous occlusive inflammation.

Tabes dorsalis is a myelopathy associated with atrophic, degenerated, and demyelinated dorsal nerve roots and posterior spinal columns and appears 10 to 20 years after the initial infection. A triad of symptoms (lightning pains, dysuria, and ataxia) and a triad of signs (Argyll-Robertson pupil, areflexia, loss of proprioception) are the characteristics of this disorder. The Argyll-Robertson pupil, seen in both tabes dorsalis and general paresis, is a small, irregular pupil that accommodates but does not react to light.

MR imaging typically demonstrates brain atrophy associated with hyperintense signal intensity on T2-weighted images and contrast enhancement in the posterior spinal cord and dorsal nerve roots.

26.-----e

Posterior and superior to the trigones that are variably hyperintense on T2-weighted images are normal in patients in their first and second decades. Hyperintense foci on T2-weighted images exist in virtually all normal patients anterior and lateral to the frontal horns. This region displays ependymitis granularis, which refers to a focal breakdown of the ependymal lining with adjacent astrocytic gliosis.

27.---e

CADASIL—cerebral autosomal dominant arteriopathy with subcortical infarcts and leukoencephalopathy—is a genetically determined form of cerebral vascular disease due to a mutation affecting the notch three gene.

This mutation affects roughly 500 families worldwide. The condition is characterized by degeneration of vascular smooth muscle in arterioles. MRI is characterized by typical white matter hyperintensities plus white matter hyperintensities in the temporal stem and corpus callosum, which distinguish this condition from garden variety white matter disease. Evidence of multiple areas of cerebral hemorrhage is also characteristic of this condition.

Amyloid angiopathy is a condition characterized by infiltration of the arterial wall by amyloid protein. This results in lobar hemorrhages, which have a tendency to affect the occipital lobe more frequently than other areas of the brain. The condition also results in multiple areas of cerebral microhemorrhage

A clinical syndrome associated with severe confluent white matter ischemic disease has been termed Binswanger syndrome. The clinical expression is a decline in cognition, gate apraxia, and urinary incontinence

Cerebral vascular disease is regarded by some to be the second-most-common cause of dementia in the elderly after AD.

28.---d

In contrast to MSA-C, in which atrophy and abnormal hyperintense signal on long-TR images in seen within the inferior olivary nuclei, there is sparing of the inferior olivary nuclei in FXTAS . Although both disorders result in pontine atrophy and abnormal pontine signal, MSA-C shows characteristic loss of the ventral bulge of the basis pontis . In contrast, the atrophic basis pontis in FXTAS maintains its oval shape. Whereas both disorders result in cerebellar atrophy, there is relative sparing of the cerebellar vermis in FXTAS . The extensive supratentorial cerebral white matter and corpus callosal signal abnormalities seen in FXTAS are not seen in MSA-C .

29.---b

The SENs have been reported to have variable patterns of enhancement. On CT, the SEN enhancement has been viewed as diagnostic of the conversion of the hamartoma into a neoplasm, the SGCA. On MR, however, multiple SENs show gadolinium enhancement, often clustered about the foramen of Monro . Because multiple SGCAs are distinctly uncommon, it is unlikely that all the enhancing SENs are undergoing neoplastic transformation into SGCAs because these are usually solitary tumors.

30-.---b

The quadrigeminal plate is stretched inferiorly and posteriorly, resulting in the characteristic "beaked" shape tectum

Stenogyria--- multiple small gyri within a cortex of normal thickness

31.---c

The trigones, occipital horns, and posterior temporal horns of the lateral ventricles are almost always enlarged (colpocephaly) as a result of the accompanying hypoplastic corpus callosum.

32.---d

ACs and epidermoids: FLAIR and diffusion sequences usually allow distinction of these entities: On these sequences, arachnoid cysts follow the CSF signal and show no restricted diffusion; epidermoids show high signal on FLAIR compared to CSF and restricted diffusion.

ACs and the mega cisterna magna. Distinct pathogenetically, these two entities may be quite difficult to differentiate on imaging. The AC may involve mass effect on the vermis and cerebellar hemispheres and may be associated with hydrocephalus. CT cisternography may also be useful in the evaluation of cysts of the posterior fossa .

33-.—d

The persistent Blake's pouch (PBP) is a cystic malformation of the posterior fossa believed to derive from persistence and expansion of the normally transient Blake's pouch that arises from the AMI and normally regresses during the weeks 5 to 8 of gestation. According to this model, the PBP is in communication with the fourth ventricle and separate from the subarachnoid spaces. Because it involves failure of regression of Blake's pouch, it is consistently associated with hydrocephalus. Because cerebellar development does not appear morphogenetically to involve the AMI, there is no malformation of the cerebellum proper.

34.—b

Most cases of osteochondroma occur in the thoracic or lumbar region; the cervical spine is only rarely the primary site.

The incidence of malignant degeneration is 1% in cases of solitary osteochondroma and 5% to 25% in cases of multiple hereditary exostosis; rapid growth of the tumor should prompt suspicion of malignancy

Factors favoring benignity include cortical margins that are contiguous with the adjacent bone, well-defined lobular surfaces, lack of adjacent bone involvement, and a thin cartilaginous cap (usually less than 1 cm) .

35.-----d

Hemangioblastomas involving the spinal cord tend to be single (79%).In spinal hemangioblastomas, the thoracic cord is most often involved (51%), followed by the cervical cord (41%)

36.---e

Multiple sclerosis lesions are peripherally located, and generally do not respect boundaries between white and gray matter.

The spinal cord is frequently involved in MS, with cord lesions found in up to 99% of autopsy cases . Although MS affects more frequently the brain and the spinal cord together, isolated involvement of the spinal cord

may occur in 5% to 24% of cases. Most lesions are smaller than two vertebral body segments, do not alter cord morphology, are hyperintense on T2-weighted images, and are not hypointense on T1-weighted images. On axial MRI the laterally located lesions tend to be wedge shaped and the centrally located lesions rounded. Lesions are associated with spinal cord swelling in 6% to 14% of cases and with atrophy in 2% to 40% of cases.
Cord swelling is usually only found in the relapsing-remitting form of MS.
Just over half of the plaques (56%) in patients referred for imaging with spinal cord MS symptoms enhance with intravenously administered gadolinium
Lesions within the cord are relatively more common in the dorsal horns
Both magnetic transfer gradient echo and fast short-TI inversion recovery (fast-STIR) sequences depict more cervical cord MS lesions than the fast spin echo sequence, with fast-STIR having the best sensitivity
Magnetization transfer– and diffusion tensor–derived measures are emergent modalities that seems well suited for evaluating normal-appearing white matter.

37.---a
The distal spinal cord forms by the process of secondary neurulation (Canalisation and retrogressive differentiation)
The position of the tip of the conus medullaris is of significance in the diagnosis of the caudal spinal anomalies and the occult dysraphisms
A conus that lies at or below L-3 is best regarded as abnormal until study demonstrates that it is not anchored or "tethered" in an abnormally low position by a bone spur, a fibrous band, or a terminal mass such as lipoma. Conversely, patients with appropriate signs and symptoms (with or without cutaneous stigmata) may have a clinically significant tethering of the cord, even if the tip of the conus falls within the normal range of position.

38.----b
Type I shows massive fusion of most of the cervical and upper thoracic spine.
Type II shows fusions of one or two interspaces, most often at C2-3 and next most often at C5-6. In 75% of cases, fusions occur from C-3 cephalad.
Type III fusions involve cervical vertebrae and lower thoracic or lumbar vertebrae.
The VATER association is a nonrandom occurrence of multisystem congenital malformations, specifically vertebral anomalies, anal atresia, esophageal atresia with tracheoesophageal fistula, and radial anomalies.
The OEIS complex is a nonrandom combination of omphalocele, exstrophy of the cloaca, imperforate anus, and spinal defects
The Currarino triad is an

association of (partial) sacral agenesis, anorectal stenosis (or other low anorectal malformation), and presacral masses, including meningocele, teratoma, enteric cyst, or a combination of these . The sacrum is partially deficient and often assumes a scimitar shape

39.---d

Superior extension into the suprasellar cistern is particularly well delineated because of the superb image contrast between the adenoma against the markedly hypointense CSF. The optic nerves, chiasm, and tracts are directly visualized as they are draped over the tumor. The presence of T2 hyperintensity in the optic nerves has been correlated with the degree of chiasm compression and the degree of visual impairment.

40.---d

SPECT radiopharmaceuticals are taken up into intracranial tumours areb ^{201}Tl chloride, ^{99m}Tc MIBI, ^{123}I α-methyl tyrosine and ^{111}In octreotide.

41.---d

In children, most of astrocytic tumours are relatively benign tumours (pilocytic or low-grade astrocytomas); in young adults low-grade astrocytomas predominate, whereas anaplastic astrocytomas have a peak incidence around 40 years and GBM usually occurs after 40 years.

42.---e

There may be a linear, contrast-enhancing 'dural tail' extending from the tumour along the dura mater. The 'dural tail sign', once thought to be pathognomonic for meningioma can also be seen with other tumours such as schwannoma or metastasis. Vasogenic oedema is not infrequently associated with meningiomas. The extent of the vasogenic oedema does not correlate with the size of the meningioma and, as with metastases, even small lesions can cause quite extensive oedema

43---e

Cervical and sometimes intracranial angiography is often important after stroke and in most circumstances conventional catheter angiography has been replaced by noninvasive methods

44..---d

Treatment response may be better assessed with DWI than conventional MRI; low signal on DWI correlates with a good clinical response whilst increasing signal implies reaccumulation of pus

45.—e

In meningiomas, the important differential of fibrous dysplasia, sclerosis is often more marked than expansion, and extension from the sphenoid bones into the facial skeleton is much less common-

46.----c

MRI changes commonly extends over multiple segments in scute myelitis

47-----b

Subependymal heterotopia are smooth and ovoid, with their long axis typically parallel to the ventricular wall, quite different from subependymal hamartomas in tuberous sclerosis which are irregular and have their long axis perpendicular to the ventricular wall.

48.----a
Favourable prognostic factors of medulloblastoma include complete surgical resection, lack of CSF dissemination at presentation, onset in the second decade, female gender and lateral location within the cerebellar hemisphere.

49..---b
The prevertebral soft tissues should not exceed two-thirds of the width of the C2 vertebral body

50.---d
Dehydrated alcohol (98%) exert sclerosing effect by causing dehydration and desaturation of peptides .

51.----b
Neonates and young infants may also show unusually thin skull vaults in addition to suture diastasis and large heads. They may show craniolacunae when the raised pressure is associated with meningocele.
Sellar erosiont is a late sign and implies longstanding chronic pressure..I n children under 10, sellar erosion without suture diastasis is likely to be due to a local erosive lesion rather than raised pressure. Above this age sellar changes are more likely to be due to raised pressure .

52.----e
53.---c
54.---e
Anaplastic astrocyroma constitute 20% to 25% of all glimas

55.—c
Medulloblastoma is hyperdense on NECT

56.---e
No capsule seen in Toxoplasmosis Gondii. .Basal ganglia and cerebral hemishphere near the corticomedullary junction are the most common site

57.---e
58.---b
59.---c
No hydrocephalus is seen in Joubert 's syndrome

60---b
90% of the white matter lesion in NFI show no mass effect and no contrast enhancement.

TEST PAPER 10

1. All are true regarding magnetization transfer sequences except
a. involves irradiating the tissue with off-resonance RF
b. a decrease in detectable water signal after the MTC pulse implies absence of macromolecules
c. may enhance the contrast obtained in imaging intracerebral hemorrhage
d. may be useful in the detection of demyelination
e. useful in reducing background signals in MR angiography of the brain

2. All are true regarding contrast in acute infarction except
a. progressive arterial enhancement persisting for the first 5 to 7 days after acute infarction
b. dense cortical contrast enhancement begin at 5 to 7 days after the acute infarction
c. may be early cortical enhancement due to sufficient collateral inflow
d. early cortical enhancement suggests more poor clinical outcome
e. contrast is not used routinely in acute stroke evaluation

3. All are true regarding the "artery of Percheron" except
a. a dominant posterior thalamoperforating artery
b. a dominant anterior basal-perforating artery
c. supplies the thalamus bilaterally
d. a single vessel
e. also known as the paramedian thalamic artery

4. All enhance the effective magnetic field B_{eff} except
a. paramagnetic
b. antiferromagnetic
c. ferromagnetic
d. superparamagnetic
e. diamagnetic

5. An elderly patient undergoes MRI of brain which reveal peripherally located multiple heamorrhages (more in perietooccipital location) of varing ages and spares the basal ganglia What is the most likely diagnosis?
a. hypertensive hemorrhage
b. amyloid angiopathy
c. Cavernous angioma
d. Contusion
e. Diffuse axonal injury

6. All are true regarding intracranial hemorrhage in AVMs except
a. the most common initial feature
b. heralds the existence of the AVM in about 15% of patients
c. most often occurs during the second /third decade
d. most often intraparenchymal
e. common cause of nontraumatic SAHs

7. All are true regarding MR angiography except
a. Gradient refocused limited-flip-angle techniques form the basis of TOF and PC MRA

b. Regions of flowing blood are most often demonstrated as low signal intensity on TOF and PC MRA
c. TOF and PC MRA clarify flowing blood in subependymal vessels or vessels near cortical margins
d. The presence of major venous sinus occlusion accompanying the AVM can be clarified with MRA techniques.
e. The search for dural vessels involved in AVMs is a clear indication for supplemental MRA rather than MR alone.

8. All are true regarding cavernous angioma except
a. encapsulated
b. no muscularis /elastic in sinusoidal vascular channels
c. the absence of interposed brain tissue
d. a rim of gliotic brain with hemosiderin pigment
e. subacute-to-chronic clotted blood

9. The pathognomonic MR signs of partially thrombosed giant intracranial aneurysms is
a. well-circumscribed mass lesion containing mixed signal intensities
b. evidence of blood flow within the patent portion of the residual lumen
c. usually periluminal hyperintensity around the patent residual lumen
d. flow void in the parent vessel anatomically related to the aneurysm
e. Perianeurysmal hemorrhage and intraparenchymal edema

10. Correctly matched variety of multiple sclerosis is
a. Classic ---Charcot type
b. Acute ---Schilder type
c. Diffuse cerebral sclerosis ---- Marburg type
d. Concentric sclerosis ---Devic type
e. Neuromyelitis optica ---Balo type

11. All are true regarding Multiple sclerosis variant except
a. Acute MS (Marburg type) typically has rapid progression to death within months.
b. acute onset of optic neuritis and transverse myelitis develop at approximately the same time in Devic type
c. extensive, confluent, asymmetric demyelination of both cerebral hemispheres noted in Schilder type
d. Concentric sclerosis (Balò type) is more common in the Philippines
e. seizures, signs of pyramidal tract involvement, ataxia, and psychiatric symptomatology noted in Balo type

12. All are true regarding Cerebral autosomal dominant arteriopathy with subcortical infarcts and leukoencephalopathy (CADASIL) except
a. manifest as subcortical dementia of the Binswanger type
b. the notch 3 gene involved
c. symmetric and confluent areas of high signal intensity on the T2 W in the subcortical and periventricular white matter
d. most lesions in the occipital and parietal lobe
e. patients typically younger than

individuals with subcortical arterial sclerotic encephalopathy.

13. Frontal white matter predominance is noted in
a. Alexander disease
b. Adrenoleukodystrophy (late onset) and MLD (late onset)
c. Alexander disease and Adrenoleukodystrophy (late onset)
d. Alexander disease and MLD (late onset)
e. Alexander disease, Adrenoleukodystrophy (late onset) and MLD (late onset)

14. All are true regarding hippocampal sclerosis except
a. associated with temporal lobe complex partial seizures
b. associated with pyramidal and granule cell neuronal loss
c. the cornu ammonis and dentate sections of the hippocampus involved
d. abundance of interneurons
e. anterior temporal lobectomy--- the most commonly performed surgery

15. All are true regarding abnormal neuronal migration disorder except
a. often have genetic origin and may be sex linked
b. bilateral periventricular nodular heterotopia may be X-linked
c. bilateral periventricular nodular heterotopia to a mutation involving filamin 1 gene
d. X-linked lissencephaly manifests as subcortical laminar heterotopia in males
e. X-linked lissencephaly is due to defect in DCX/XLIS gene

16.. Frequently cystic tumour are all except
a. medulloblastoma
b. ependymoma (supratentorial)
c. craniopharyngioma
d. ganglion cell tumour
e. pilocystic astrocytoma

17. All are true regarding anaplastic astrocytoma except
a. highly malignant
b. The peak incidence is in the fifth decade.
c. lack of the necrosis and degree of vascular proliferation in comparison to glioblastoma
d. The high-intensity abnormality on T2W with vasogenic edema
e. intense homogenous contrast enhancement

18. All are true regarding noninfiltrative astrocytic tumors except
a. common tendency to be well circumscribed
b. more differentiated than infiltrative astrocytoma
c. relatively favorable prognosis
d. limited capacity for invasion and spread
e. more tendency to progress into more malignant forms

19. All are true regarding PCNL (parenchymal) except
a. involve the deep gray matter structures, periventricular regions, and corpus callosum
b. up to 75% of lesins in contact with ependyma, meninges, or both
c. enhancement along perivascular spaces on MR imaging
d. Lymphomatous masses do not calcify and hemorrhage is highly common

e. deep and periventricular lesions are often isointense to gray matter on all spin echo sequences

20. All are true regarding acoustic schwannoma except
a. most frequently arise from the vestibular portion of the eighth cranial nerve.
b. typically bilateral in NF 1
c. generally involve the intracanalicular portion of the nerve
d. compact texture in Antoni type B tissue
e. mucinous and microcystic change frequent in the Antoni type B tissue

21. All are true regarding imaging of acoustic schwannoma except
a. thin-section (3 mm) axial T1-weighted images reveal most tumors
b. mild hypointensity noted on T1W
c. significant heterogeneity with cystic and/or hemorrhagic regions on MR
d. The widening of the internal auditory canal usually appreciated best on coronal images
e. erosion of the posterior wall of the canal best appreciated in the axial view

22. All are primitive neuroectodermal tumors except
a. Medulloblastoma
b. pineoblastoma
c. haemangioblastoma
d. central neuroblastoma
e. retinoblastoma

23. All are true regarding dysembryoplastic neuroepithelial tumor except
a. frequently have a gyriform configuration
b. the most common site---the temporal lobe
c. The strong association with dysplasia
d. no contrast-enhancement
e. show strong restriction on diffusion

24. A 60 yrs old patient presents with rapidly progressive dementia, myoclonic jerks, and periodic sharp-wave EEG tracing. CJD is suspected. MR of brain was advised as MR is highly sensitive and specific for the detection of CJD abnormalities. All are true regarding CJD except
a. Lesions do not enhance and do not demonstrate mass effect
b. DWIs is superior to over any T2-weighted images in the assessment of CJD
c. DWI changes have been observed as early as 1 month after the onset of symptoms
d. hyperintensity on DWI found in the cortex and basal ganglia
e. primary sensorimotor cortex is almost always involved

25. All are true regarding empyema (SDE) except
a. subdural empyema is aoften complication of purulent meningitis in adult
b. MR imaging is the preferred method for evaluating patients with a suspected empyema
c. SDE is most commonly located over the cerebral convexity and is often bilateral,
d. epidural empyema is

continuous across the midline and has a hypointense margin on both T1- and T2W
e. Empyema appear hyperintense to CSF but hypointense relative to brain parenchyma on T1W

26. All are true regarding neurosyphilis except
a. Vascular neurosyphilis usually appears around 5 to 10 years after primary infection
b. Heubner endarteritis is the most common form of syphilitic arteritis, affecting small arteries
c. Syphilitic gummas occur 3 to 10 years after infection
d. General paresis usually presents 10 to 20 years after the initial infection
e. hyperintense signal on T2W and contrast enhancement in the posterior spinal cord and dorsal nerve roots.

27. All are true regarding the parietopontine tracts of the posterior limb of the internal capsule except
a. On axial images at the level of the velum interpositum
b. medial to the distal putamen near the junction of the posterior limb and retrolenticular portion of the internal capsule
c. oval, and symmetric low signal intensity on T2W
d. do not demonstrate intravenous contrast enhancement.
e. not seen in patients younger than the age of 10 years

28. All are true regarding Alzheimer disease except
a. decrease value of the ADC
b. decrease of fractional anisotropy values
c. tempo-parietal decrease in cerebral blood flow on MR perfusion
d. Positive PIB uptake on amyloid imaging
e. PIB has great potential value in the differential diagnosis of dementia syndromes

29. All are true regarding imaging features except
a. asymmetric occipito-parietal lobar atrophy is noted in CBD
b. midbrain atrophy and periaqueductal signal alterations is noted in PSP
c. atrophy of the putamen more than the caudate is noted in multiple system atrophy–P
d. the "hot cross bun" sign in pons is noted in multiple system atrophy–C
e. . the "hot cross bun" sign in pons is noted in Wolfram syndrome

30. All are true regarding cortical tuber in tuberous sclerosi except
a. prone to calcification.
b. contain unusually large cells
c. the "gyral core" appearance on T2W and the "sulcal island" on T1W
d contrast enhancement rare
e. seen in cerebellum

31. All are true regarding The Chiari II malformation except
a. displacement of the brainstem and lower cerebellum into the cervical spinal canal
b. The fourth ventricle is caudally displaced and extends below the foramen magnum
c. nearly all associated with thoracic myelomeningoceles.

d. enlargement of the massa intermedia
e. small posterior fossa

32. All are true regarding arachnoid cyst except
a. developmental cavities of the subarachnoid space
b. associated with malformations of cortical development, and cerebellar hamartomas
c. associated with anomalous venous drainage, hypogenesis of the corpus callosum.
d. the associations with ADPKD and Walker-Warburg syndrome
e microcephaly and intracranial hypertension--the most common presentations in children

33. All are true regarding Dandy-Walker malformation except
a. completely absent vermis in 75%
b. cerebellum hypoplastic and splayed anterolaterally against the petrous bones
c. hydrocephalus in about 75% of patients by the age of 3 months
d. hypogenetic corpus callosum in about 25% of patients
e. Polymicrogyria or gray matter heterotopias in approximately 10% of patients

34. All are true regarding vertebral haemangioma except
a. solitary in 66%
b. 60% in the thoracic region
c. "jail bar" appearance on plain films.
d. tend to have increased signal intensity on T1W and T2W images
e. Compression fractures in hemangiomas very common

35. All are true regarding myxopapillary ependymoma except
a. large, soft, expansile masses
b. always found in the region of the filum terminale
c. presence of fat spaces
d. generally hyperintense
e. may be found in brain

36. All are true regarding acute transverse myelitis except
a. centrally located increased signal intensity on T2WI
b. usually involve more than two thirds of the cross-sectional area of the cord
c. extend more than three to four vertebral segments in length
d. abnormal gadolinium enhancement of the spinal cord
e. Cord expansion in all cases

37. Concurrent malformations associated with spinal lipoma are all except
a. Dermal sinuses may concur in up to 20% of cases
b. Dermoids and teratomas are seen in 3% to 7% of patients
c. diastematomyelia in 1% to 6%,
d hydromyelia in 2.5% to 24%
e. The cord lay abnormally low in 9% of lipomas

38. All are true regarding vertebral anomaly except
a. Persistence of separate ventral and dorsal ossification centers for each centrum produces coronal cleft vertebrae
b. Failure of bony union of the two neural arches posteriorly leads to spina bifida occulta
c. In block vertebrae, the intervertebral disk is absent or rudimentary
d. the most common sites of unfused spinous processes are L-5

and S-1
e. block vertebra show wide sagittal diameter and concave configuration

39. All are true regarding pituitary macoadenoma except
a. mostly nonfunctional
b. hypointense on T1W
c. more often hyperintense on T2W than microadenomas
d. enlargement of the sella
e. consistency accurately predicted by MR signal intensities

40. All are true except
a. The diffuse or multifocal lesions of the basal meninges are noted in sacrcoidosis
b. The Tolosa-Hunt syndrome refers to a painful ophthalmoplegia caused by an inflammatory lesion of the cavernous sinus
c. triad of diabetes insipidus, exophthalmos, and lytic bone lesions is referred as the Hand-Schüller-Christian syndrome
d. Acute degeneration in a pituitary adenoma is termed "pituitary apoplexy
e. the sella is of smaller size in Sheehan Syndrome

41. All are true regarding dynamic susceptibility contrast (DSC) MRI except
a. The TTP map is a measure of the delayed arrival of contrast
b. a larger TTP is a sign of abnormality
c. cerebral blood volume (CBV) maps the area under the concentration versus time curve
d. Calculation of the CBV is not susceptible to motion-related noise
e. MTT is a refined version of the TTP, but it is not identical to it

42. All are true regarding MRS except
a. The acquisition of long echo time data allows the detection of N-acetylaspartate (NAA), creatine (Cr/PCr) and choline (Cho) in normal brain
b. The methyl resonance of NAA produces a large sharp peak at 2.01 p.p.m
c. choline produce resonance at 3.22 p.p.m
d. the acquisition of long echo time data provides spectra with better signal to noise ratio
e. the acquisition of short echo time data detects resonance of myo-inositol, glutamate and glutamine

43. The pre-operative localization of eloquent cortical regions is done by
a. DWI
b. PWI
c. MRS
d. BOLD –functional MRI
e. proton-density MRI

44. All are true regarding meningioma except
a. flat, infiltrating lesions referred as 'en plaque' lesions
b. mostly correspond to WHO grade II
c. most frequent site ---the parasagittal region
d. On CT, 60 per cent hyperdense on CT
E. usually intense and uniform enhancement on CT

45. All are true regarding role of DWI in infarction except

a. high sensitivity in the first few hours after infarction
b. high signal in acute infarct due to restricted diffusion
c. acute infarct dark on the ADC (high ADC)
d. small infarcts can be masked during pseudonormalization
e. low signal on DWI and bright on the ADC map after 5-14days of infarct

46.All are true regarding brain abscess except
a. Abscesses are more likely to show small satellite lesions than tumour
b. enhancing rim typically has a smooth inner margin and shows thinning of its medial aspect
c. the abscess rim is relatively hyperintense on T2W
d. high signal in centre of abscess on DWI
e. lower relative cerebral blood volume in their enhancing rim than gliomas

47.All are true regarding hematoma except
a. the temporoparietal convexity is the most common site for extradural hematoma
b. extradural hematoma cross cranial sutures
c. Dilatation of the contralateral ventricle is a bad prognostic sign in subdural hematoma
d. 'rabbit's ear' configuration of frontal horn may be noted in bilateral subdural hematoma
e. The interhemispheric subdural haematoma may appear comma shape on axial CT sections

48.All are true regarding intramedullary tumour except

a. Spinal capillary haemangioblastomas nearly always involve the anterior columns of the spinal cord
b. About 70 per cent of intramedullary tumours are associated with cysts
c. Unlike the brain, the great majority of spinal cord gliomas enhance at least partially
d. Spinal angiography often provides definitive diagnosis of spinal haemangioblastoma,
e. syringomyelia in intramedullary tumour is probably most frequent with haemangioblastoma

49.All are true regarding malformations of neuronal migration and cortical organization except
a. Schizencephaly is a cleft lined by grey matter and leptomeninges.
b. pachygyria and polymicrogyria may be distinguished more easily on volumetric T1W imaging.
c. lissencephaly is likely to be reliably diagnosed on early fetal MRI
d. Cobblestone lissencephaly is the result of overmigration of neurons
e. Walker–Warburg syndrome may show 'cobblestone lissencephaly'

50.All are true regarding medulloblastoma except
a. associated with Li–Fraumeni syndrome
b. hyperdensity on CT
c. presence of restricted diffusion
d. midline vermian mass abutting the roof of the fourth ventricle in children

e. T2 hyperintensity on MRI

51. All are true regarding ADEM except
a. a monophasic disease with multiple lesions
b. No cortical abnormality
c. more frequent involvement of deep grey matter thanMS
d. increased free diffusion within the lesions on DWI
e. multiple asymmetrical areas of demyelination

52. All are true regarding Trisacryl gelatine microsphere (embosphere) except
a. Non-absorbable material
b. less deeper penetratation than PVA particles
c. donot aggregate
d. deformable
e. longer occlusive effect

53. The first and most prominent feature of raised intracranial pressure in infants and children is
a. suture diastasis
b. thin skull vaults
c. large heads.
d. craniolacunae
e. increased convolutional markings

54. All are true regarding MRI of spine except
a. FLAIR is a highly sensitive sequence to spine pathology
b. MRI may be used to acquire CSF flow related data
c. MR neurography uses diffusion weighted imaging
d. phased array coils permit the whole spinal cord to be imaged in one acquisition
e. diffusion imaging have proven insensitive to pathology shown by T1 and T2W imaging

55. Common normal variants of Circle of Willis are all except
a. hypolasia of one or both posterior communicating artery
b. hypoplastic/absent A1 anterior cerebral artery segment
c. fetal origin of the posterior cerebral artery
d. absent P1 segment
e. infundibular dilatation at the PCoA origin from ICA

56. All are true regarding intracranial aneurysm except
a. female preponderance
b. 1 to 2 % multiple
c. 90% on circle of Willis /MCA bifurcation
d. average size larger in children than adult
e. posterior fossa and peripheral cortical vessels involvement common in children

57. All are true regarding pineal gland except
a. pineal gland.lies behind the third ventricle
b. pineal gland lies below the posterior commissure
c. a recess of third ventricle lies above the pineal gland
d. the quadrigeminal plate lies behind the pineal gland
e. the velum interpositum lies above the pineal gland

58. All are features of normal meningeal enhancement except
a. thin
b. smooth
c. continuous
d. most prominent near vertex
e. less intense than cavernous sinus

59. All are true regarding pineal cell tumours except

a. germinoa engulfs a calcified pineal gland
b. teratoma is the most common pineal region tumour
c. pineoblastoma show uniform strong enhancement
d. endodermal sinus tumour show elevated alpha-fetoprotein levels
e. alpha-FT and HCG are elevated with embryonal cell carcinoma

60. All are true regarding HIV encephalopathy except

a. no mass effect
b. infection by HIV virus itself
c. cerebral atrophy –most common finding
d. frontal lobes ----most common sites
e. typically involve both gray and white matter

TEST PAPER 10 (ANSWER)

1.----b
A decrease in detectable water signal after the MTC pulse implies a magnetization exchange, which further implies the presence of macromolecules. On the other hand, the absence of significant change in detectable water signal after the MTC pulse is applied implies an absence of macromolecules.

2.---d
Early cortical enhancement suggested a more favorable clinical outcome. Contrast is not used routinely in acute stroke evaluation.

3.---b
A dominant posterior thalamoperforating artery that gives rise to a single vessel that supplies the thalamus bilaterally and is referred to as the "artery of Percheron" or the paramedian thalamic artery. (Chapter 15,,Atlas)

4.---e
Any material, when placed into a constant magnetic field, responds by generating its own magnetic field. The magnetic susceptibility of a substance (or tissue) describes this magnetic response. Diamagnetic materials respond to an applied field with a very weak induced field (approximately 10^{-6} × the magnitude of the applied field) and in a vector direction that opposes that of the applied field. Paramagnetic materials have a larger induced field (approximately 10^{-2} to 10^{-4} × the magnitude of the applied field), which is in the same vector direction as the applied field. Superparamagnetic and ferromagnetic materials generate a very large induced field, equal to or even greater than the applied field, and, as with paramagnetic substances, the induced field is in the same vector direction as the applied field.
Diamanetic substance reduces the effective magnetic field B_{eff}.

5.---b.

6.—b
Intracranial hemorrhage heralds the existence of the AVM in 30% to 55% of patients and most often occurs during the second or third decade

7.---b
Regions of flowing blood are most often demonstrated as high signal intensity on TOF and PC MRA

8.—a
On microscopic examination, cavernous angioma shows a honeycomb of multiple, partially collagenized, endothelial-lined sinusoidal vascular channels that varies in caliber. The walls of these channels may be thin, irregularly thickened and hyalinized or partially calcified Although virtually always well demarcated by a rim of gliotic brain stained by hemosiderin pigment from prior hemorrhages or diffusion of red cell pigment from prior intracavernous

sequestration, the lesions are not encapsulated
Absent muscularis /elastica in vessel walls and the absence of interposed brain tissue in the lsion differentiate cavernous angioma from AVMs.
Adjacent parenchymal atrophy and gliosis may be found

9.—b
The presence of three specific MR characteristics allows differentiation of partially thrombosed giant aneurysms from isolated intracerebral hematomas: flow phenomena with the patent portion of the lumen (usually flow void), laminated thrombus of mixed stages in the clotted portion of the lumen, and recognition of the anatomic relationship of signal void in the parent vessel.
Rapidly flowing blood through the patent portion of the lumen appears as an area of signal void on SE images
Flow phenomena, especially ghost image pulsation artifacts, arising from the intraluminal signal can be used to prove the vascular nature of lesions

10.—a
Multiple sclerosis variety---
　Classic (Charcot type)
　Acute (Marburg type)
　Diffuse cerebral sclerosis (Schilder type)
　Concentric sclerosis (Balò type)
　Neuromyelitis optica (Devic type)

11.----e
Schilder type, or myelinoclastic diffuse sclerosis refers to an entity consisting of extensive, confluent, asymmetric demyelination of both cerebral hemispheres with involvement of the brainstem and cerebellum. It is usually seen in children presenting with seizures, signs of pyramidal tract involvement, ataxia, and psychiatric symptomatology. .Typically, there is a rapid progression of disease over the course of 1 to 2 years, but the demyelinating process may be fulminant. Late in the disease, Wallerian degeneration and cavitation can be seen.

12.---d
Most lesions CADASIL are seen in frontal, temporal, and insular lobes.

13.----e

14.---d
Hippocampal reorganization and changes in energy metabolism are associated with hippocampal sclerosis and may be the result of a brain insult occurring during brain maturation .Findings of reorganization include abnormal axonal sprouting and loss of interneurons, which is thought to change the balance of neuronal excitation and inhibition.

15.---d
Classic lissencephaly is either X-linked or associated with LIS1 gene on chromosome 17 . X-linked lissencephaly (defect in DCX/XLIS gene) has several phenotypes. Although it appears similar to LIS1 lissencephaly in males, it manifests as subcortical laminar heterotopia (double cortex) in females .

16.---a
Frequently Cystic Tumors
Colloid cyst
Craniopharyngioma
Desmoplastic infantile ganglioma
Dermoid
Ependymoma (supratentorial and spinal)
Epidermoid
Ganglion cell tumors
Glioblastoma (cystic necrosis)
Hemangioblastoma
Pilocytic astrocytoma
Pleomorphic xanthoastrocytoma
Rathke cleft cyst

17.---e.
Contrast enhancement is extremely variable in anaplastic astrocytomas in both extent and pattern.
Intratumoral hemorrhage may be seen on MR . The type of enhancement is variable and can be focal and nodular , homogeneous, or ringlike.
Intratumoral focal regions of signal void due to prominent neovascularity can occasionally be seen but are not as common in anaplastic astrocytoma .

18.---e
Localized (noninfiltrative) astrocytic tumors are pilocytic astrocytoma, pleomorphic xanthoastrocytoma (PXA), and subependymal giant cell astrocytoma. The better outlook for patients harboring these lesions is due to a limited capacity for invasion and spread and a limited tendency to progress into more malignant forms.

19.—d
Lymphomatous masses do not calcify and hemorrhage is distinctly uncommon on imaging studies.
 Enhancement after intravenous contrast occurs in most cases and can be dense and homogeneous,but necrotic lesions can show ring enhancement
The detection of enhancement along perivascular spaces on MR imaging should put PCNSL at the top of the differential diagnosis, with sarcoidosis representing the only other consideration.
Reports indicate that lymphoma in AIDS patients more commonly appears as multifocal lesions with ring enhancement and with more prominent edema than in the general population

20.---d
Antoni type A tissue has a compact texture composed of interwoven bundles of bipolar spindle cells

21---d
The widening of the internal auditory canal is usually be appreciated best on axial images, which demonstrate the entire length of the canal on a single slice, in contrast to the coronal image , which generally does not reveal the entire length of the canal on a single section.

22---c

23.----e
Dysembryoplastic neuroepithelial tumor (DNET) is an uncommon, slow-growing, quasi-hamartomatous tumor that occurs in the older child.
A classic DNET involves just the cortex and does not contrast-

enhance. A less typical tumor involves not only the cortex, but also the subadjacent white matter, and shows contrast enhancement. On CT, DNETs appear as hypodense masses. On MRI on T1-weighted sequence they show focal punctate hypointensities within the substance of the mass, seen as cystlike areas on T2-weighted images. These tumors frequently have a gyriform configuration. On FLAIR these may be hyperintense lesions. On diffusion, they do not restrict, but rather show increased motion of water. When they are superficially located, remodeling of bone in the overlying calvarium may be present. The differential diagnosis includes ganglioglioma, low-grade cortical astrocytoma, and oligodendroglioma.

24.----e
Symmetric increased signal in T2-weighted images in the caudate nuclei, putamen, thalamus and cortex, basal ganglia, periventricular white matter, and occipital lobes are noted in CJD. Primary sensorimotor cortex is almost always spared, even when extensive abnormalities are found in the frontal and parietal cortex.
The mechanism of hyperintensity on DWI found in the cortex and basal ganglia is poorly understood, although it correlates with deposition of abnormal prion protein, vacuolation, neuronal loss, and gliosis. DWI changes have been observed as early as 1 month after the onset of symptoms and may show modifications 6 months prior to T2-weighted images and 4 months prior to FLAIR images

25.---a
In infants, subdural empyema is a complication of purulent meningitis. In older children and young adults, it is often secondary to otorhinologic infection, which accounts for 65% to 90% of cases. The frontal and ethmoidal sinuses are most often involved. The pathophysiologic mechanism of empyema may be due to direct spread from the extraaxial space and/or retrograde thrombophlebitis via bridging emissary veins

26.---b
Two types of vascular involvement have been described in neurosyphilis—Heubner endarteritis and Nissl-Alzheimer endarteritis.
The Heubner type is the most common form of syphilitic arteritis, affecting large and medium-sized arteries. Pathophysiologically, there is fibroblastic proliferation of the intima, thinning of the media, and adventitial fibrous and inflammatory changes, resulting in an irregular luminal narrowing and ectasia
. Less frequently, the Nissl-Alzheimer type of arteritis is present, primarily involving small vessels in which a luminal narrowing occurs as a consequence of intense proliferation of endothelial and

adventitial cells. Both types of arteritis may lead to vascular occlusion. Moreover, syphilis can be associated with a venous occlusive inflammation.

Tabes dorsalis is a myelopathy associated with atrophic, degenerated, and demyelinated dorsal nerve roots and posterior spinal columns and appears 10 to 20 years after the initial infection . A triad of symptoms (lightning pains, dysuria, and ataxia) and a triad of signs (Argyll-Robertson pupil, areflexia, loss of proprioception) are the characteristics of this disorder .

The Argyll-Robertson pupil, seen in both tabes dorsalis and general paresis, is a small, irregular pupil that accommodates but does not react to light.

MR imaging typically demonstrates brain atrophy associated with hyperintense signal intensity on T2-weighted images and contrast enhancement in the posterior spinal cord and dorsal nerve roots.

27.---c

In certain locations, elevated signal intensity on conventional and FLAIR T2-weighted images is a normal finding even in young individuals .The parietopontine tracts of the posterior limb of the internal capsule is one such location.Here foci are well circumscribed, round or oval, and symmetric, and they appeared comparable to cortical gray matter on T2 and iso- or hypointense on proton-density images.

28.----a

Increase of value of ADC noted in AD.

Pittsburgh Compound B, commonly referred to as PIB has been most extensively studied for amyloid imaging.

PIB uptake is greatest in the frontal lobes, the posterior cingulate/precuneus, and the temporal parietal association cortex. Binding is typically low in the sensorimotor cortex and primary visual cortex. PIB binding is typically not present in the cerebellum, and therefore the cerebellum is used as a reference region. PIB uptake is typically significantly greater, on the order of two times, in affected cortical areas in AD patients relative to controls.

In addition to its utility as a tool for early and definitive diagnosis of AD, PIB has great potential value in the differential diagnosis of various dementia syndromes, particularly in differentiating AD from frontotemporal lobe dementia. Of equal or greater importance is the potential use of PIB as an outcome measure in therapeutic studies aimed at reduction of brain amyloid load. PET imaging tracers approved by FDA for amyloid imaging are , florbetaben F18 injection (*Neuraceq*, Piramal Imaging).,florbetapir (*Amyvid*, Eli Lilly and Company) and flutemetamol (*Vizamyl*, GE Healthcare),

29.---a

Asymmetric fronto-parietal lobar atrophy is noted in CBD.
The most useful imaging findings for distinguishing CBD from PSP are the presence of midbrain atrophy and periaqueductal signal abnormalities in PSP and the presence of asymmetric frontoparietal lobar atrophy in CBD . Asymmetric frontoparietal lobar atrophy on MRI is a mandatory exclusion criterion for the diagnosis of PSP according to the NINDS and SPSP diagnostic criteria for PSP.
On conventional MRI, MSA-P shows characteristic putaminal atrophy and hypo- and/or hyperintense signal changes on T2-weighted images whereas PD spares the putamen
Changes in diffusivity within the putamen and/or middle cerebellar peduncles can help to differentiate MSA-P from PD and other parkinsonian syndromes.
A recent diffusion tensor MRI investigation found a significant increase in mean diffusivity in the midbrain of PSP patients compared with PD and MSA patients.
On MR of MSA-C the midline sagittal section shows selective pontine atrophy with flattening of its inferior part and loss of the normal pontine bulge . Atrophy of the middle cerebellar peduncles, the cerebellum (hemispheric greater than vermian), and the inferior olives is also well seen on MR . On long-TR sequences and FLAIR sequences hyperintense signal involves the pontocerebellar pathway and the olives . Adjacent tracts not involved in the pontocerebellar pathway (i.e., the tegmentum, pyramidal tracts, and superior cerebellar peduncles) are spared pathologically and on MR . The result is an abnormal hyperintense cruciform pattern consisting of the transverse pontine fibers coursing mediolaterally and the pontine raphe coursing anteroposteriorly . . Schrag et al. coined the very descriptive term the "hot cross bun" sign, likening this cruciform imaging finding to the hot cross bun baked for the last Thursday before Easter.

30-.---c
The cortical tuber show "gyral core" appearance on T1-weighted MR and the "sulcal island" on T2-weighted
The abnormal hamartomatous tissue of the cortical tubers usually has prolonged T1 and T2, and so they are bright on T2-weighted images.
The characteristic gyral core is an isointense expanded gyrus of gray matter surrounding a central hypointense white matter center
The sulcal island is both a geometric and signal intensity inversion of the gyral core—the subcortical white matter is abnormally bright and surrounds a sulcus with its gray matter borders of normal intensity

31---c
The Chiari II malformation is nearly all associated with lumber myelomeningoceles

32.—e
In children, the most common presentations are macrocephaly (49%) and intracranial hypertension (36%)

33.---a
There is a spectrum of deformity of the vermis in Dandy-Walker malformation. In 25% of cases it is completely absent. In the 75% of cases where there is a residual vermis, the inferior portion is hypoplastic and the residual vermis and superior medullary velum are rotated anterosuperiorly and in severe cases may become attached to the tentorium.

34.---e
Compression fractures in hemangiomas are unusual because the involved vertebrae usually have thickened vertical trabeculae, which tend to work against axial collapse.

35.---c
Mucin accumulation around vessels and between cells surrounding vessels is characteristic of myxopapillary ependymoma.

36.—e
The spinal cord may be of normal caliber or slightly expanded, which in the latter case may even suggest a neoplasm. Cord expansion is found in up to 47% of cases.

Conditions that may Present with a Transverse Myelopathy Picture
Demyelinating diseases: multiple sclerosis, acute disseminated encephalomyelitis, Devic syndrome
Infections: syphilis, Lyme disease, *Mycoplasma*, viral infections
Vaccination
Disorders of the connective tissue such as systemic lupus erythematosus, sarcoidosis, Behçet disease, Sjögren syndrome, mixed connective tissue disorder
Paraneoplastic syndromes
Venous ischemia secondary to radiculomedullary fistulas
Spinal cord infarction due to occlusion of the anterior spinal artery
Acute compression due to disc herniation or fracture

37.---e
The cord lay abnormally low in 94.8% of lipomas.

38.----e
In block vertebrae, the intervertebral disk is absent or rudimentary. The combined vertebrae may be normal in height or tall. Deficient growth at the fusion site leads to narrow sagittal diameter and concave configuration of the block. Scalloping of the posterior surface may result from associated dural ectasia or (rarely) congenital mass.

39.---e
Consistency of pituitary macroadenomas could not be accurately predicted based on MR signal intensities. However, a significant direct correlation has recently been shown between tumor consistency (hardness) and apparent diffusion coefficient (ADC) values
Large pituitary adenomas virtually

always enlarge the sella due to their slow growth and late presentation, whereas other intrinsic pituitary lesions, such as pituitary metastasis and inflammatory lesions, do not.

40.—e
The MR appearance of Sheehan Syndrome is similar to that of pituitary apoplexy, except that the sella is of normal size and there is no evidence of an adenoma.

41.----d
Calculation of the CBV is very susceptible to motion-related noise.

42.---d
The acquisition of long echo time data (TE = 270 ms, TR = 3 ms) allows the detection of N-acetylaspartate (NAA), creatine (Cr/PCr) and choline (Cho) in normal brain, and lactate in areas of abnormality. The methyl resonance of NAA produces a large sharp peak at 2.01 p.p.m. and acts as a neuronal marker as it is almost exclusively found in neurons in the human brain, where it is found predominantly in the axons and nerve processes. The creatine peak (3.03 p.p.m.) arises from both phosphocreatine- and creatine-containing substances in the cell and choline (3.22 p.p.m) is thought to arise from choline-containing substances in the cell membrane.

The acquisition of short echo time data (TE = 30 ms, TR = 2s) has become the standard spectroscopy sequence and has the advantage of reduced effects from T2 losses and therefore provides spectra with better signal to noise. In addition, it detects additional resonances from metabolites with complex MR spectra such as myo-inositol, glutamate and glutamine .

43.----d

44.----b
Most of meningioma correspond to WHO grade I.
Of meningiomas, 90 per cent are supratentorial arising, in decreasing order of frequency, from the parasagittal region, cerebral convexities, sphenoid ridge and olfactory grove. Infratentorial meningiomas are most frequently located on the posterior surface of the petrous bones and clivus and can mimic acoustic neuromas

45.---c
Restricted diffusion in acute infarcts (low ADC) returns high signal on DWI and appears dark on the ADC map
Chronic lesions with very long T2 relaxation times may appear high signal on DWI due to 'T2 shine through', but in comparison to acute infarcts they will also appear bright on the ADC map.
Another potential pitfall of DWI is acute haemorrhage, which can return high signal resembling an infarct

46.---c
A thick, irregular rind of enhancement is more suggestive of tumour.
On magnetic resonance imaging, the signal of the abscess centre is between that of cerebrospinal

fluid (CSF) and white matter on T1W images, and iso- or slightly hyperintense to CSF on T2W images. On T2W images the abscess rim is relatively hypointense; it may be slightly hyperintense to white matter on T1W images. The pattern of rim enhancement is similar to that shown by CT. Surrounding vasogenic oedema is of low signal on T1W and high signal on T2W images. The abscess centre is high signal on diffusion-weighted imaging (DWI) and low signal on maps of apparent diffusion coefficient (ADC), because of restricted diffusion in the viscous pus.

47.----b
Extradural hematoma tend not to cross cranial sutures

48.---a
Spinal capillary haemangioblastomas nearly always involve the posterior columns of the spinal cord and abut against a pial surface. Most are solitary.

49.----c
In complete lissencephaly the brain surface is smooth and the Sylvian fissures are wide and vertically orientated. The cortex is thin; there is a 'cell-sparse zone' of white matter adjacent to it and a broad band of grey matter, the 'arrested neurones' that have failed to migrate to the cortex, deep to it .
The gyral pattern of the brain resembles the appearance of the 23–24-week normal fetal brain. So lissencephaly is unlikely to be reliably diagnosed on early fetal MRI.

50.---e
The typical appearance of the childhood medulloblastoma on CT is of a hyperdense midline vermian mass abutting the roof of the fourth ventricle, with perilesional oedema, variable patchy enhancement and hydrocephalus. The brainstem is usually displaced anteriorly rather than directly invaded. Cystic change, haemorrhage and calcification are frequently seen. On MRI, the mass is hypointense or isointense compared to grey matter. The CT finding of hyperdensity and MRI finding of T2 hypointensity, supported by the presence of restricted diffusion on diffusion-weighted imaging, are the most reliable observations in prospectively differentiating medulloblastoma (and atypical rhabdoid tumour which on imaging appears identical to medulloblastoma) from ependymoma or other posterior fossa tumours
Atypical rhabdoid tumour imaging feature akin to medulloblastoma

51.---b
On MRI multiple asymmetrical areas of demyelination seen as increased signal intensity on T2-weighted imaging with swelling occur within the subcortical white matter of both hemispheres and may also involve the cerebellum and spinal cord. Cortical and deep grey matter may also be involved but to a lesser extent

Periventricular and callosal lesions (such as Dawson's fingers) are more in keeping with MS lesions while cortical abnormality is not seen with MS and deep grey matter involvement, though seen in both, is more frequent in ADEM.

52.---b
Trisacryl gelatine microsphere (embosphere) show deeper penetration into vascular system than PVA particles.

53.---a
In infants and children suture diastasis is the first and most prominent result of raised intracranial pressure, and the younger the child the more marked is the sign. The coronal and sagittal sutures are most markedly affected.

54.---a
FLAIR is of disappointing sensitivity to spine

55.---e

56.---b
15 to 20% of aneurysm are multiple

57.----b
Pineal gland lies above the posterior commissure, cerebral aqueduct and ductal plate

58-.---c
Normal meningeal enhancement is discontinuous .**59.—c**
Pineoblastoma show strong but heterogenous enhancement

60.---e
HIV encephalopathy typically spare of gray matter.

TEST PAPER 11

1. All are true regarding MR contrast except
a. related to the density of mobile protons
b. T1 relaxation times increase 25% to 40% with every doubling of the magnetic field strength
c. Cerebrospinal fluid TI--4,000(ms), T2---2,200(ms)
d. order of relative T1 times --CSF » white matter > gray matter.
e. Proton densities follow the order of white matter < gray matter < CSF

2. All are true regarding acute infarction except
a. loss of flow void in the arteries of the circle of Willis and arteries within cortical sulci.
b. loss of flow void in the arteries may precede any parenchymal water accumulation
c. Spin echo images and T2-images may show thrombosis/slow flow
d. Mass effect peaks at 3 to 4 days after infarction
e. Fast spin echo sequence preferred to detect acute hemorrhage

3. Posterior cerebral artery supply all except

a. the brainstem and thalamus
b. the medial geniculate body
c. the medial and posterior portion of the temporal lobe
d. the posterior medial portion of the parietal lobe and the occipital lobe
e. the anterior limb of the internal capsule

4. All are true regarding contrasts except
a. antiferromagnetic augment the the applied magnetic field but lessr than paramagnetic substance
b. the antiferromagnetic substance becomes paramagnetic above the Néel temperature
c. ferromagnetic materials possess a magnetic field even in the absence of an applied magnetic field
d. superparamagnetic produces a greater enhancement of the applied magnetic field compared with paramagnetic substances.
e. Superparamagnetic materials retain their magnetic field when removed from an applied field.

5. All are true following diseases except
a. Clusters of hyperintensity on T1W with peripheral circumferential rims of hypointensity on T2W is noted in cavernous angioma
b. pons is favored location for cavernous angioma
c. Multiple hemorrhages of differing ages is noted in amyloid angiopathy
d. Lamellated hematoma with different stages of blood clot is noted in thrombosed aneurysm
e. Hematoma in white matter or at gray–white junction is noted in arterial infarction

6. All are true regarding intracranial hemorrhage in AVMs except

a. the most common initial symptom
b. heralds the existence of the AVM in about 15% of patients
c. most often occurs during the second or third decade
d. most often intraparenchymal
e. common cause of nontraumatic SAHs

7. True regarding posttherapy MRI of AVMs is/are
a. A significant reduction in nidus size is usually clearly recognized on MR
b. Significant evidence of reductions in AVM flow generally does not occur until at least 12 months after the initial treatment
c. Changes of transient vasogenic edema and radiation necrosis in the surrounding parenchyma have been noted as early as 3 months after treatment
d. Symptomatic radiation necrosis is seen as high intensity with mass effect and irregular enhancement
e. the region of the N-butyl cyanoacrylate "glue" cast appear hyperintense on conventional images

8. All are true regarding cavernous angioma except
a. the second-most-common type of vascular malformation to be symptomatic
b. Seizures are the most common symptom
c. Seizures associated with cavernous angiomas are most often focal
d. the risk of hemorrhage is in the range of 0.1% to 1.1% /yr for each lesion
e. Extension of hemorrhage into subarachnoid or intraventricular space is common

9. All are true regarding giant aneurysm except
a. most commonly found in middle-aged women
b. usually present with signs more indicative of a mass lesion
c. Mostly related to the extradural internal carotid within the cavernous sinus or MCA
d. Basilar giant aneurysms are associated with particularly poor outcomes
e. the apex of the basilar artery is a rare site for giant aneurysm

10. All are true regarding subdural hematoma except
a. typically caused by stretching and tearing of bridging veins
b. mostly found along the supratentorial convexity
c. Interhemispheric and tentorial leaf subdural hematomas specific for child abuse
d. crescentic collection of blood between the brain and the falx
e. MR signal appearance varies with the age of the lesion

11. Features of plaques that strongly suggest the diagnosis of multiple sclerosis are all except
a. a multiple in number
b. different stages
c. variable size and shape
d. markedly symmetric involvement
e. subpial cortical plaques

**12. An old patients of 50yrs was on immunosuppressive therapy after organ transplantation. He developed headaches, decreased alertness, altered mental

functioning, seizures, and visual loss .There was acute acute elevation of blood pressure about 3-4 days before the onset of symptom.All are features of Reversible Posterior Leukoencephalopathy except
a. lesions usually in regions supplied by the posterior circulation
b. Confluent areas of high signal abnormality on T2W, normal / increased diffusion
c. lesions typically seen in a bilateral asymmetric pattern
d. lesions may be limited to the subcortical white matter
e. Mild mass effect with sulcal effacement is usually seen

13. ALL shows delayed myelination (hypomyelinative leukoencephalopathies) except
a. Pelizaeus-Merzbacher disease
b. Alexander disease
c. Canavan disease
d. Krabbe's disease
e. Infantile GM1 / GM2 gangliosidosis

14. Which surgery is indicated in Hippocampal sclerosis ?
a. anterior temporal lobectomy
b. Lesionectomy
c. Nonlesional cortical resection
d. Corpus callosotomy
e. Hemispherectomy

15. All are true regarding abnormal neuronal migration disorder except
a. often have a genetic origin and may be sex linked
b. bilateral periventricular nodular heterotopia may be X-linked
c. bilateral periventricular nodular heterotopia to a mutation involving filamin 1 gene
d. X-linked lissencephaly manifests as subcortical laminar heterotopia in males
e. X-linked lissencephaly is due to defect in DCX/XLIS gene

16. Causes of high intensity in tumors on T1W are all except
a. Subacute-chronic blood (methemoglobin)
b. Melanin
c. Very low (nonparamagnetic) protein concentration
d. Fat
e. Flow-related enhancement in tumor vessels

17. All are true regarding astrocytoma except
a. calcification in approximately 20% of astrocytomas on CT
b. the microcysts found in astrocytoma are typically filled with clear fluid
c. relatively homogeneous mass lesions of the cerebral hemisphere
d. hyperintense on T2-weighted images
e. significant peritumoral edema

18. All are true regarding pleomorphic xanthoastrocytoma except
a. PXA ---WHO grades II and III
b. found in young adults
c. The frontal lobe is the most common location
d. large cyst immediately deep to very superficial solid mass on MR
e. The solid component usually enhances and is calcified in about 50%

19. All are true regarding Primary CNS lymphoma (PCNSL) except
a. 10-fold rise in incidence over

the last two decades

b. nearly all PCNSL is of the Hodgkin type
c. The peak age of incidence in the non-AIDS population is the sixth decade
d. Focal intracerebral masses are the most common initial presentation of PCNSL
e. the subarachnoid space is an extremely common site for recurrent disease

20. All are true regarding chordoma except
a. usually highly vascular with frequent focal calcifications
b. usually hyperintense with considerable heterogeneity on T2W
c. relationship to the clivus, usually with bone changes
d. more laterally centered lesions
e. typically enhance with intravenous contrast

21. All are true regarding following lesions except
a. postoperative evaluation of a patient with a cerebellar astrocytoma is generally performed beyond 24 hours of surgery
b. the most sensitive postoperative technique to detect residual tumor is MRI
c. Fibrillary astrocytomas are infiltrating and poorly defined tumors
d. meningiomas may occur a decade or more after the completion of radiation therapy
e. bilateral and multiple sites of high T2 signal in cerebellar dentate nuclei may be noted in NF1

22. All are true regarding Pleomorphic Xanthoastrocytomas except
a. most commonly seen in the firtst decade of life
b. large superficial hemispheric masses with frequent cyst.
c. involve the temporal and frontal lobes most frequently
d. the desmoplastic infantile ganglioglioma like appearance on MRI
e. WHO as grade II

23. All are true regarding subdural collection except
a. effusions are isointense to CSF, whereas empyemas show greater signal intensity than CSF on T1-weighted and FLAIR images
b. Postgadolinium images show a thickened enhancing membrane associated with an empyema but not with a simple effusion
c. H. influenzae meningitis in children usually show crescentic collections adjacent to the frontal and parietal lobes
d. Lack of restricted diffusion in pyogenic effucsion ---a definite distinguishing feature from empyema
e. The presence of signal alterations in the cortex subjacent to an extraaxial collection more likely indicates empyema than a simple effusion

24. All are true regarding normal aging process except
a. cerebral atrophy leading to prominence of the ventricles, cisterns, and sulci
b. hyperintense areas on T2/FLAIR images in the hemispheric

white matter
c. increase in the signal intensity of the extrapyramidal nuclei
d. predominant atrophy of white matter
e. regions of decreased anisotropy noted with increasing age

25. All are true regarding Alzheimer disease except
a. the regions of greatest loss is in the medial temporal lobe on voxel-based morphometry
b. Rates of atrophy of the hippocampus are in the 4% to 6% per year
c. relative sparing of the sensorimotor and visual cortices over time
d. decrease in N-acetylaspartate
e. decrease in myo-inositol

26. All are true regarding imaging of Progressive supranuclear palsy except
a. abnormal hypointense signal on T2-weighted MR images of the superior collicular
b. thinning of the superior colliculus on sagittal T1W midline images
c. loss of the normal convexity of the superior midbrain tegmentum on sagittal T1W midline images
d. abnormal convexity of the lateral margin of the midbrain tegmentum on axial long-TR images
e. abnormal hyperintense signal on the long-TR sequences of the periaqueductal gray matter

27. All are true regarding SEN of tuberous sclerosis except
a. the SEN is due to migrational disorder
b. The SENs are are smaller than tuber in size
c. the SEN arise primarily in the striothalamate groove
d. The SENs do not appear to grow
e. virtually 100% of SEN are hyperdense due to calcification by the age of 10yrs

28. All are true regarding septooptic dysplasia (SOD) except
a. overrexpression of dorsalizing gradient genes
b. optic nerve hypoplasia and deficiency of the septum pellucidum
c. HESX1 gene implicated
d. concurrent schizencephaly in 50% of patients
e. hypoplasia of the hypothalamus

29. All are true regarding schizencephaly except
a. abnormal white matter–lined clefts
b. type II the cleft is filled with CSF
c. a ventricular dimple
d. may be Features of SOD
e. associated polymicrogyria

30. All are true regarding Dandy-Walker malformation except
a. microcephaly with dolicocephaly
b. The angle between the superior sagittal sinus and the straight sinus increased to 90 to 150^0
c. widened incisura
d. absent the falx cerebelli
e. cystic dilation of the fourth ventricle

31. All are true regarding extradural tumour in spine except
a. uninvolved marrow appears of low signal on T2W in case of the

anemia of chronic disease
b. T1W sequences are ideal for showing impingement on the thecal sac
c. lower signal intensity of bone marrow is noted on T1W image in neoplastic collapse
d. DWI is very important to differentiate benign and neoplastic collapse
e. postcontrast imaging for spinal column lesions should be combined with fat suppression.

32. All are true regarding imaging of spinal cord ependymomas except
a. erosion of the pedicles or of the posterior surface of the vertebral bodies
b. typically heterogeneous on T2-weighted images
c. tend to enhance intensely but irregularly
d. often have ill defined
e. areas of hemorrhage

33. All are true regarding MRI finding of arachnoiditis except
a. peripheral adherent roots
b. Segmentally clumped roots centrally located
c. Empty thecal sac
d. Peripheral thickening of the thecal sac
e. calcification related to ligaments

34. All are true regarding Spinal Lipoma except
a. the most common type of occult spinal dysraphism
b. Dermal sinuses may concur in up to 20% of cases of spinal lipoma
c. Spinal lipomas are nearly always single lesions
d. Spinal lipomas with Intact Dura typically lies ventral or ventrolateral to the cord
e. Spinal lipomas with Deficient Dura constitute 84% of spinal lipoma

35. All are true spine regarding
a. The last lumbar vertebra is sacralized in 6% of patients
b. S-1 is lumbarized in 12% of cases
c. the T-12 vertebra may lack ribs in 2% of patients
d. the first lumbar vertebra may carry ribs in 6% to 11% of cases
e. Errors in the Hox code can lead to malsegmentation of the vertebrae

36. All are true regarding pituitary incidentalomas except
a. due to the presence of asymptomatic coincidental cysts or microadenoma
b. due to artifactual hypointensities caused by magnetic susceptibility–induced signal distortions in the gland
c. usually less than 1 mm in size.
d. greater than 2 mm are nearly always either pituitary adenomas or Rathke cleft cysts from autopsy studies
e. greater than 2 mm found in 5.8% to 8.3% of all subjects older than the age of 30 years at autopsy

37. All are true regarding pituitary lesions except
a. thickening of the pituitary stalk may be seen in Langerhans cell granulomatosis
b. presence of an air-fluid level may be seen in pituitary abscess
c. The basal meninges in and around the suprasellar cistern are

susceptible to tuberculous
d. Lymphocytic hypophysitis occurs almost exclusively in men
e. diffuse enlargement of the anterior lobe in lymphocytic hypophysitis on CT and MR

38.All are true regarding dynamic susceptibility contrast (DSC) MRI except
a. The transit time through the vascular system in the brain is on the order of 4 seconds
b. requires much tighter bolus and much higher temporal resolution imaging to measure perfusion
c. the image intensity fully returns to the original intensity
d. TTP map is provides a clean measure of the arrival time of the bolus in the tissue
e. a typical range of TTP for normal tissue is less than 5 seconds

39. All are physiological intracranial calcification except
a. pineal gland
b. habenular commissure
c. choroid plexus
d. petroclinoid ligaments
e. all

40.All are true regading MR Spectroscopy except
a. Choline is a reflection of the turnover of cell membranes
b. Lactate (Lac) is a marker of hypoxia in tumour tissue
c. mobile lipids are thought to reflect tissue necrosis
d. MRS with a short TE has the advantage of demonstrating additional metabolites
e. Long echo times lead to a increase of signal to noise

41.All are true regarding extra-axial neoplasm except
a. meningiomas represent the commonest nonglial intracranial neoplasm
b. meningioma account for approximately 20 per cent of all primary intracranial tumours
c. Multiple meningiomas and cranial nerve tumours are found in neurofibromatosis type 1
d. dermoid cysts and schwannomas tend to cause bone thinning
e. meningiomas tend to induce a hyperostotic bone reaction

42.All are true regarding perfusion-weighted imaging in infarction except
a. TTP provides a qualitative overview of brain perfusion
b. A threshold of 8 s delay in TTP correlates with a CBF of under 20 ml 100 g^{-1} min
c. a CBV deficit seems to be the best predictor of initial infarct
d. a CBV deficit seems to be the best predictor of final size if successfully reperfused
e.. The MTT and CBF indicate tissue at risk (the final infarct volume)

43.All are true regarding Intracranial vascular malformations except
a. arteriovenous shunting is present in cerebral (or subpial) arteriovenous malformation and dural fistulae
b. . Cavernous angiomas and telangiectasias are angiographically occult or 'cryptic' vascular malformations.
c. Dilated feeding arteries and early opacification of draining

veins are the angiographic hallmarks of AVMs
d. spin-echo sequences are the most sensitive to detect cavernoma
e. typical 'caput medusa' appearance on the venous phase of conventional angiograms is noted in Developmental venous anomalies.

44. All are true regarding white matter diseases except
a. Mutations in the *ATP7B* gene cause Wilson disease
b. The commonest MRI finding is high signal in the putamen on T2W images
c. lesions of multiple sclerosis is commonest in the periventricular white matter
d. Lesions of the corpus callosum in multiple sclerosis is best shown on sagittal T2W images
e. Lesions of multiple sclerosis is aligned with the transverse axis of the cord

45. All are true regarding spinal lesions except
a. the most common extradural tumours are metastases
b. neurinomas and meningiomas are the commonest lesions in intradural extramedullary location
c. 80 per cent of meningiomas occur in the lumber region in middle aged women
d. hyperostosis is uncommon with meningiomas of the spine
e. most of intramedullary tumours are gliomas

46. All are true regarding cerebral cortex formation except
a. neuroblasts that are generated in the germinal matrix
b. The migration of the neuroblasts starts at about week 7 of gestation
c. The migration of the neuroblasts, is most intense during weeks 15–17
d. The migration of the neuroblasts starts is largely complete by weeks 23–24
e. the youngest neurones of cortex lies adjacent to the subcortical white matter

47. All are true regarding craniosynostosis except
a. MRI is more sensitive and specific than plain radiographs for detecting craniosynostosis
b. CT venography may be helpful to assess the jugular foramina
c. The sutures should be assessed on both the axial 2D CT anc 3D CT
d. bicoronal synostosis is seen in Apert syndrome
e. Crouzon's syndrome demonstrate a complex syndromic synostosis

48. All are true regarding gelfoam except
a. prepared from pork-skin gelatin
b. used for occlusion of distal vessels
c. no significant sclerosing
d. recanalises within approx. 6weeks
e. pliable material

49. The first and most prominent feature of raised intracranial pressure in infants and children is
a. suture diastasis
b. thin skull vaults
c. large heads.
d. craniolacunae
e. increased convolutional markings

50. All are true regarding skull trauma except
a. The cephalhaematoma lies under the periosteum
b. leptomeningeal cysts is congenital in nature
c. pneumocephalus most commonly result from fractures involving the frontal/ethmoid sinuses
d. CT cisternography may be required for accurate localization for CSF rhinorrhoea
e. CSF otorrhoea may follow fractures involving the petrous bone

51. A complete circle of Willis is seen in
a. 20%
b. 45%
c. 55%
d. 65%
e. 75%

52. All shows increased incidence of intracranial aneurysm except
a. anomalous vessels
b. aortic dissection
c. polycystic kidney disease
d. fibromuscular dysplasia
e. Down syndrome

53. All are true regarding brain tumour in adult except
a. 70% of gliomas are astrocytoma
b. the second most common primary brain tumour is meningioma
c. intraaxial posterior fossa tumour in adult are very common
d. metastases is the most common intraaxial posterior fossa tumour
e. hemangioblastoma and brainstem glioma are most common tumour in infratentorial location

54. All are common causes of multiple "holes in the skull" except
a. normal structures
b. multiple burr holes/surgical defects
c. age-related osteoporosis
d. hyperparathyroidism
e. metastases

55. All are true regarding pineal cell tumours except
a. germinoma engulfs a calcified pineal gland
b. teratoma is the most common pineal region tumour
c. pineoblastoma show uniform strong enhancement
d. endodermal sinus tumour show elevated alpha-fetoprotein levels
e. alpha-FT and HCG are elevated with embryonal cell carcinoma

56. All are true regarding hepes simplex encephalitis except
a. predilection for limbic encephalitis
b. sequential bilaterality
c. haemorrhage –highly suggestive
d. haemorrhage ---early finding
e. spare putamen

57. All are true regarding Pelizaeus-Merzbacher disease except
a. due to lack of lipophilin
b. patchy demyelination with sparing of perivascular white matter
c. preserved internal capsule and subcortical U fibres
d. diffuse low signal on T2w
e. hypointense basal ganglia and thalamus on T2W

58. All are true regarding normal anatomy of spine except
a. the conus tip is normally at

about the L1-L2 level
b. the thoracic spinal cord space measures 12 to 13 mm in sagittal diameter
c. Ligamentum flavum is seen on axial CT as V-shaped
d. the cervical subarachnoid space is widest at the craniovertebral junction
e. there is abundant epidural fat in cervical region

59. All are true regarding lissencephaly except
a. type I has figure of eight appearance of sylvian fissure
b. type II has well-formed cortex
c. Miller-Dieker syndrome is associated with type I lissencephaly
d. Walker-Warburg syndrome is associated with type II lissencephaly
e. hypoplastic cerebellum is seen in type III lissencephaly

60. All are true regarding posterior fossa malformation except
a. high tentorial insertion is noted in Dandy-Walker malformation
b. megacisterna magna is opacified on intrathecal contrast
c. arachnoid cyst in posterior fossa show intense contrast enhancement
d. enterogenous cyst is noted posterior to brainstem
e. epidermoid cyst is irregular and frond-like

TEST PAPER 11(ANSWER)

1.---d
Relative longitudinal relaxation(T1) times follow the order CSF » gray matter > white matter.

2.---e
In fast spin echo imaging, the detection of acute hemorrhage is reduced by virtue of lower sensitivity to magnetic susceptibility changes. So, the MR evaluation of stroke patients should be supplementd with with gradient echo imaging, which is highly sensitive to susceptibility variations that accompany intraparenchymal hemorrhage. Intravenous contrast was used in the past to help characterize cerebral infarction in the acute time period .Early arterial enhancement without significant early parenchymal enhancement was seen in most patients with a completed stroke while early cortical enhancement(due to sufficient collaterals) suggested a more favorable clinical outcome.

3.---e
The thalamogeniculate arteries ,a branch of the posterior cerebral artery supply the medial geniculate body, the pulvinar of the thalamus, and the posterior rim of the internal capsule (not anterior).

4.----e
Superparamagnetic materials do not retain their magnetic field when removed from an applied field.
The alignment pattern in antiferromagnetic substances can be disrupted if the thermal energy is increased, and initially the response to an applied field is enhanced as the temperature is increased. Above a critical temperature, known as the Néel temperature, adjacent spin pairing is disrupted, and the antiferromagnetic substance becomes paramagnetic.

5.---e
Hematoma in white matter or at gray–white junction is noted in venous infarction. Hemorrhage in arterial infarction is localized to cortex.

6.—b
Intracranial hemorrhage heralds the existence of the AVM in 30% to 55% of patients and most often occurs during the second or third decade

7.---e
MR imaging of patients after staged transarterial flow-directed embolization with N-butyl cyanoacrylate demonstrated the region of the "glue" cast as mixed regions of alternating high and low signal on conventional images.

8.---e
Extension of hemorrhage into subarachnoid or intraventricular space is not common. Progressive neurologic deficit is an uncommon manifestation of supratentorial cavernous angiomas but occurs more often with those in the infratentorial space

9.---e

Most giant aneurysms are related to the extradural internal carotid within the cavernous sinus or MCA, but a high percentage occur at the apex of the basilar artery. Basilar giant aneurysms are associated with particularly poor outcomes.

10.---c

Interhemispheric and tentorial leaf subdural hematomas are commonly found in children who are victims of nonaccidental injury due to violent shaking (shaken-baby syndrome). Although these hematomas are not completely specific for child abuse, their presence should always alert one to the possibility of this syndrome.

11.----d

In general, a combination of multiple plaques in different stages, plaques of variable size and shape, markedly asymmetric involvement, and subpial cortical plaques strongly suggest the diagnosis of multiple sclerosis

12.----c

In reversible posterior leukoencephalopathy, Confluent areas of signal abnormality are typically seen in a bilateral symmetric pattern that may be limited to the subcortical white matter but frequently also involves the overlying cortex
The mechanism underlying the syndrome is likely a brain-capillary leak syndrome with regions of vasodilation and vasoconstriction, particularly in arterial boundary zones. Sympathetic innervation to the vasculature has been shown to initiate vasoconstrictive protection to the brain from marked increases in blood pressure. Because the anterior circulation is better supplied with sympathetic innervation than the posterior circulation, it is theorized to be better protected during elevation of systemic blood pressure.

13.---d

14.---a

15.---d

Classic lissencephaly is either X-linked or associated with LIS1 gene on chromosome 17. X-linked lissencephaly (defect in DCX/XLIS gene) has several phenotypes. Although it appears similar to LIS1 lissencephaly in males, it manifests as subcortical laminar heterotopia (double cortex) in females.

16.----c

Causes of High Intensity in Tumors on T1-Weighted Magnetic Resonance Images

Paramagnetic effects from --- hemorrhage-	Subacute-chronic blood (methemoglobin)
Paramagnetic material without – hemorrhage	Melanin Naturally occurring ions associated with necrosis of calcification Manganese Iron Copper
Nonparamagnetic effects-----	Very high (nonparamagnetic) protein

concentration
Fat
Flow-related enhancement in tumor vessels

17.---e
Astrocytoma usually lack significant peritumoral "edema," which distinguishes it from more malignant astrocytic tumors on MR.
The most common glial neoplasm with calcification is the astrocytoma, despite the fact that oligodendrogliomas have the highest frequency of calcification.
Cortical involvement by astrocytoma is best seen on MR imaging as thickening of the cortical mantle.
However the lesion does not obey a vascular territory and lacks the restricted diffusion as seen in arterial infarctions
The well-differentiated astrocytoma has a variable appearance after contrast administration but classically shows no significant contrast enhancement.

18.----c
The temporal lobe is the most common location. On MR imaging, the differential diagnosis includes pilocytic astrocytoma and ganglion cell tumor.

19.---b
Nearly all PCNSL is of the non-Hodgkin type. Organ transplant recipients, congenital immunodeficiency syndromes, AIDS are risk factors.
The supratentorial compartment is involved in approximately 75% to 85% of patients at initial presentation. Multiplicity is very common and has been noted in up to one half of cases

20.---d
On MR, sagittal T1-weighted images demonstrate chordoma tumor best. It is manifested by a moderately hypointense lesion that replaces the hyperintense clival fatty marrow. On T2-weighted images, it is usually hyperintense, with considerable heterogeneity.
The diagnosis in these cases hinges on the identification of relationship to the clivus, usually with bone changes. A midline location favors chordoma, whereas the presence of more laterally centered lesions (near the petroclival ridge) favors chondrosarcoma

21.---a
Postoperative evaluation of a patient with a cerebellar astrocytoma is generally performed within 24 hours of surgery. The reason for this is to avoid postoperative contrast enhancement at the site of reactive granulation tissue, which could be misinterpreted for residual tumor. Several days after surgery, granulation tissue starts to form, with disturbance in the BBB, and enhancement occurs at the margins of the resection whether there is or is not residual tumor.

22----a
Pleomorphic xanthoastrocytoma (PXA) is a tumor of mixed

neuronal and glial origin that is most commonly seen in the second decade of life

23.---d

Pyogenic empyema shows restricted diffusion, a definite distinguishing feature from effusions

24.—c

The three most common MRI-detectable abnormalities typically ascribed to "normal" aging are atrophy, hyperintense areas on T2 or fluid-attenuated inversion recovery (FLAIR) images in the hemispheric white matter, and decrease in the signal intensity of the extrapyramidal nuclei attributed to iron deposition.

The study has shown statistically significant decreases in diffusion anisotropy with increasing age in the periventricular white matter, frontal white matter, genu, and splenium of the corpus callosum, despite the absence of signal abnormalities in the white matter on visual inspection of conventional images.

Enlarged ventricles and subarachnoid spaces(transient) may be seen in paediatrics patient due to steroids

25.---e

NAA is found in neurons, and a decrease in NAA follows logically from the neuron loss associated with AD. Myo-inositol is located primarily in astrocytes. It is elevated in AD and Down syndrome;

Patients with more-atrophic hippocampi have a greater risk of progressing to AD within a finite follow-up than do patients with less-atrophic hippocampi

Patients with greater rates of brain shrinkage and ventricular expansion have a greater risk of subsequently progressing from aMCI to AD than do patients with lesser of rates of brain shrinkage and ventricular expansion.

One of the most common voxel-based techniques is voxel-based morphometry (VBM), which compares groups of subjects and identifies differences in the patterns of gray matter density across the whole brain

VBM studies in AD have shown that the regions of greatest loss are in the medial temporal lobe, but there is also extensive atrophy throughout the basal temporal lobe, lateral temporal and parietal neocortex, posterior cingulate and percutaneous, insula, temporal parietal association neocortex, and prefrontal cortex . Structures in the central gray matter are also involved that include the caudate putamen, thalamus, and hypothalamus

26.---a

Pathologic and neuroimaging studies have documented focal midbrain atrophy in PSP. PSP shows abnormal concavity of the lateral margin of the midbrain tegmentum on axial long-TR images (the morning glory sign).

27.---e

Virtually 100% of SEN are hyperdense due to calcification by the age of 20yrs

The cortical tubers are large, potato- or tuberlike, misshapen gyri. . The cortical hamartomas of TS contain unusually large cells. The presence of calcification allows SENs to be distinguished from the otherwise similar-appearing subependymal gray matter heterotopias

28.---a
Neural Tube Dorsalizing Gradient Mutations are divided into those that involve overexpression of dorsalizing gradient genes, such as duplication of the dorsal horns of the spinal cord, duplication of dorsal brainstem structures, and the dorsal interhemispheric variant of HPE, and those that involve underexpression of dorsalizing gradient genes, such as septooptic dysplasia (SOD).

29.---a
Schizencephaly describes abnormal gray matter–lined clefts that extend through the cerebral hemisphere.

30.---a
Classically, there is macrocephaly with dolicocephaly, thinning and protuberance of the occiput, widening of the lambdoid sutures, and scalloping of the inner table of the occipital bone and the petrous pyramids .

31---d
Utility of DWI in making benign and neoplastic collapse distinction is controversial.
When gadolinium compounds are given for spinal lesions, enhancement is extremely variable.
Because low-intensity lesions tend to enhance after the administration of gadolinium, they often become isointense with surrounding marrow and are less easily detectable . In fact, gadolinium can even obscure some lesions. For this reason, if the detection of vertebral body lesions is a consideration, scans should be performed without contrast; postcontrast imaging for spinal column lesions should be combined with fat suppression.

32.---d
Although ependymoma are characteristically quite heterogeneous and astrocytomas are characteristically more homogeneous, it often is very difficult to differentiate these tumors from astrocytomas by imaging criteria. There are a few suggestive criteria, however.
First, ependymomas occur far more often in the lower cord and conus than astrocytomas.
Second, astrocytomas tend to arise eccentrically within the cord, especially posteriorly. Ependymomas arise from ependymal cells in the central canal and tend to be central
Third, ependymomas are more frequently hemorrhagic than astrocytomas.
Fourth, regions of low intensity reflecting hypercellularity are more common in ependymomas.
Finally, because of the thin pseudocapsule that surrounds ependymomas, it may be possible on very thin sections to identify a plane separating the ependymoma from the cord, unlike astrocytomas, which tend to be infiltrative and have poorly

defined borders.
33.---e

Myelographic Diagnosis of Arachnoiditis---

Lack of filling of one or more root sleeves
Segmental nerve root fusion
Irregularities of the contrast column
Lack of discrete roots in the thecal sac
Defects on the contrast column
Mass of fibrotic nerve roots filling the thecal sac
Myelographic block
Calcification related to a nerve root or defect
Rests of oily contrasts
There is a near-perfect agreement between myelographic and MR findings.
Magnetic Resonance Imaging Diagnosis of Arachnoiditis

Centrally clumped or peripheral adherent roots
Segmentally clumped roots centrally located
Empty thecal sac
Peripheral thickening of the thecal sac
Soft tissue masses into the thecal sac
Cysts and loculations in the subarachnoid space
   (more common in the thoracic spine)
Syringomyelia
Rests of oily contrast
Variable enhancement of nerve roots
34.--d

Spinal Lipomas with Intact Dura typically lies dorsal or dorsolateral to the cord
35.---b
S-1 is lumbarized in 2% of cases
36.---c
Most of these incidental "lesions" are small—usually less than 3 mm in size.
37.----d
Features that may favor an abscess over an adenoma include presence of an air-fluid level, meningeal enhancement, cerebritis, sphenoid sinus effusion, sella or sphenoid sinus bony destruction, absent posterior pituitary bright spot, and cavernous sinus thrombosis. Lymphocytic hypophysitis occurs almost exclusively in women and particularly during late pregnancy or in the postpartum period. The diagnosis should be considered in a female patient who is in the peripartum period with a pituitary mass, particularly when the degree of hypopituitarism is greater than that expected for the size of the mass. CT and MR demonstrate diffuse enlargement of the anterior lobe, usually without evidence of any focal abnormality or change in internal characteristics of the gland
38----c
Prior to the contrast arrival, the image intensity is stable, but once the agent starts to enter the vasculature of the tissue, the signal intensity drops rapidly. Depending on the contrast agent used, the sequence parameters, and the volume of the blood

vessels in the tissue, the signal intensity can drop by from a few percent to more than a factor of two. Eventually the signal rises again after the bolus washes through the tissue, but usually before the signal can recover to zero, the bolus returns after circulating through the heart and lungs again. This second bolus is strongly attenuated because of further spreading of the bolus as well as absorption into the permeable tissues outside of the brain. Usually a third recirculation is hard to detect, but the image intensity never fully returns to the original intensity because the arterial concentration of contrast agent remains significant for many minutes after the injection.

39.---e

Pineal gland (60 per cent of adults)
Habenular commissure (30 per cent)
Choroid plexus (10 per cent)
Dura mater falx cerebri (7 per cent) and superior sagittal sinus
Tentorium dural plaques (frequently parasagittal)
Petroclinoid (12 per cent) and interclinoid ligaments
Diaphragm sellae
Pituitary gland (rare)
Carotid arteries (in elderly patients)

40.---e

The choice of echo time (TE) is an important technical consideration for performing MRS. It can be short (20–40 ms), intermediate (135–144 ms) or long (270–288 ms).

MRS with a short TE has the advantage of demonstrating additional metabolites, which may improve tumour characterization, such as myo-inositol, glutamate/glutamine (Glx) and lipids but is hampered by baseline distortion and artefactual NAA peaks.
Intermediate echo times have a better defined baseline and quantification of NAA and Cho is more accurate and reproducible. Long echo times lead to a decrease of signal to noise

41.---c

Multiple meningiomas and cranial nerve tumours are found in neurofibromatosis type 2

42.----b

TTP provides a qualitative overview of brain perfusion. A threshold of 4 s delay seems to indicate tissue at risk and correlates with a CBF of under 20 ml 100 g^{-1} min^{-1} [30]. However proximal vessel stenosis can delay TTP even if CBF via collaterals is normal and tissue viability not threatened. As outlined earlier, within an area of prolonged MTT (or TTP), moderate ischaemia may cause increased CBV, however reduced CBV indicates inadequate collateral supply and high risk of infarction.

43.---d

On MRI cavernoma appear multilobular with mixed signal intensity centrally surrounded by a dark haemosiderin rim.
So, gradient-echo sequences are the most sensitive technique to detect

44.---e
Lesions of multiple sclerosis is aligned with the long axis of the cord
45.---c
80 per cent of meningiomas occur in the thoracic region in middle aged women
46.---e
The six layers of the cortex are formed with the youngest neurones on the surface and the oldest ones adjacent to the subcortical white matter
47.---a
CT is more sensitive and specific than plain radiographs for detecting craniosynostosis
48.---b
Gelfoam is used for occlusion of more proximal vessels, frequently following embolisation of distal vessels with PVA. It has no significant sclerosing effect
49.---a
In infants and children suture diastasis is the first and most prominent result of raised intracranial pressure, and the younger the child the more marked is the sign. The coronal and sagittal sutures are most markedly affected.
50.—b
Leptomeningeal cysts is acquired in nature following the trauma to skull

When a fracture in an infant or child involves the meninges, cerebrospinal fluid may escape from the subarachnoid space and form a cyst beneath the fracture. Atrophy of the overlying bone margins may result and quite large bone defects can follow.
51.----a
52-.---e
53.---c
Intraaxial posterior fossa tumour in adult are rare
54.---d
55.—c
Pineoblastoma show strong but heterogenous enhancement
56.----d
Hemorrhage is not the early finding
57.---d
Severe cases of Pelizaeus-Merzbacher disease show near – total lack of normal myelination with diffuse high signal on T2W image that extends peripherally to involve the arcuate fibres.
58.---e
There is sparse epidural fat in cervical region
59.---b
Type II lissencephally has agryric, severely disorganized unilayered cortex
60.---d
Enterogenous cyst is noted anterior to brainstem

TEST PAPER 12

1. As per Rose Criterion, what should be of the order of contrast-to-noise ratio (CNR) for the radiological images to have sufficient contrast and be easily interpretable
a. 1:1
b. 2:1
c. 4:1
d. 4:1
e. 5:1

2. All are true regarding acute infarction except
a. the T2 signal is often normal in the first 8 hours after infarction
b. approx. 90% of patients show changes in the T2-weighted sequence at 24 hrs
c. the white matter often does not show appreciable change in this first 24-hour period
d. subcortical white matter hypointensity on T2W is most likely due to haemorrhage
e. signal changes seen in the first 24 hours are best appreciated in gray matter

3. All are true regarding MRI except
a. nuclear magnetization is the origin of the signal used to construct the MR image
b. the magnetic properties of tissue are determined chiefly by the electronic configuration
c. Materials that reduce the magnitude of an applied magnetic field are termed diamagnetic
d. greater than 99% of human tissue is paramagnetic
e. Materials that increase the magnitude of an applied magnetic field are termed diamagnetic

4. All are features of intratumoural hemorrhage except
a. heterogeneous and markedly complex signal pattern
b. rapid temporal evolution of MR intensity patterns
c. lack of a well-defined, complete, markedly hypointense rim
d. the persistent perilesional high intensity on T2W in chronic hemorrhage
e. enhancement

5. All are true regarding Moyamoya disease except
a. progressive symmetric occlusion involving the bifurcations of the internal carotid arteries (ICAs) and the proximal anterior and middle cerebral arteries
b. development of an extensive network of enlarged basal, transcortical, and transdural collateral vessels.
c. presence of the expected flow void within the cavernous and supraclinoid portions of the ICAs
d. The angiographic appearance of the innumerable tiny collateral vessels, termed "puff of smoke" or "moyamoya" in Japanese.
e. Moyamoya disease has a bimodal age presentation, with the first peak occurring in the first

decade of life, associated with cerebral infarction

6. All are true regarding cavernous angioma except
a. familial pattern in 10% to 15% of patients
b. the peak incidence of symptom onset is between the first and second decades of life
c. approx. 20% to 30% of cases multiple
d. superficial location with proximity to the subarachnoid space /ventricle is common.
e. The pons is the most common brainstem location.

7. An adult female patients complain of isolated pain in right eye with features of ptosis, diplopia, pupillary dilation, and strabismus. The symptom persist with no evidence of improvement. The clinician suspected of intracranial aneurysm and so the patient was advised for CT ANGIORAPHY. The most likely site of aneurysm in such case is

a. The junction of the anterior cerebral and anterior communicating arteries
b. the posterior communicating artery
c. the bifurcation of the MCA
d. the posterior cerebral artery
e. the bifurcation of the ICA

8. All are characteristics of venous epidural hematoma except
a. usually due to laceration of a dural sinus by occipital, parietal, or sphenoid bone fractures
b. more variable in shape than those of arterial origin
c. always lie adjacent to a dural sinus that is transgressed by a fracture line
d. often lie both above and below the tentorium like a subdural hematoma
e. expand more slowly than arterial lesions

9. All are features of multiple sclerosis lesions except
a. multiple
b. well-defined lesions
c. usually in the same stage of disease progression
d. the plaques often oval in shape and oriented lengthwise in the spinal cord
e. volume loss and atrophy of the optic nerve and optic chiasm.

10. All are true regardin following diseases except
a. Marchiafava-Bignami disease cause demyelination and necrosis primarily in the corpus callosum
b. SCD changes is confined to the dorsal column of the cervical and thoracic cord
c. carbon monoxide tend to selectively affect the globus pallidus
d. pathologic findings with toluene toxicity is similar to adrenoleukodystrophy
e. heroin pyrolysate involve the anterior limb and subcortical white matter on MR image.

11. Deep gray matter involvement (± white matter) is feature of which Leukoencephalopathy
a. Mitochondrial disorders
b. Pelizaeus-Merzbacher disease
c. Alexander disease
d. Canavan disease

e. MLD

12. All are indication of hemispherectomy except
a. Sturge-Weber syndrome
b. Rasmussen encephalitis
c. hemimegalencephaly
d. hemiatrophy
e. Hippocampal sclerosis

13. All are abnormal neuronal migration disorder except
a. Lissencephaly
b. pachygyria
c. subcortical laminar heterotopias
d. tuberous sclerosis
e. subependymal heterotopia

14. Frequently cystic tumour are all except
a. medulloblastoma
b. ependymoma (supratentorial)
c. craniopharyngioma
d. ganglion cell tumour
e. pilocystic astrocytoma

15. All are true regarding astrocytoma except
a. necrosis and vascular endothelial proliferation noted in glioblastoma
b. anaplastic astrocytoma belongs to WHO grade III
c. infiltrative astrocytomas are derived typically from the prtotoplasmic astrocytoma
d. cerebellar astrocytoma is more commonly infiltrative than pilocytic in adult
e. infiltrative astrocytomas overall have a poor prognosis

16. All are true regarding subependymal giant cell astrocytoma except
a. Calcification is extremely rare
b. hyperintense, somewhat heterogeneous masses on T2W
c. generally enhance with intravenous contrast
d. central regions of marked hypointensity on gradient echo images
e. located in the region of the foramen of Monro

17. All are true regarding colloid cyst except
a. benign, epithelial-lined mass lesions
b. may produce intermittent and positional hydrocephalus
c. location at the posterosuperior aspect of the third ventricle
d. believed to be derived from the embryologic paraphysis
e. contain dense, turbid, mucoid material

18. All are true regarding chordoma except
a. tumors of notochordal tissue remnants
b. most frequently affect the sacrum
c. clival chordoma very prone to invade the nasopharyngeal region
d. clival chordoma commonly invade the brain directly
e. The peak age for clival chordomas appear is 20 - 40 years

19. All are true regarding pilocystic astrocytoma except
a. cystic with mural nodules in 50%
b. Calcification is uncommon
c. contrast enhancement on CT and MRI
d. Twenty-five-year survival rate -- on the order of 90%
e. decreased apparent diffusion coefficient (ADC) values

20. All are true regarding desmoplastic infantile

ganglioglioma except
a. large frontoparietal tumors
b. the solid portion of the tumor lies centrally within the mass
c. avid contrast enhancement on CT and MRI
d. invade the leptomeninges
e. originates superficially from pia and cortex

21. All are true regarding imaging of meningitis except
a. leptomeningeal enhancement is better seen on MRI than CT
b. A dural, pachymeningeal, enhancement follows the inner contour of the calvaria
c. T2W sequences are superior to other MR images to show meningeal inflammatory changes
d. FLAIR shows hyperintense signal intensity in the subarachnoid space
e. DWI is of great value in demonstrating any associated acute brain infarction

22. All are true regarding intraventricular neurocysticercosis except
a. most commonly found in the fourth ventricule
b. may enhance,
c. scolices are usually found
d. 3D-CISS demonstrate the intraventricular cysts
e. MR better than CT

23. All are true regarding Alzheimer disease except
a. beta amyloid is a component of the microtubule system
b. Neurofibrillary tangles consist of pathologic aggregates of tau protein
c. Neuritic plaque consists of a dense central β-amyloid core
d. The most promising biomarker appear to be CSF Aβ$_{1-42}$ protein levels
e. the neurofibrillary pathology of AD begins in the transentorhinal area

24. All are true regarding Wilson disease except
a. abnormal copper deposition
b. most pronounced involvement in the liver and brain
c. results from excessive function of the copper transport protein
d. autosomal recessive
e. peak age at presentation is between 8 and 16 years

25. The retinal lesion of van der Hoeve' phakoma can be differentiated from retinoblastoma by all except
a. not necrotic
b. do not hemorrhage
c. do not fungate
d. nor grow into the vitreous
e. No calcification

26. All are true regarding alobar holoprosencephaly except
a. absence of the interhemispheric fissure and falx cerebri
b. frequently associated with severe midline facial deformities
c. TThe corpus callosum and anterior commissure usually absent
d. crescent-shaped holoventricle
e. the septum pellucidum present

27. All are true regarding polymicrogyria except
a. perirolandic extension of the sylvian fissures in perisylvian polymicrogyria
b. inverted appearance of bodies of lateral ventricles in perisylvian

polymicrogyria
c. thickened cortex with poorly developed sulci
d. an irregular margin at the cortical–white matter junction
e. Prenatal HSV infection may be associated with polymicrogyria

28.All are true regarding Dandy-Walker malformation except
a. cerebellar dysgenesis
b. cystic dilatation of the 4th ventricle,
c. large posterior fossa
d. superior displacement of tentorium
e. a defect in development of the area membranacea superior

29.-All are true regarding technique of extradural tumour of spine except
a. Unenhanced MR scans generally are delineate extradural tumors superbly
b. MR is more sensitive than bone scan for marrow abnormalities
c. Fast spin echo (FSE) sequences increase visualization of a spinal bone tumor
d. Normal marrow is generally is of high signal intensity on T1W
e. Tumors usually are hypointense on T1W and hyperintense on T2W

30.All are true regarding spinal cord ependymoma except
a. the myxopapillary form-- particularly common in the conus and filum
b. often tend to be central in location
c. cylindrical, elongated masses
d. calcification extremely common
e. Cyst formation in 50% of the cases

31.All are true regading healing spondylodiscitis except
a. persistent disc space narrowing
b. hypointense disc on T2-weighted images
c. fusion of the adjacent vertebral bodies
d. resolution of the high signal intensity in the adjacent endplates
e. low signal intensity on T1W from a previously infected vertebra

32.All are true regarding dorsal dermal sinus except
a. the points of attachment of skin and cord are segmental or metameric
b. the sinus ostium is typically midline
c. the the dermal sinus tract extends into the spinal canal in one half to two thirds of cases
d. Approx.25% of all spinal epidermoids are associated with dermal sinuses
e. Thoracic and cervical dermal sinuses are usually associated with tethering of the spinal cord

33.All are true regarding development of vertebrae except
a. fissures of von Ebner form between the two half-sclerotomes
b. Chondrification begins in the lumber region
c. central ossification centers for the centra first appear at about 9 weeks' gestation
d. interpediculate distance at L1-4 is 70% of adult size at birth
e. A secondary ossification center for the tip normally fuses with the dens by age 12 years

34.All are true regarding pituitary

microadenoma except
a. unenhanced T1W Spin –echo is the primary imaging sequence for the pituitary gland
b. a plain scan followed by a repeat T1W coronal sequence immediately after i.v. contrast is the best imaging technique
c. delayed images (30 to 60 minutes after injection) is useless effort to detect microadenoma
d. The major limitation of MR of pituitary is the detection of very small adenomas (3 to 4 mm)
e. ACTH-secreting adenomas are the smallest and the most difficult to detect.

35. All are true regarding intracranial lesions except
a. The most common site of Intracranial schwannomas is the vestibular division of the eighth cranial nerve
b. The fifth cranial nerve is the second-most-common site of intracranial neuroma
c. the most frequent cranial nerve tumor to cause a parasellar mass is the fifth cranial nerve
d. Suprasellar arachnoid cysts arise from an imperforate membrane of Liliequist
e. Tuber Cinereum Hamartoma is isointense to gray matter on T1W and show strong enhancement

36. All are true regarding dynamic susceptibility contrast (DSC) MRI except
a. T2 and T2* are increased relative to normal physiologic value
b. the contrast agent is usually injected as a rapid bolus
c. images are acquired rapidly to monitor the signal change on time scales of 2 seconds or less
d. the tighter the bolus, the better
e. rapid the transit time of contrast through the tissue is a big challenge of DSC MRI

37. All are true regarding optic canal except
a. contents---Optic nerve and sheath; ophthalmic artery
b. present in basisphenoid
c. 6 mm diameter 8 mm long
d. 2 mm difference in size suspicious
e. keyhold and figure of eight variants

38. All are true regarding Diffusion-weighted imaging (DWI) except
a. the lower the ADC ---- the greater the signal loss on DW images
b. ADC is an indicator of disruption of tissue microstructure, cellular density and matrix
c. ADC measurements correlate inversely with the histological cell count of gliomas
d. DWI and ADC measurements assess the overall freedom of water-movement
e. DTI provides information about the direction of water diffusion

39. All are true regarding intraventricular lesions except
a. fourth ventricular ependymomas frequently extend through the foramina of Magendie and Luschka
b. Central neurocytomas shows susceptibility artefact from calcification and grey-matter-isointense nodules

c. Choroid plexus papilloma is as an iso- to hyperdense mass with punctate calcification and homogeneous enhancement
d. colloid cyst is characteristically hyperdense on unenhanced CTs
e. ependymoma is the commonest cause of a mass in the trigone of the lateral ventricle after the first decade of life

40. All are true regarding Haemorrhagic transformation except
a. due to secondary bleeding into reperfused ischaemic tissue
b. occurs during the first 2 weeks
c. in up to 55 per cent of infarcts on MRI
d. often seen in the basal ganglia and cortex
e. severity correlates with degree of contrast enhancement in the early stage

41. The method of choice for the investigation of cerebral AVMs and dural fistulae
a. Intra-arterial angiography
b. CTA
c. MRA
d. usg
e. none

42. All are true regarding HIV-related CNS disease except
a. Toxoplasmosis typically shows multiple lesions at the corticomedullary junction and in the basal ganglia
b. lesions of Primary cerebral lymphoma abut the ependyma, leptomeninges or both in 75 per cent.
c. A single enhancing mass lesion in AIDS is more likely to be lymphoma
d. Thallium-201 SPECT and FDG-PET show greater uptake in lymphoma than toxoplasmosis
e. commonest site of PML lesion in the brain is in the temporal regions

43. All are true regarding imaging of degenerative changes of spine except
a. a minimum midsagittal diameter of the cervical canal of less than 10 mm (tube-film distance around 2 m) indicates that cord compression is probably present.
b. the cross-sectional area of the canal of about 100 mm^2 or less show a consistent association with clinical cauda equina entrapment.
c. the MR signal returned from degenerate discs is usually higher than from healthy discs
d. signal change in the spinal cord do not always indicate permanent damage
e. Compression of the spinal cord is generally assessed best on axial imaging

44. All are true regarding cerebral malformation except
a. Alobar holoprosencephaly is the severest form
b. semi-lobar holoprosencephaly has single ventricle
c. de Morsier's syndrome includes the triad of hypopituitarism, hypoplasia of the optic nerves and absence of the septum pellucidum
d. a small or absent genu or body, with an intact splenium and rostrum, indicates congenital cause

e. callosal abnormalities are seen in Aicardi's syndrome

45. All are true regarding craniosynostosis except
a. The most common type of primary craniosynostosis is simple sagittal synostosis.
b. the Towne's view may be used to assess lamdoid and sagittal sutures
c. Skull growth decreases parallel to the suture and increases perpendicular to it.
d. Bicoronal synostosis produce 'harlequin' deformity,
e. Metopic synostosis causes trigonocephaly or 'keel deformity'

46. All are true regarding following diseases except
a. 3DFT-CISS imaging may be more sensitive than CT to the changes of labyrinthitis ossificans
b. restricted diffusion is noted in the central region of abscess
c. the racemose form of neurocysticercosis shows multilobular cysts with scolex within the subarachnoid space
d. The anterior temporal and inferior frontal cortical regions are a classical location for herpes encephalitis.
e. Thalamic and upper brainstem involvement is a feature of Japanese encephalitis

47. All are true regarding polyvinyl alcohol (PVA) except
a. particulate embolic material
b. supplied in sizes ranging from 50 to 1000 μm
c. diluted in radiopaque contrast medium
d. 15-150 micrometer particle more effective in inducing tumour necrosis
e. 15-150 micrometer particle carry lower risk of cranial nerve damage

48. All are true regarding skull except
a. Dolichocephalic---skull abnormally long in relation to relation to their transverse diameter
b. Bathrocephaly ---occipital bone overlaps the parietal bones at the lambdoid suture
c. Trigonocephaly---due to premature in utero fusion of metopic suture
d. scaphocephaly –due to premature fusion of the sagittal suture.
e. Plagiocephaly ----- due to bilateral premature fusion of the lambdoid and coronal sutures

49. All are true regarding skull lesions except
a. Paget's disease produce irregular mottled texture to the thickened skull hone.
b. hairbrush type of radiating linear spicules are noted in coolers anemia
c. blistering is noted in schwannoma
d. Leontiasis ossea refers to hyperostosis affecting the frontal bones and facial bones
e. normal brain growth is necessary for normal growth and moulding of the overlying skull.

50. All are true regarding artery except
a. the right vertebral artery originates as the first right

subclavian artery
b. the right vertebral aretery is the dominant vertebral artery in about 25% of cases
c. the right carotid artery typically bifurcates around the C3 to C5 level
d. the right and left vertebral artery are equal in size in approx. 25%
e. the middle meningeal artery has hairpin turn on angiogram

51. A complete circle of Willis is seen in
a. 20%
b. 45%
c. 55%
d. 65%
e. 75%

52. All are true regarding diffuse cerebral edema except
a. more in trauma of children than adult
b. severe edema usually takes 24—48 hrs to develop after trauma
c. -most reliable early imaging finding-- effacement of the surface sulci and the suprasellar and perimesencephalic sulci
d. cerebellum relatively hyperdense than cerebral hemishphere
e. hypodensity of thalamus ,brainstem and cerebellum compared to the cortex and deep white matter

53. All are true regarding brain tumour except
a. meningiomas are the most common mesenchymal neoplasm
b. Schwannomas show a definite predilection for motor nerves
c. teratoma is the most common intracranial;l tumour in the neonatal period
d. the optochiasmatic – hypothalamic area is the most common location for astrocytoma in childhood
e. about one third of posterior fossa neoplasm in children are crebellar astrocytoma

54. All are common causes of "holes in the skull" except
a. dermoid
b. eosinophilic granuloma
c. metastases
d. surgical
e. epidermod

55. All are true regarding heamangioblastoma except
a. 60% --cystic with nodule
b. 50% ---occur with VHL
c. 80% to 85% --in cerebellum
d. 60---show calcification
e. approx 45% of VHL develop haemangioblastoma

56. All are causes of ring enhancing lesions except
a. anaplastic astrocytoma
b. metastatic brain tumour
c. resolving hematoma
d. infarct
e. arachnoid cyst

57. All are causes of low signal in both basal ganglia(T2W) except
a. normal aging
b. long standing MS
c. hypoxic insults in children
d. parkinsonian syndrome
e. mitochondrial cytopathy

58. All are associated with absence of septum pellucidum except
a. aqueductal stenosis
b. Chiari II malformation
c. cephalocoele

d.porencephaly
e.lissencephaly
59. All are true regarding Alexander and Canavan disease except
a. massive deposition of Rosenthal fibres is noted in Alexander disease
b.frontal lobe hyperintensities on T2W image is seen in Alexander disease
c.canavan disease preferentially involves the subcortical U fibres
d.Canavan disease is also known as van Bogaert Bertrand disease
e.Low N-acetylaspartic acid is noted in Canavan disease
60.Associated anomalies with myelomeningocele are all except
a.Chiari II (virtually 100%)
b.syringohydromyelia(30% to 75%)
c.hydreocephalus (80%)
d.diastematomyelia (90%)
e.intracanalicular spinal lipoma (about 75%)

TEST PAPER 12(ANSWER)

1.—d
2.—d
At 24 hours approximately 90% of patients with infarction show changes in the T2-weighted sequence as compared with approximately 50% on T1-weighted images
Subcortical white matter hypointensity on T2-weighted images has been ascribed to iron, free radicals, sludging of deoxygenated red blood cells, or even incidental magnetization transfer effects. This hypointensity in acute cortical infarction is located within the subcortical white matter and therefore is most likely not due to hemorrhage, which characteristically is situated in the affected cortex.

3.----d
Greater than 99% of human tissue is diamagnetic. Materials that have no intrinsic magnetic field in the absence of an applied magnetic field but augment an applied magnetic field on exposure to it are termed paramagnetic. Naturally occurring paramagnetic substances include copper, iron, and manganese.

4.---b
The temporal evolution of MR intensity patterns in hemorrhagic malignancies is often delayed or different from those seen in benign intracranial hemorrhage. An important role for intravenous contrast is in distinguishing hemorrhagic tumor from hematomas without underlying lesions. This diagnosis can be revealed by any of the following findings: (a) intrahematoma enhancement in a presumed acute hematoma whereas benign hematomas do not show enhancement until they evolve into the subacute stage, when a thin rim of peripheral enhancement is seen; (b) irregular or nodular enhancement outside the area of the hemorrhage or (c) within a focal portion of the hematoma itself, regardless of age.

5.—c
Moyamoya disease has a bimodal age presentation, with the first peak occurring in the first decade of life, associated with cerebral infarction as progressive carotid occlusion develops. Adult patients most often present in the fourth decade with intracranial hemorrhage arising from the rupture of the delicate network of collateral vessels
Absence of the expected flow void within the cavernous and supraclinoid portions of the ICAs is a consequence of narrowing and ultimately occlusion of these vessels
There is increased incidence of moyamoya changes in patients with Down syndrome.

6.—b

Cavernous angioma is believed to be congenital, but the peak incidence of symptom onset is between the third and fifth decades of life.

7.-b

8.---d

A venous epidural, unlike a subdural hematoma, often lie both above and below the tentorium. Due to the lower pressure of the injured vein lesions may expand more slowly than arterial lesions and therefore may be delayed in onset.

9.---c

Different lesions in a brain are usually not in the same stage of disease progression. In the spinal cord, the plaques are often oval in shape and are oriented lengthwise. Other common changes include volume loss and atrophy of the optic nerve and optic chiasm, cerebral white matter, brainstem, and spinal cord . Hydrocephalus is present in about 5% to 10% of longstanding cases

10.----e

Heroin pyrolysate (obtained after heating the drug on aluminum foil; also called "chasing the dragon") produces a particular leukoencephalopathy with spongiform changes and characteristic involvement of the cerebellar white matter and posterior limb of the internal capsule, sparing the anterior limb and subcortical white matter on MR image.

11.----a

12.----e

13.-----d

14.---a

Frequently Cystic Tumors------
Colloid cyst
Craniopharyngioma
Desmoplastic infantile ganglioma
Dermoid
Ependymoma (supratentorial and spinal)
Epidermoid
Ganglion cell tumors
Glioblastoma (cystic necrosis)
Hemangioblastoma
Pilocytic astrocytoma
Pleomorphic xanthoastrocytoma
Rathke cleft cyst

15.---c

Infiltrative astrocytomas are derived typically from the fibrillary, which is found in cerebral white matter, as opposed to the protoplasmic astrocyte found in gray matter.

16.----a

Calcification is extremely common. Central regions of marked hypointensity can be seen on T2-weighted MR imaging and on gradient echo images due to susceptibility-induced signal loss from calcification and accompanying iron. Giant cell astrocytomas generally enhance with intravenous contrast , but the lack of enhancement cannot be used as exclusionary proof of this diagnosis. Moreover, the presence of enhancement in a subependymal nodule does not necessarily prove the diagnosis of giant cell astrocytoma.

17.---c

Colloid cyst is located at the anterosuperior aspect of the third ventricle, between the columns of the fornices.

One of the distinguishing features of colloid cysts from other neuroepithelial cysts, aside from location, is the composition of the cyst contents. Colloid cysts contain dense, turbid, mucoid material with numerous constituents, including old blood, hemosiderin within macrophages, cholesterol crystals, CSF, and various ions (sodium, magnesium, calcium, copper, silicon, aluminum, iron, and phosphorus).

18.----d

Besides invading the dura, clival chordoma may extend into the subarachnoid space but rarely invade the brain directly.

19.----e

Diffusion studies show increased motion of water within both the cystic and the solid portions of the tumor, with increased apparent diffusion coefficient (ADC) values –a point of difference from the solid component of cystic PNET

Cerebellar astrocytomas are hypointense on T1 and hyperintense on T2, proton density, and FLAIR . The solid portion of the tumor is typically more hyperintense than the solid component of otherwise similarly appearing cystic PNET

The cystic portions of the tumor often show only elevated lactate and a lack of other metabolites. The presence of lactate in the cystic portion of the tumor has nothing to do with the tumor being aggressive, as in the case of malignant glioma, where it reflects anaerobic metabolism. Lactate in the cyst fluid of low-grade astrocytoma reflects the byproducts of metabolism that seep into the cysts. There is a low incidence of blood products in the wall of the cyst

Cerebellar astrocytomas do not present acutely as hemorrhagic masses, a finding that, when present, suggests a more aggressive tumor such as a PNET, atypical teratoid rhabdoid tumor (ATRT), or a tumor with a tendency to hemorrhage such as an ependymoma

20.---b

Desmoplastic infantile ganglioglioma (DIG) is a WHO grade I variant of the ganglioglioma that arises in infants.

The tumor originates superficially from pia and cortex, so that the solid portion of the tumor lies peripherally within the mass and the typically large cyst remain located deep to the solid tumor.

21.---c

FLAIR sequences are superior to other MR images in depicting meningeal inflammatory changes, showing hyperintense signal intensity in the subarachnoid space contrasting against the normal CSF portrayed as black. A dural, pachymeningeal, enhancement follows the inner contour of the calvaria, and a pial-subarachnoid, leptomeningeal, enhancement extends into the cerebral and cerebellar sulci and fissures

22.----b

Intraventricular neurocysticercosis generally does not enhance.

Three-dimensional constructive interference in a steady-state MR sequence (3D-CISS) is able to better demonstrate not only the intraventricular cysts. Diffusion-weighted imaging demonstrates signal intensity similar to CSF, without restricted diffusion . This fact can be helpful in the differential diagnosis with a brain abscess that has characteristically restricted diffusion caused by the viscous pus content , whereas cysticercosis lesions do not have hyperperfusion. Perfusion imaging can be used to establish the differential diagnosis with brain neoplasms . MR spectroscopy analysis shows decreased NAA and creatine peaks and increased lactate, alanine, succinate, and choline levels .

23.---a

The major pathologic features that characterize AD are senile plaques, neurofibrillary tangles, decreased synaptic density, neuron loss, and cerebral atrophy .

Neurofibrillary tangles consist of pathologic aggregates of tau protein--- component of the microtubule system is tau protein It is well established that the neurofibrillary pathology of AD begins in the transentorhinal area and progresses to the hippocampus, to paralimbic and adjacent medial-basal temporal cortex, to neocortical association areas, and lastly to primary sensory-motor and visual areas The second pathologic lesion associated with AD is the senile (neuritic) plaque. Neuritic plaque consists of a dense central β-amyloid core with inflammatory cells and dystrophic neurites in its periphery.

24.---c

The Wilson results from loss of function of the copper transport protein ATP7B.

The differential diagnosis of unexplained hepatic disease in a young patient should include WD . Neurologic and/or psychiatric manifestations more commonly present in young adults aged 19 to 20 years.

The Kayser-Fleischer ring, a granular deposit of copper in Descemet's membrane of the cornea, is virtually diagnostic of WD . The definitive diagnosis is made biochemically, with low levels of serum ceruloplasmin, increased rate of urinary copper excretion, and elevated hepatic copper levels

once the diagnosis is established in symptomatic patients with WD, screening of all first-degree relatives (siblings and children) is necessary to detect presymptomatic patients who would benefit from treatment to prevent hepatic and cerebral disease and to detect asymptomatic carriers who would benefit from genetic counseling.

25.---e

The retinal lesion of TS (van der Hoeve' phakoma may be similar to retinoblastoma in location (retina) and age at presentation (childhood), are frequently multiple and often bilateral, and have the common presence of calcification within the hamartoma. However, unlike retinoblastoma, they are not necrotic, do not hemorrhage, do not fungate, nor grow into the vitreous or invade through the retina into the surrounding choroid or sclera.

26.---e

The septum pellucidum is absent in alobar holoprosencephaly

27.---e

Prenatal CMV may be associated with polymicrogyria

28.---d

The Dandy-Walker Malformation may be defined as a cystic malformation of the posterior fossa resulting from a defect in development of the area membranacea superior, and exhibiting the common phenotypic triad of cerebellar dysgenesis, cystic dilatation of the 4th ventricle, and a large posterior fossa with superior displacement of the dural sinuses and tentorium.

29.—c

Fast spin echo (FSE) sequences must be used with caution because the persistent high signal of surrounding fat on T2-weighted images may decrease visualization of a tumor.

Two objectives exist in the MR evaluation of spinal tumors in the epidural space: (a) the detection of vertebral body lesions, even if there is no suspicion of epidural impingement; and (b) the delineation of possible thecal sac impingement.

Unenhanced MR scans generally are superb at delineating extradural tumors, whether they are primary or secondary

30.---d

Ependymoma is the most common primary cord tumor of the lower spinal cord, conus medullaris, and filum terminale. Ependymomas often tend to be central in location and exhibit centrifugal growth.

Ependymomas are cylindrical, elongated masses that cause localized fusiform expansion of the spinal cord. They are brownish red to blue in color, depending on their blood content. Although ependymomas in the brain frequently calcify, calcification is extremely uncommon in spinal ependymomas.

The most common lesion of the filum terminale is the myxopapillary type, in which mucinous change also is seen. This type especially is prone to hemorrhage and can present as an unexplained subarachnoid bleed

31.---e

The finding of high signal intensity on T1-weighted images from a previously infected vertebra reflects replacement of cellular marrow by fat, indicating healing. Once adequate antibiotic treatment has been instituted, the clinical symptoms improve dramatically, whereas the MR findings evolve much more slowly

32.---e
Lumbosacral dermal sinuses are usually associated with tethering of the spinal cord and low position of the conus (80%).
Thoracic and cervical dermal sinuses do not appear to influence conal position
Some 15% to 20% of patients with dermal sinus have concurrent lipoma, and vice versa, presumably because both lesions result from deranged disjunction of cutaneous from neural ectoderm.

33.---b
Chondrification begins in the cervicothoracic region and extends outward from there both cranially and caudally
The axis (C-2) usually develops from four primary ossification centers: one for the dens, one for the body, and two for the neural arches. These primary centers fuse by ages 3 to 6 years. A secondary ossification center for the tip of the dens normally appears at ages 3 to 6 years and fuses with the dens by age 12 years.

34.---c
In a small number of cases, the dynamic study will demonstrate an adenoma that is otherwise occult. If these images are all negative or equivocal, delayed images (30 to 60 minutes after injection) can in some instances demonstrate reversal of this image contrast because of the accumulation of Gd-DTPA in the adenoma and washout from the normal gland.

35.---e
The most frequent presenting complaint of Tuber Cinereum Hamartoma is that of precocious puberty.
Hamartomas have been consistently reported as isointense to gray matter on T1-weighted MR.
Contrast enhancement should not occur because hamartomas should possess an intact blood–brain barrier, equivalent to that of normal brain tissue.
Contrast enhancement in any hypothalamic mass is highly atypical for hamartoma and would suggest another diagnosis.

36.---a
When contrast agent is present in high concentration in the vasculature, T2 and T2* are decreased relative to normal physiologic values. Smaller T2 or T2* means that the signal intensity on T2- and T2*-weighted images is decreased relative to normal

37.----d
I mm difference in size of optic canal is suspicious

38.---a
Diffusion-weighted imaging (DWI) measures Brownian motion of water molecules within the tissue. Isotropic-trace-weighted DW images are obtained by measuring the signal loss on typically T2W images following the application of diffusion gradients. The signal loss depends on several factors

including the gradient strength and apparent diffusion coefficient (ADC), which describes water diffusibility in tissue.

The more mobile the water molecules are, the higher the ADC and the greater the signal loss on DW images

The tendency of water to move in some directions more than others is called anisotropy and can be quantified using parameters such as fractional anisotropy (FA). Compact white matter tracts show normally a high degree of anisotropy, which can be lost if they are infiltrated by tumour cells, which destroy the ultrastructural boundaries formed by myelin sheaths.

39.------e

Meningiomas is the commonest cause of a mass in the trigone of the lateral ventricle after the first decade of life

Central neurocytomas are s relatively benign tumours and probably the commonest lateral ventricular masses in in the second and third decades of life .

40.---c

Haemorrhagic transformation is shown in up to 80 per cent of infarcts on MRI, appearing hyperintense on T1-weighted and hypointense on T2-weighted images. It is often seen in the basal ganglia and cortex, where it can assume a gyriform pattern . The occurrence and severity of haemorrhagic transformation correlates with the size of the infarct and degree of contrast enhancement in the early stage.

41.----a

42.----e

Commonest site of PML is in the parieto-occipital regions. MRI shows multifocal, asymmetric bilateral white matter lesions that are of high signal on T2W and low signal on T1W images . Extension to the subcortical U-fibres gives the lesions a characteristic 'scalloped' appearance

43.----c

The MR signal returned from degenerate discs is usually lower than from healthy discs and best appreciated on T2W images.

44.---d

The anterior part (posterior genu and anterior body) is formed before the posterior part (posterior body and splenium). Thus a small or absent genu or body, with an intact splenium and rostrum, indicates secondary destruction rather than abnormal development. The structure develops between about 7 and 20 weeks gestation

There are many well-defined syndromes in which callosal abnormalities feature, including Aicardi's syndrome characterized by seizures, intellectual impairment and brain abnormalities. Callosal agenesis is a feature of oculocerebrocutaneous syndrome or Delleman's syndrome .

Dysgenesis of the corpus callosum is frequently seen in fetal alcohol syndrome.

45.---c

Skull growth decreases perpendicular to the suture and

increases parallel to it.

46.---c
In the racemose form of neurocysticercosis, there are multilobular cysts without a scolex within the subarachnoid space, typically in the cerebellopontine angles, suprasellar region and basal cisterns and Sylvian fissures.
Labyrinthitis ossificans is the most common cause of acquired deafness in childhood. High-resolution T2-weighted MRI (e.g. performed with 3DFT-CISS imaging) may be more sensitive than CT to the changes of labyrinthitis ossificans, and T2 signal drop-off may detect the fibrous stage before ossification when children are still suitable for cochlear implantation.

47.---e
15-150 micrometer particle carry higher risk of cranial nerve damage or skin damage.

48.---e
Plagiocephaly (oblique or slanting skull) describes a skull that is markedly asymmetric due to unilateral premature fusion of the lambdoid and coronal sutures. Microcephaly *is* associated with a generalised premature fusion of all the skull sutures and the skull vault is abnormally small Oxycephaly (pointed skull), acrocephaly (peak or summit skull) and turricephaly (tower skull) are all terms used to describe the brachycephalic skull which results from premature fusion of the coronal and lambdoid sutures.

49.---c
Normal brain growth is necessary for normal growth and moulding of the overlying skull.
With meningiomas arising in the region of the jugum or anterior clinoid, a rare manifestation is local bone expansion with pneumatisation, so-called ` blistering.

50.---e
Superficial temporal artery has hairpin turn on angiogram

51.----a

52.----e
Normal density of thalamus, brainstem and cerebellum compared to the cortex and deep white matter (the reversal sign) and relatively hyperdense cerebellum than cerebral hemishphere (white cerebellum sign) are features of diffusecerebral edema.

53.---b
Schwannomas show a definite predilection for sensory nerves

54.----e

55.---b
10% to 20% haemangioblastoma occur with VHL

56.---e

57.---e
High signal in both basal ganglia on T2W is seen in venous infarcts, HIE, toxic encephalopathy and mitochondrial cytopathy.

58.---e

59.—b
High N-acetylaspartic acid is increased in urine, plasma and brain in Canavan disease

60.---d

Diastematomyelia is seen in 30% to 45%)

TEST PAPER 13

1. Who were jointly awarded the Nobel Prize in Physiology or Medicine (2003) "for their discoveries concerning magnetic resonance imaging"
a) Lauterbur and Sir Peter Mansfield
b) Bloch and Purcell
c) Ernst and Anderson
d) Jackson and Damadian
e) Aberdeen and Nottingham

2. Conventional MR findings in acute infarction are all except
a. Lesion in the arterial distribution
b. High intensity FLAIR and T2-weighted images
c. Gyri swollen, sulci effaced
d. Absence of arterial flow void
e. lack of intravascular contrast enhancement

3. Possible etiologies of arterial infarction in Older Children and Young Adults is/are
a. cyanotic congenital heart disease
b. mitochondrial disorders
c. lysosomal disorders
d. organic acidurias
e. all

4. All are features of hemorrhage on MRI of Hemorrhagic neoplasm except
a. Multiple stages of hematoma in same lesion
b. Debris–fluid levels
c. Persistent deoxyhemoglobin absent hemosiderin
d. identification of nonneoplastic tissue
e. hemosiderin present significantly

5. The most common clinically symptomatic cerebrovascular malformation is
a. AVM
b. cavernous angioma
c. capillary telangiectasia
d. venous angioma
e. the dural AVM (DAVM)

6. Causes of cryptic AVMs(angiographically occult small AVMs) is/are
a. compression of the lesion by adjacent hematoma
b. vasospasm
c. extremely slow flow
d. thrombosis
e. all

7. All are true regarding venous angioma except
a. a spoke wheel–appearing collection of small, tapering veins arranged in a radial pattern
b. normal arterial and capillary phases
c. opacification of the lesion usually remain opacified through the late venous phase
d. typically intimately associated with the lateral ventricle and draining into a subependymal vein
e. MRA is necessary in most cases.

8. The Guglielmi detachable coil (GDC) is composed of
a. platinum
b. silver
c. tungsten
d. zirconium
e. roententium

9. The size of giant intracranial aneurysm exceeds
a. 1.5 cm
b. 2.5 cm
c. 3.5 cm
d. 4.5 cm
e. 5.5 cm

10. All are true regarding epidural hematoma except
a. most commonly of arterial origin
b. usually arise from direct laceration or tearing of the middle meningeal artery
c. fracture is present in 85% to 95% of cases
d. arterial epidurals typically occur in the temporal or temporoparietal region
e. dura is visualized as a thin line of low signal intensity between the brain and the crescentric-shaped hematoma

11. All are true regarding multiple sclerosis except
a. most periventricular plaques are seen anatomically related to subependymal veins
b. periventricular plaques are predominantly near the angles of the lateral ventricles
c. MS plaques are never seen entirely within gray matter
d. show multiple well-defined lesions scattered throughout white matter
e. Different lesions in a brain are usually not in the same stage of disease progression

12. An old alcoholic patient developed spastic quadriparesis, pseudobulbar palsy, and changing levels of consciousness after rapid correction of hyponatremia. On suspicion of Osmotic demyelination syndrome, MRI of brain was done. All the findings favour osmotic demyelination except
a. involvement of pons, external capsule and deep gray matter
b. sparing of corticospinal tracts in pons
c. the bilateral asymmetric involvement of the central pons
d. high signal intensity on the T2-weighted sequences and restricted diffusion
e. sparing of the peripheral pial and ventricular surface

13. The "tigroid" pattern of demyelination is seen in
a. Pelizaeus-Merzbacher disease
b. Canavan disease
c. Alexander disease
d. Vanishing white matter disease
e. Zellweger Syndrome

14. The most commonly performed neurosurgical procedures for refractory complex partial seizures is
a. anterior temporal lobectomy
b. Lesionectomy
c. Nonlesional cortical resection
d. Corpus callosotomy
e. Hemispherectomy

15. All are true regarding malformation of cortical development except
a. dysembryoplastic neuroepithelial tumor is a glial abnormalities
b. tuberous sclerosis shows abnormal neuronal proliferation
c. hemimegalencephaly has contralateral ventricular enlargement,
d. cortical thickening and radial

bands extending toward the ventricle is noted in tuberous sclerosis
e. balloon cell focal cortical dysplasia of Taylor appears hyperintense on T2W

16. Causes of high intensity in tumors on T1W MR are all except
a. Subacute-chronic blood (methemoglobin)
b. Melanin
c. Very low (nonparamagnetic) protein concentration
d. Fat
e. Flow-related enhancement in tumor vessels

17. All are true regarding brain tumour except
a. The gliomas comprise nearly half of all intracranial tumors
b. almost half of gliomas are glioblastoma multiforme
c. Most adult gliomas are supratentorial
d. the incidence ---- astrocytoma 20.5%, ependymoma 6%,
e. infiltrative astrocytomas comprise approximately 25% of astrocytic tumors of the CNS

18. All are true regarding imaging of oligodendroglioma except
a. usually heterogeneous but isointense to gray matter on T2W
b. the cortical infiltration and marked cortical thickening
c. Conventional spin echo MR imaging highly sensitive to calcification of tumour
d. edema is usually not a significant feature of lower-grade oligodendrogliomas
e.. Contrast enhancement in about one half of cases

19. All are true regarding pineoblastoma except
a. typically found in children
b. Hemorrhage –uncommon
c. Calcification---common
d. Enhancement---dense
e. tendancy to disseminate through the subarachnoid pathways

20. All are true regarding intracranial lymphoma except
a. propensity for leptomeningeal involvement
b. extend along the Virchow-Robin spaces
c. Subarachnoid involvement usually not identified with CT
d. hypointense to gray matter on T2W
e. Contrast-enhanced images usually reveal more extensive meningeal spread

21. All are true regarding cerebellar astocytoma in paediatric age group except
a. the most common cerebellar hemispheric tumor of glial origin
b. The most frequent astrocytoma is the pilocytic (85%) and fibrillary (15%)
c. The pilocytic astrocytoma belongs to grade II of WHO classification
d. The juvenile pilocytic astrocytomas are unencapsulated
e. Glioblastomas of the cerebellum may be radiation induced

22. All are true regarding Ganglioglioma except
a. characterized by slow growth
b. most frequently located in the temporal and frontal lobes
c. 50% are cystic and 50% are

solid
d. 50% show calcifications
e. 50% show contrast enhancement

23. All are true regarding brain abscess except
a. MRS pattern derived from the central portion of an abscess appears to be fairly characteristic
b. MRS can be of some use in the etiologic classification of brain abscesses
c. DWI can be of great use in the evaluation of treatment response
d. Spectroscopy can be useful in the assessment of response to treatment
e. MR perfusion sequences usually display higher rCBV values in the brain abscess capsule

24. All are true regarding racemose variety of neurocysticercosis except
a. frequently infiltrates the basal cisterns and sylvian fissure
b. Scolices are usually not seen in subarachnoid cysts
c. may cause ventriculitis and obstructive hydrocephalus
d. usually does not calcify after degeneration
e. subarachnoid cysts is easily identified MRI

25. All are true regarding risk factor of Alzheimer disease except
a. increasing age and positive family history
b. Carriers of the apolipoprotein e2 allele
c. the amyloid precursor protein gene on chromosome 21
d. the presenilin-1 gene on chromosome 14
e. the presenilin-2 gene on chromosome 1

26. All are true regarding imaging of brain in hepatic encephalopathy except
a. abnormally increased signal on T1W (hyperintense relative to white matter) within extrapyramidal nuclei
b. Hyperintense signal on T1W in the anterior pituitary gland, the quadrigeminal plate, and the hemispheric white matter.
c. The hyperintense signal on T1W is believed to be due to deposition of manganese
d. abnormal hyperintense gray and/or white matter foci on long-TR sequences
e. increase of ml, choline, glutamine and glutamate

27. All are true regarding spinocerebellar Ataxias except
a. SCA2 shows "hot cross bun" sign
b. Friedreich ataxia is the commonest hereditary ataxia
c. the basis pontis and the cerebellum is preserved in Friedrich ataxia
d. Ataxia Telangiectasia is characterized by atrophy of the cerebellar vermis and cerebellar hemispheres
e. Vit E causes ataxia

28. All are true regarding Motor neurone disease except
a. Motor neuron diseases cause the degeneration of the upper and/or lower motor neurons
b. Amyotrophic lateral sclerosis (ALS) is the most frequent type of motor neuron disease

c. hyperintense signal in the corticospinal tract of FLAIR in ALS
d. Hypointense signal on the T2W and FLAIR sequences in the motor cortex in ALS
e. an increase in mean diffusivity and a increase in fractional anisotropy of the corticospinal tract in ALS

29. Polymicrogyria are associated with all except
a. the Adams-Oliver
b. Aicardi
c. Kallman
d. Goldberg-Shprintzen
e. Warburg

30. All are true regarding intracranial lipoma except
a. subarachnoid choristomas,--- congenital malformations
b. due to maldifferentiation of the meninx primitive
c. most common location ---36% pericallosal, 25% quadrigeminal/superior cerebellar cisterns
d. intracranial vessels and cranial nerves often course around lipomas
e. interhemispheric lipomas are nearly always associated with hypogenesis of the corpus callosum

31. All are true regarding spinal tumour except
a. In intradural extramedullary masses, the subarachnoid space is widened and caps the lesion
b. The most common diagnosis in the scenario of a lesion occupying two compartments is meningioma
c. metastases are far more common in the extradural space
d. primary tumors are relatively common in the intradural etramedullary space
e. primary tumors are far more common than metastases in the intramedullary space

32. All are true regarding imaging of astocytoma of spinal cord
a. associated with reactive and neoplastic cysts
b. low signal intensity on T1W.
c. almost always cord enlargement (marked)
d. the margins --- well defined
e. enhancement nearly always present in some part of the lesion

33. All are true regarding The MR findings of spondylodiscitis except
a. Near endplates or near whole vertebrae: low intensity on T1W and high intensity on T2W
b. High intensity and loss of the internuclear cleft on T2W
c. Loss of a margin between disc and vertebral bodies
d. Irregularities and destruction of the vertebral endplates
e. Osseous and extraaxial abscesses show no restricted diffusion with dark appearance on ADC map

34. All are true regarding associated feature of Myelocele and myelomeningocele except
a. Hydromyelia is observed at necropsy in 30% to 50% of patients with myelomeningocele
b. Lipomas are found in 6% of newborn untreated myelomeningoceles
c. Diastematomyelia is seen in 31% to 46% of patients with myelomeningocele
d. Overall, 80% of patients with

myelomeningocele have scoliosis by age 10 years
e. Myelocele and myelomeningocele are nearly never associated the Chiari II malformation

35.All are true regarding vertebral development except
a. Rostrocaudal patterning of the somites appears to be controlled by the Hox code
b. Pax6 is not expressed in the open neural tube
c. Noggin stimulate BMP-4
d. low noggin expression is related to emigration of the neural crest cells
e. The expression of BMP-4 is homogeneous along the length of the embryo

36.All are true regading pituitary microadenoma except
a. ACTH-secreting microadenomas are on average the smallest of all adenomas
b. prolactin and growth hormone microadenomas have a predilection to a lateral position within the gland
c. Growth hormone microadenomas tend to demonstrate infrasellar extension rather than suprasellar extension
d. T2 hypointensity is seen more commonly in sparsely granulated GH-secreting adenomas
e. Tilt of the stalk is a poor lateralizing sign of intrapituitary pathology

37.All are true regarding intracranial pathology except
a. Almost all cranial chordomas are found in relation to the clivus
b. Ecchordosis refers to a nodule of benign cells of notochordal origin
c. Pituicytoma and Granular Cell Tumors is situated anteriorly within the gland
d. Pituicytoma and Granular Cell Tumors are extremely vascular
e. chordomas are histologically benign but locally invasive and destructive

38.All are true regarding dynamic susceptibility contrast (DSC) MRI except
a. injection of a bolus of magnetic contrast agent
b. bolus tracking
c. usually performed using T2* or T2 contrast
d. no exogenous contrast agents
e. meant for perfusion study

39.All are true regarding the apparent diffusion coefficient (ADC) except
a. Quantitative analysis (ADC) requires sequences with at least two different b-values
b. ADC maps are solely based on differences of tissue diffusion
c. The ADC in the normal brain ranges from 2.94×10^3 mm
d. Areas with a decreased ADC appear dark on ADC maps
e. ADC maps are dependent on T2 effects

40.All are true regarding permeability imaging (K^{trans})except
a. Microvascular permeability of brain tumours can be quantified by measuring the transfer coefficient K^{TRANS}
b. T1W steady-state method of K^{TRANS} can be combined with DSC perfusion imaging

c. T1W steady-state has a higher spatial resolution and is more accurate than first-pass T2*W gradient-echo technique.
d. T1W steady-state requires longer acquisition times and more complicated post-processing than first-pass T2*W gradient-echo technique.
e. K^{TRANS} correlates with tumour grade

41. All are correctly matched typical location of intraventricular tumour except
a. Colloid cyst--- Foramen of Monro/third ventricle
b. Meningioma--- third ventricle
c. Choroid--- Fourth ventricle
d. Neurocytoma--- Lateral ventricles (involving septum pellucidum)
e. Ependymoma---Lateral ventricle and fourth ventricle

42. All are true regarding subacute phase of infarct except
a. low attenuation on CT and T2 hyperintensity on MRI involving both gray and white matter
b. Contrast enhancement on CT and MR
c. swelling usually increases during the first two week
d. Lack of enhancement of large cortical lesions on MRI suggests alternative diagnoses
e. gyriform enhancement is most characteristic of a cortical infarct

43. All are true regarding intracerebral haemorrhage except
a. The preferential sites of hypertensive haemorrhage is cerebellum and medulla
b. Peripheral / lobar haemorrhages in the elderly are suggestive of amyloid angiopathy,
c. may be caused by cocaine and ecstasy
d. blood–fluid level may to be noted in haemorrhage from coagulopathies
e. a haemorrhage in the basal ganglia in a young, normotensive patient may be due to AVM

44. All are true regarding cryptococcosis in AIDS except
a. second commonest opportunistic CNS infection in AIDS
b. dilatation of perivascular spaces, most often in the basal ganglia
c. cryptococcomas lack surrounding oedema
d. cryptococcomas do not show restricted diffusion
e. cryptococcomas show very prominent enhancement

45.--- All are true regarding degenerative changes of spine except
a. the commonest site of protrusion is located posterioriorly
b. type 1 reactive changes yield high signal on T1W and high on T2W
c. Ossification OPLL involves the mid- and lower cervical region in over 90 per cent of cases
d. Retro-odontal pseudotumour refers to thickened transverse ligament of the atlas and associated ligaments
e. 'snake eyes' appearance within the spinal cord on axial images is seen in Cervical spondylotic

myelopathy

46. All are true regarding Chiari II malformation except
a. inferior displacement of the cerebellum
b. an inferiorly displaced and elongated fourth ventricle
c. beaking of the tectum
d. enlarged the massa intermedia of the thalami
e. tube-shaped foramen magnum

47. All are true regarding Disorders of heavy metal metabolism except
a. Hyperintensities on T2W are seen in the basal ganglia, midbrain and pons, thalami and claustra in wilson disease
b. subdural haematomas is noted in Menke's disease
c. a 'panda face' in mid brain with involvement of the substantia nigra and tegmentum is noted in Krabbe's disease
d. MELAS shows cerebral infarcts in nonvascular territories and symmetrical basal ganglia calcification.
e. periventricular germinolytic cysts, peri-Sylvian polymicrogyria are seen in Zellweger's syndrome

48. All are true regarding venous infarcts except
a. often bilateral
b. frequently haemorrhagic.
c. parasagittal in the superior sagittal sinus involvement
d. basal ganglia in vein of Galen involvement
e. temporal lobe in vein of Labbé involvement

49. All are true regarding Chiari II malformation except
a. large posterior fossa
b. lacunar skull
c. beaked tctum
d. hydrocehalus
e. medullary spur and kink

50. All are true regarding angioplasty and stenting of exctracranial vessels except
a. primary stenting is the endovascular technique of choice for carotid artery stenosis,
b. The majority of major strokes after carotid PTA are the result of dissection of the carotid artery.
c. Carotid stenting is generally performed under general anaesthesia
d. filters and occlusion balloons are used to catch any embolic material released during stenting
e. The self-expandable stent adapts to the different diameters of the common and internal carotid arteries

51. All are causes of high signal in both basal ganglia(T1W) except
a. hepatocellular degeneration
b. Leigh disease
c. calcification
d. NF
e. Mn toxicity

52. All are true regarding anatomy of skull except
a. The optic canal is 4-9 mm long and 4-6.5 mm in maximum diameter
b. A length of l 1 -16 mm and a depth of 8-12 mm of pituitary fossa are regarded as within normal limits
c. The J-shaped sella is seen in children with 'gargoylism',
d. The calcification in habenular commissure is typically L-shaped
e. The posterior fontanel closes at

3-6 months

53. All are true regarding skull lesions except
a. Glioma of the optic canal cause expansion of the optic foramen
b. syphilis of the skull vault produces an extensive `moth-eaten' appearance
c. Large retro-orbital aneurysm may cause erosion of the optic strut
d. NF may produce congenital defect in the occipital bone
e. miliary osteoporosis of skull may be seen in hypoparathyroidism

54. All are true regarding imaging the dopamine transporter system except
a. 23 1-FP-CIT (ioflupane) for demonstrating the presynaptic dopamine transporter
b. 1-beta-CIT for demonstrating the presynaptic dopamine transporter
c. '3 1-iodobenzamide (IBZM) for demonstrating the presynaptic dopamine transporter
d. with '- 3 1-FPCIT images can be obtained on the same day as injection
e. SPELT imaging may be abnormal 3 years or more before the onset of clinical symptoms

55. All are true of congenital HIV except
a. maternally transmitted
b. diffuse cerebral atrophy
c. basal ganglia calcification
d. progressive encephalopathy in 30 to 50% cases
e. good prognosis

56. All are true regarding descending transtentorial herniation except
a. medial displacement of the uncus and parahippocampal gyrus
b. effacement of ipsilateral suprasellar cistern
c. enlargement of ipsilateral cerebellopontine angle cistern
d. periaqueductal necrosis
e. medullary hemorrhage (Duret hemorrhage)

57. All are true regarding brain tumour except
a. primary neoplasm account for approx. two-thirds of all brain tumours
b. pilocystic astrocytoma occur in the hypothalamus and visual pathways
c. cortical involvement is common in oligodendroglioma
d. cellular ependymoma occur exclusively in the spinal cord
e. choroid plexus tumour are mostly found in the atrium of lateral ventricle

58. All are common causes of thick skull except
a. chronic dilantin therapy
b. microcephalic brain
c. shunted hydrocephalus
d. osteogenesis imperfect
e. fibrous dysplasia

59. Lesions that may mimic meningiomas are all except
a. cavernous angioma
b. dermoid cyst
c. hemangiopericytoma
d. metastases
e. extramedullary hematopoiesis

60. All are true regarding septooptic dysplasia (SOD) except
a. overrexpression of dorsalizing gradient genes

b. optic nerve hypoplasia and deficiency of the septum pellucidum
c. HESX1 gene implicated
d. concurrent schizencephaly in 50% of patients
e. hypoplasia of the hypothalamus

TEST PAPER 13(ANSWER)

1.----a
2.---e
Intravascular contrast enhancement is noted in acute infarction.
3.---e
4.---e
Inappropriate enhancement with acute hematoma, perihematoma "edema" and mass effect in late hemorrhage are other features of hemorrhagic neoplasm. There is marked heterogeneity, due to mixed stages of hemorrhage, debris fluid (intracellular-extracellular blood) levels, edema + tumor + necrosis with blood. There is delayed evolution of blood-breakdown products. Absent, diminished, or very irregular hypointense rim representing iron storage forms is noted
5.---a
6.---e
7—e
MRA is unnecessary in most cases. GRE imaging can occasionally show marked hypointensity within venous angiomas. This should not be mistaken for hemorrhage; it is simply a reflection of the paramagnetic deoxyhemoglobin within venous blood.
8.—b
GDCs are composed of platinum and therefore are nonferromagnetic, and thus magnetic susceptibility artifact and signal loss should be minimal when endovascularly treated aneurysms are imaged with MR techniques
9.---b
10.---e
In epidural hematoma, the dura can often be seen to be displaced away from the inner table of the skull. It is visualized as a thin line of low signal intensity between the brain and the lenticular-shaped hematoma. Visualization of the dura on MR scans allows one to be absolutely certain of the diagnosis of an epidural hematoma.
11.---c
Although MS plaques are typically situated within white matter, gray matter lesions are not uncommon on pathologic examination. In the study of Brownell and Hughes 74% of plaques were found to be distributed in the deep white matter, whereas 17% were entirely within gray matter. Typically, MS lesions go through different stages, including an acute "active" stage, followed by a subacute stage with plaques with radially expanding "active rims" and plaques with "smoldering rims," and finally reach the "inactive" gliotic stage.
12.—c
The key to the MR diagnosis is the bilateral symmetric involvement of the central pons and deep and capsular white matter, often

accompanied by abnormalities in the thalami and basal ganglia.
The pontine lesion is central, with characteristic sparing of the peripheral pial and ventricular surface . Gadolinium contrast enhancement is occasionally seen in the periphery of the signal abnormality.
On gross examination, the classic pontine demyelinating lesions appear as triangular or butterfly-like areas of symmetric gray discoloration along the midline of the basis pontis . A rim of normal white matter typically surrounds the area of demyelination, and the tegmentum is usually not involved.

13.---a
Pelizaeus-Merzbacher disease is an X-linked disease affecting males.Itresults from a mutation of the proteolipid protein (PLP) gene on Xq21.33-22 that leads to abnormal PLP and DM20 proteins, the two most abundant proteins in the myelin sheath.
The brain is usually atrophic, and the condition is particularly severe in the posterior fossa (cerebellum and brainstem)

14.----a
Anterior temporal lobectomy and selective amgdalohippocampactomy are the most commonly performed neurosurgical procedures for refractory complex partial seizures is

15.---c
Features of hemimegalencephaly include hemispheric enlargement (or a portion of it), white matter hyperintensity, ipsilateral ventricular enlargement, heterotopia, and thickened cortex.
Glial abnormalities consist of developmental neoplasms such as dysembryoplastic neuroepithelial tumor , ganglioglioma, and gangliocytoma. These abnormalities are usually cortical in location and appear as focal lesions on MR, often with a cystic component.
 Abnormal neuronal proliferation is typified by disorders with "balloon cell" proliferation , such as tuberous sclerosis, balloon cell focal cortical dysplasia of Taylor, and hemimegalencephaly.
Balloon cells are large progenitor cells with both neural and glial characteristics.
The imaging findings in balloon cell focal cortical dysplasia(type II focal cortical dysplasia) and tuberous sclerosis are similar . Both have hyperintense cortical lesions on T2-weighted images, often with cortical thickening and radial bands extending toward the ventricle.
However, unlike tuberous sclerosis, the balloon cell focal cortical dysplasia is not associated with multiplicity of cortical lesions, subependymal nodules, or systemic manifestations (such as the cardiac, renal, and dermatologic abnormalities found in tuberous sclerosis).
Because of focal hyperintensity on T2-weighted images, balloon cell cortical dysplasia may mimic a tumor. Other features of balloon

cell dysplasia (i.e., cortical thickening, homogeneous bright signal in subcortical white matter, and radial bands) facilitate the distinction. This differentiation may be crucial for surgical management.

16.----c
Causes of High Intensity in Tumors on T1-Weighted Magnetic Resonance Images

Paramagnetic effects from hemorrhage	Subacute-chronic blood (methemoglobin)
Paramagnetic material without hemorrhage	Melanin Naturally occurring ions associated with necrosis of calcification Manganese Iron Copper
Nonparamagnetic effects	Very high (nonparamagnetic) protein concentration Fat Flow-related enhancement in tumor vessels

17.---e
Astrocytic brain tumors can be divided into two major groups : the infiltrative fibrillary, or "diffuse," astrocytomas (WHO grades II to IV) and the localized, noninfiltrative astrocytomas (WHO grade I and sometimes II). Infiltrative astrocytomas comprise approximately 75% of astrocytic tumors of the CNS, and localized tumors make up the remainder.

Most of childhood gliomaa are infratentorial.

18.---c
Gradient echo imaging (not Conventional spin echo) MR imaging is highly sensitive to calcification. Linear or nodular tumoral calcification on CT has been reported in 50% to 90% of oligodendrogliomas, which are the intracranial tumors with the highest frequency of calcification. Pronounced thickening of cortex in a heterogeneous intraaxial mass should prompt the consideration of oligodendroglioma.
Calvarial erosion is seen

19.---b
Pineoblastoma often shows focal hemorrhage and microscopic necrosis. A rare variant of pineoblastoma is the "trilateral retinoblastoma," the term used for a pineoblastoma in a patient with bilateral retinoblastoma. This is most often an inherited syndrome, and the diagnosis should be sought in any patient with bilateral retinoblastoma.

20.—c
Subarachnoid involvement is usually not identified with CT
Lymphoma is typically of relatively low signal intensity on T2-weighted images (i.e., isointense to gray matter), reflecting its hypercellularity. This signal pattern is also seen in prostate metastases and sarcoidosis, making it virtually impossible to distinguish among these entities by MR alone

21.---c

The pilocytic astrocytoma falls under the World Health Organization (WHO) classification as grade I, meaning extremely benign and generally curable if it can be completely resected. Although unencapsulated, they remain remarkably circumscribed and do not undergo malignant differentiation with time.

22.---d
Thirty-three percent show calcifications.
Ganglioglioma (GG) is classified by the WHO as type 1 tumor in the vast majority of cases.
The mean age at presentation is around 9.5 years. The age range is from 6 months to 80 years.
The tumor is characterized by slow growth, resulting in a long clinical history, with seizures being the most common symptom. Gangliogliomas have been found to be the structural lesions underlying chronic temporal lobe epilepsy in up to 20% to 40% of patient cohorts undergoing neurosurgery.
It is the combination of the long history of seizures and the benign appearance on imaging that enables the radiographic diagnosis.

23.----e
MR perfusion sequences usually display lower rCBV values in the brain abscess capsule than those in the solid rim of high-grade neoplasms.
Diffusion tensor imaging may demonstrate regions of elevated FA values within a brain abscess cavity.

24.---e
MR imaging may show enhancement of the basal cisterns and enlargement of the ventricles.
On CT and MR, subarachnoid cysts may be difficulty to identify because they are isodense/isointense to CSF and do not enhance. Larger racemose cysts can produce significant distortion of the subarachnoid spaces. Noninvasive MR cisternography has been described in performing FLAIR sequences after the inhalation of 100% O_2. As a result, the CSF in the subarachnoid space becomes hyperintense, enabling subarachnoid cyst detection.

25-.----b
Alzheimer disease (AD) is the most common cause of dementia in the elderly.
AD is characterized clinically by a progressive dementia, which typically begins with an isolated memory impairment.
Increased educational attainment and higher job complexity may reduce risk for late-onset AD.
The rare early-onset cases of AD present in individuals younger than the age of 65 years, some as young as the 30s.
The majority of individuals with autosomal dominant transmitted AD have mutations in one of three genes---the amyloid precursor protein gene on chromosome 21, the presenilin-1 gene on chromosome 14, and the presenilin-2 gene on chromosome 1. These known autosomal

dominant mutations are involved in metabolism of amyloid protein, which implicates disordered amyloid protein in the causal pathway leading to AD.
The ε4 allele of apolipoprotein E (APOE), however, increases the risk of developing AD and also lowers the mean age at onset of the disease . APOE is a component of lipoproteins . Three normally occurring alleles of APOE have been identified: ε2, ε3, and ε4.
APOE ε3 is the most prevalent allele in the general population, with a frequency of roughly 80%. The APOE ε3/4 genotype confers a roughly threefold increase in risk of developing AD, whereas ε4/4 confers an eightfold-increased risk of developing AD compared to the risk associated with the ε3/3 genotype. The ε2 allele decreases the risk of developing AD; however, this protective effect is not as strong as the risk conferred to carriers of ε4 allele.

26.---e
Hyperintense signal on T1-weighted images within the extrapyramidal nuclei has been reported in association with congenital portal systemic shunt without intrinsic liver disease and in patients who received long-term parenteral nutrition. Decrease of mI and choline (Cho) with increased levels of glutamine and glutamate are spectroscopic findings appear to be unique to HE.

27.---a
SCA3 (Machado-Joseph disease) shows abnormal signal of the transverse pontine fibers (with the "hot cross bun" sign) together with atrophy of the pons, middle cerebellar peduncles, and cerebellum, similar to MSA-C. Differences exist, however. SCA3 shows neuropathologic and MRI findings not seen in MSA-C, including atrophy of the superior cerebellar peduncles, frontal and temporal lobes, and globus pallidi and abnormal linear hyperintense signal along the medial margins of the internal segments of the globus pallidi bilaterally on long-TR and FLAIR images . The latter imaging finding correlates pathologically with degeneration of the lenticular fasciculus, a major outflow of the internal segment of the globus pallidus.
Gross pathology and MRI of Friedreich Ataxia reveal atrophy of the spinal cord . Spinal cord atrophy has been variably reported to affect the cervical spinal cord and/or along the length of the entire cord, from the cervicomedullary junction through the conus medullaris. These atrophic changes are due to degeneration with myelin loss and gliosis of the posterior columns and roots and spinocerebellar and corticospinal tracts .
The absence or milder nature of the cerebellar atrophy in Friedreich ataxia serves as a useful differential diagnostic feature on MRI and contrasts with the imaging findings in primary

cerebellar degenerative processes.

28.---e
Advanced MR techniques, particularly DTI and MRS, are more sensitive than conventional MRI in detecting upper motor neuron degeneration, particularly early in the disease. When compared with normal controls, ALS patients show an increase in mean diffusivity and a decrease in fractional anisotropy of the corticospinal tract . Mean diffusivity correlated with disease duration, whereas fractional anisotropy correlated with disease severity.

29.----c
Galloway-Mowat, Zellweger, and oculocerebrocutaneous syndromes, thanatophoric dysplasia, and the cobblestone complexes are also associated with polymicrogyria.

30.—d
Intracranial vessels (e.g., pericallosal arteries) and cranial nerves often course through, rather than around, lipomas .It is important to remember that intracranial lipomas are congenital malformations and not neoplasms
lipomas are frequently apposed to malformed brain. . intracranial vessels and cranial nerves often course through lipomas
The prepontomedullary cisterns are the first subarachnoid cisterns to be created (Osaka)

31.---b
The most common diagnosis in the scenario of a lesion occupying two compartments is a neurofibroma extending into both the extradural and the intradural extramedullary spaces .Two lesions with identical pathology may occur in different compartments. For example, metastastases may occur in any of the three compartments, including the intramedullary space.

32.---d
After contrast administration,astrocytoma almost always enhance, but because of the infiltrative nature of the tumor, without a capsule or cleavage plane between the lesion and the spinal cord, the margins of the lesion often are poorly defined and irregular.

33.---e
There is enhancement following magnetic resonance imaging signal changes; annular enhancement indicates abscess formation.
Osseous and extraaxial abscesses show restricted diffusion on diffusion-weighted imaging and dark appearance on diffusion-weighted maps.
Differential Diagnosis of Infectious Spondylodiscitis
------Postoperative disc changes
Degenerative changes
Dialysis-related arthropathy
Pseudoarthrosis, neuropathic arthropathy
Richter syndrome (among other neoplastic conditions)

34--e
Myelocele and myelomeningocele are nearly always associated the

Chiari II malformation
35-.—c
Noggin inhibits BMP-4. Noggin inhibits BMP-4. Where noggin expression is high, BMP-4 activity is low, and the neural crest cells do not migrate. Where noggin expression is low, BMP-4 activity is high, and the neural crest cells may emigrate

36.-d
GH-secreting adenomas are histologically classified as densely or sparsely granulated. T2 hypointensity is seen more commonly in GH-secreting adenomas, and this finding is almost exclusive to the densely granulated type.

ACTH, thyroid-stimulating hormone, and luteinizing hormone/follicle-stimulating hormone microadenomas tend to be centrally located

37----c
The specific anatomic site of the mass is the most telling feature of Pituicytoma and Granular Cell Tumors ,in fact, the diagnosis should be suspected when the pituitary mass is situated posteriorly within the gland and the normal posterior lobe hyperintensity cannot be identified. Of course, the most common posteriorly situated pituitary tumor is still the adenoma.

38.—d
Dynamic contrast enhancement (DCE) MRI uses the T1 properties of contrast agent. The arterial spin labeling (ASL) technique requires no exogenous contrast agents. In this technique, the spins in the inflowing arteries are perturbed with radiofrequency pulses, and the effect of these perturbed spins on image intensity after they flow into the slice is measured.

39.---e
ADC maps are solely based on differences of tissue diffusion, independent of any T2 effects. The ADC in the normal brain ranges from $2.94 \times 10^3 mm^2 s^1$ for CSF to $0.22 \times 10^3 mm^2 s^1$ for white matter; grey matter lies in between with a ADC of $0.76 \times 10^3 mm^2 s$. Areas with a decreased ADC appear dark on ADC maps, which is the converse to diffusion-weighted images where areas of decreased diffusion appear bright.

40.---b
First-pass $T2^*W$ gradient-echo technique can be combined with DSC perfusion imaging.

41.----b
Intraventricular lesions

Tumour	Typical site
Colloid cyst	Foramen of Monro/third ventricle
Meningioma	Trigone of lateral ventricle
Choroid	Fourth ventricle
Ependymoma	Lateral ventricle (more common in children) and fourth ventricle
Neurocytoma	Lateral ventricles (involving septum pellucidum)
Metastases	Lateral ventricles, ependyma and choroid plexus

42.---d
The severity and duration of brain swelling depends on infarct size. It

usually increases during the first week, persists during the second week and then regresses. Other diagnoses such as tumour or infection should be considered if there is extensive white matter oedema without cortical involvement or prolonged brain swelling.

43.----a
The preferential sites of hypertensive haemorrhage are the basal ganglia, thalamus and ponsHaemorrhage in a young, normotensive patient warrants further investigation with angiography to exclude an AVM. Peripheral or lobar haemorrhages in the elderly are suggestive of amyloid angiopathy

44.---e
Enhancement of cryptococcomas or the leptomeninges is rare because these patients are profoundly immunocompromised The earliest imaging manifestation is dilatation of perivascular spaces, most often in the basal ganglia but also in the brainstem and cerebral white matter . These spaces are distended by mucoid material, organisms and inflammatory cells, and appear as multiple small foci of high signal on T2W image

45.---b
Modic described three types of reactive changes in the cancellous bone adjacent to the vertebral end-plates: (type 1) in the acute stage of disc disease there is invasion of the cancellous spaces by fibrovascular reactive tissue; in time this leads to (type 2) fatty replacement of red marrow; eventually this leads to (type 3) bony sclerosis. These changes are exquisitely shown by MRI: (A) type 1 changes yield low signal on T1W and high on T2W; (B) type 2 changes yield high signal on T1W and T2W (unless fat suppressed, when they will yield low signal); (C) type 3 changes yield low signal on all sequences.

46.---e
The foramen magnum is enlarged and 'shield-shaped'

47.---c
A 'panda face' in mid brain with involvement of the substantia nigra and tegmentum is noted Leigh's disease

48.---d
Venous infarcts are often bilateral, do not conform to an arterial territory but to the territory of venous drainage, and are frequently haemorrhagic. They are parasagittal when the superior sagittal sinus is involved, thalamic when the internal cerebral veins or straight sinus/vein of Galen are involved, and temporal lobe when the transverse or sigmoid sinus or vein of Labb.
On diffusion imaging there is a mixture of restricted and free diffusion even when nonhaemorrhagic.

49.---a
50.----c
Carotid stenting is generally performed under local anaesthesia

51.---b
52.---d

The *habenular commissure* lies directly anterior to the pineal at the back end of the third ventricle. It is frequently calcified but is often mistaken for the pineal, although its characteristic shape readily distinguish it. The calcification is typically C-shaped with the open part of the letter facing backward.

The *J-shaped sella* (synonyms: 'omega-shaped', 'shoe-shaped' or ' hour-glass' sella) is an elongated sella with a shallow anterior convexity which represents an exaggeration of the normal slight impression of the sulcus chiasmaticus. The latter is rarely seen in films of an adult skull, but is sometimes well shown i n those of children (about 5%,). This odd-shaped sella has also been described in glioma of the optic chiasm, in children with 'gargoylism', and in those with chronic hydrocephalus.

The *posterior fontanel* closes at 3-6 months, while the larger *anterior fontanel* closes at 15-18 months.

53.---e
Miliary /pepper pot osteoporosis of skull may be seen in hyperparathyroidism

54.---c
The preferred agent for demonstrating the presynaptic dopamine transporter is 1 23 1-FP-CIT (ioflupane). '- 3 1-beta-CIT has similar properties but its uptake into the target sites is slower, so
i maging has to he done 18-24 h after injection, while with '- 3 1-FPCIT images can be obtained on the same day as injection. For i nvestigation of the postsynaptic dopamine receptors, the favoured agent is 1 '3 1-iodobenzamide (IBZM).

55.---e
Most patients die in first year of life

56.----e
Secondary midbrain (Duret hemorrhage) and Kernohan's notch are features of descending transtentorial herniation

57.---d
Myxopapillary ependymoma occur exclusively in the spinal cord

58.---d
59.----b
60.---a
Neural Tube Dorsalizing Gradient Mutations are divided into those that involve overexpression of dorsalizing gradient genes, such as duplication of the dorsal horns of the spinal cord, duplication of dorsal brainstem structures, and the dorsal interhemispheric variant of HPE, and those that involve underexpression of dorsalizing gradient genes, such as septooptic dysplasia (SOD).

TEST PAPER 14

1. The NMR concept was first proposed in 1936 by
a) Bloch and Purcell
b) C. J. Gorter
c) Hahn
d) Lauterbur
e) Mansfield

2. All are true regarding venous infarction except
a. The single common pathway for venous infarction is venous thrombosis
b. the cortical location of hemorrhage in most venous infarctions
c. sinusitis or mastoiditis may lead to venous infarction
d. the radiologist plays the critical role in making this diagnosis
e. The most commonly involved sinus is the superior sagittal sinus

3. **Conventional Magnetic Resonance Findings in acute infarction are all except**
a. Lesion in the arterial distribution
b. High intensity FLAIR and T2-weighted images
c. Gyri swollen, sulci effaced
d. Absence of arterial flow void
e. lack of intravascular contrast enhancement

4. Possible etiologies of arterial infarction in Older Children and Young Adults is/are
a. arterial dissection
b. moyamoya disease
c. neurofibromatosis
d. intracranial infective arteritis
e. all

5. The most specific and sensitive noninvasive modality for the detection of intracranial vascular malformations of all types is
a. CT scan
b. Catheter angiography
c. MRI
d. USG
e. X RAY

6. The most common clinically symptomatic cerebrovascular malformation is
a. AVM
b. cavernous angioma
c. capillary telangiectasia
d. venous angioma
e. the dural AVM (DAVM)

7. Differential diagnosis of AVMs is/are
a. cavernous hemangioma with vascular channels in contiguity with the lesion
b. hemangioblastoma
c. Moyamoya disease and Sturge-Weber syndrome
d. progressive distal internal carotid occlusion due to neurofibromatosis
e. all

8. All are true regarding developmental venous anomalies except
a. no arterial component
b. intervening brain tissue is usually abnormal
c. may be the most common cerebrovascular malformation
d. clinically silent
e. may be associated with cortical dysplasia

9. All are true regarding dural arteriovenous malformations (DAVMs) except
a. more than half of DAVMs are in the anterior fossa
b. Approximately 35% of posterior fossa AVMs are purely dural in supply
c. represent AV shunts located within the dura or tentorium
d. Arterial supply is primarily via meningeal branches
e. drainage is into the dural venous sinuses or other dural or leptomeningeal venous channels

10. All are true regarding MR of DAVM except
a. The actual site of the fistulous communication virtually never seen on MR
b. exquisitively delineate the arterial supply to DAVMs
c. extremely useful for evaluation of DAVMs with pial venous drainage
d. suspected by presence of large draining veins and feeding vessels exclusively in superficial dural-based locations
e. suspected by presence of dilation of cortical veins in the absence of visualization of a parenchymal vascular nidus

11. The most common atraumatic cause of SAH
a. Aneurysms
b. AVMs
c. cavernous angioma
d. coagulopathy
e. amyloid angiopathy

12. Which sequence is preferred for documenting acute SAH on MRI
a. SE MR images
b. FLAIR imaging
c. GRE
d. Fat sat imaging
e. GRASS

13. All are criteria for diagnosis of multiple sclerosis (Barkhof and Tintore criteria) except
a. One gadolinium- enhancing lesion
b. seven T2-hyperintense lesions
c. At least one infratentorial lesion
d. At least one juxtacortical lesion involving the subcortical U-fibers
e. At least three periventricular lesions

14. A 50 yr old patient with AIDs presents with an insidious onset of dementia. Visual loss, weakness, ataxia, and speech disturbances are noted. Polymerase chain reaction JC virus in CSF analysis is positive. The patients died within six months. Brain biopsy shows confluent areas of demyelination, distributed throughout the cerebral white matter. Microscopically, there are multiple foci of demyelination. There are atypical oligodendrocytes containing large, swollen nuclei with basophilic / eosinophilic inclusion bodies accompanied by reactive astrocytes. What is the most likely diagnosis?
a. PML
b. lymphoma
c. toxoplasmosis
d. HIV-1 encephalopathy
e. CMV

15. All are Vacuolating Leukoencephalopathies except

a. Canavan disease
b. Alexander disease
c. Vanishing white matter disease
d. Megalencephalic leukoencephalopathy with subcortical cysts
e. Progressive cavitatory leukoencephalopathy

16. An appropriate choice in emergency setting for evaluation of new-onset seizure patients with symptomatic causes is
a. CT
b. MRI
c. PET
d. USG
e. SPECT

17. All are findings of hippocampal sclerosis except
a. hyperintense signal on T2-weighted images
b. hippocampal atrophy
c. Loss of the hippocampal internal architecture
d. ipsilateral accentuation of hippocampal head digitations
e. dilation of temporal horn of lateral ventricle

18. Most epileptogenic neoplasms occur in or adjacent to the cerebral cortex of which part of brain
a. frontal lobe
b. temporal lobe
c. occipital lobe
d. parietal lobe
e. brainstem

19. All are true regarding tumour except
a. meningiomas enhances on contrast
b. epidermoid and dermoid tumors undergoes contrast enhancement
c. extraaxial masses are most frequently malignant in nature
d. intratumoral necrosis is considered a poor prognostic sign
e. Fluid–debris intensity levels are a pathognomonic sign of cystic tissue

20. All Of followings are true regarding cyst except
a. Cyst---- sharply demarcated, round, smooth
b. Cyst ---- isointense to CSF on T1-weighted, T2-weighted
c. tumour cysts are hypointense to normal CSF on FLAIR
d. Fluid–debris intensity levels are a pathognomonic sign of cystic tissue
e. "ghost" images propagated along the phase-encoding direction on conventional images

21. All are true regarding diffusion imaging except
a. ADC values may aid in the distinction of low-grade astrocytomas from oligodendrogliomas
b. ADC has been proposed as a surrogate marker for treatment response of gliomas and metastases to radiation and chemotherapy
c. DTI provides a sensitive means to detect alterations in the integrity of gray matter structures
d. DTI has been proposed as a method for delineation of glioma margins and regions of tumor infiltration
e. DTT has been found to be beneficial in the neurosurgical planning and postoperative assessment of gliomas

22. All are true regarding

noninfiltrative astrocytic tumors except
a. common tendency to be well circumscribed
b. generally more differentiated than infiltrative astrocytoma
c. relatively favorable prognosis
d. a limited capacity for invasion and spread
e. more tendency to progress into more malignant forms

23. All are true regarding subependymal giant cell astrocytoma except
a. WHO grade I
b. a well-circumscribed mass in the region of the foramen of Monro
c. in a young adult
d. tumor of the ependyma
e. present in up to 10% of patients with tuberous sclerosis

24. All are true regarding pineal cell tumours except
a. Pineoblastoma ---WHO grade IV and
b. pineocytoma ---WHO grade II
c. may contain melanin
d. striking predilection for female
e. arise from the neuroepithelial cells of the gland

25. All are true regarding meningioma except
a. strong uptake of contrast by essentially all meningiomas
b. usually produces marked homogeneous tumor enhancement
c. contrast enhancement on MR is not identifiable in densely calcified lesion
d. meningioma capillaries have no blood–brain barrier
e. the degree of enhancement is usually more intense at 3 minutes than at 25 or 55 minutes

26. The three most common pediatric brain tumors of the cerebellum are, (in decreasing order of frequency)
a. the primitive neuroectodermal tumor (medulloblastoma), cerebellar astrocytoma, and ependymoma
b. cerebellar astrocytoma, ependymoma and the primitive neuroectodermal tumor (medulloblastoma),
c. .cerebellar astrocytoma, the primitive neuroectodermal tumor (medulloblastoma) and ependymoma
d. cerebellar astrocytoma ,the primitive neuroectodermal tumor (medulloblastoma) and the hemangioblastoma
e. ependymoma ,the primitive neuroectodermal tumor (medulloblastoma) and the hemangioblastoma

27. All are true regarding imaging of herpes encephalitis (TYPE 1) except
a. FLAIR and DWI most sensitive sequences
b. T2WI and FLAIR: hyperintense insula/temporal cortex/ subcortical white matter
c. T1WI: may show hemorrhage;
d. DWI: no restriction on diffusion
e. CBV elevated

28. The most common cause of serious fetal and neonatal encephalitis in developed countries
a. CMV
b. HSV-1
c. HSV-2

d. Toxoplasmosis
e. HIV

29. Imaging features that favour HIV encephalitis over progressive multifocal leukoencephalopathy (PML) are all except
a. pattern of diffuse centrum semiovale and periventricular white matter
b. The demyelination lesions more symmetric and central than those of PML
c. the lesions usually unapparent on T1-weighted images,
d. . frequent involvement of posterior fossa and posterior portion of brain
e. a global encephalopathy

30. All are true regarding progressive multifocal leukoencephalopathy except
a. JC polyomavirus causes infection of the astrocyte
b. PML causes death in 90% of patients within 1 year after diagnosis
c. the pathological triad ---- demyelination, giant atypical astrocytes, and oligodendrocytes with intranuclear inclusion bodies noted
d. MRI is always the procedure of choice in imaging any patient with suspected PML
e. MR spectroscopy and diffusion tensor imaging seems to contributes to avoiding interventional procedures.

31. All are true regarding toxoplasmosis of brain except
a. multiple areas of isointensity or hypodensity with a ring enhancement
b. The asymmetric target sign

c. Double-dose delayed technique extremely useful
d. Hemorrhage in Toxoplasma lesions is extremely common
e. commonly seen in the basal ganglia and frontal and parietal lobes

32. All are true regarding neurocysticercosis except
a. Ring enhancement seen in colloidal stage
b. Vasogenic edema seen in colloidal stage
c. Fluid isointense to cerebrospinal fluid on all MR sequence
d. Calcification begins in granular nodular stage
e. Mineralized lesion without surrounding edema noted in nodular stage

33. All are true regarding neuroimaging of Wilson disease except
a. diffuse / focal atrophy of the cerebrum, brainstem, and/or cerebellum
b. Gray matter nuclei involment usually bilateral and symmetric
c. lenticular nucleus typically involved
d. Cerebral lesions are hyperdense on CT
e. variable signal on MRI.

34. All are the commonest sites of involvement of Wernicke encephalopathy (WE) on MRI except
a. the peri-third ventricular medial thalami
b. the periaqueductal gray matter of the midbrain
c. the peri-fourth ventricular pons and cerebellar vermis

d. the perilateral ventricular caudate nuclei
e. the perimidline mammillary bodies

35. All are true regarding tuberous sclerosis except
a. Vogt triad: adenoma sebaceum, epilepsy, and mental handicap
b. autosomal dominant
c. The TSC1 gene is located on chromosome 13q34
d. TSC2 are often have more tubers
e. Known as Bourneville-Pringle disease

36. PHACES includes all except
a. posterior fossa malformations
b. hemangiomas
c. arterial anomalies
d. coarctation of the aorta
e. ear abnormalities

37. All are true regarding lissencephalies except
a. The most severe of the neuronal migrational anomalies
b. generalized paucity of gyral and sulcal formation
c. abnormal neuronal migration between about 8 and 14 weeks' gestation.
d. LIS1 mutations may result in the phenotypes of the Miller-Dieker syndrome
e. Band heterotopia is found most often in males

38. All are true regarding dermoids except
a. exhibit markedly increased attenuation on CT
b. may be Calcification in the wall of the lesion
c. may be fat droplets "floating" within the frontal horns
d. some component of high signal on T1-weighted images
e. Chemical shift artifact not useful in the diagnosis

39. All are true regarding the developmental venous anomaly (DVA) except
a. The most common sites of DVA are the temporal lobes and the posterior fossa
b. may be associated with the Sturge-Weber syndrome
c. sinus pericranii may be seen
d. the caput medusae is usually seen within the deep white matter
e. DVAs may drain to the superficial or deep venous system

40. All are true regarding intramedullary tumour except
a. STIR sequences are more sensitive than FSE T2-weighted sequences for the detection of intramedullary pathology
b. T2-weighted gradient recalled echo sequences have excellent sensitivity for detection of hemorrhage
c. superficial siderosis is seen as marked hyperintensity along the periphery of the cord on T2W
d. hemangioblastomas are commonly associated with syrinx cavities
e. large majority of gliomas of the cord tend to enhance

41. All are true regarding spinal cord ischemia and infarction except
a. MRI is the diagnostic study of choice
b. posterior column functions are usually preserved in ischemia involving the ASA distribution
c. cervical cord is particularly

susceptible to ischemia
d. Spontaneous aortic dissection may be the most common cause of ischemic damage to the spinal cord
e. spinal angiography carries a risk of neurologic complications in the range of 2.2% to 3.6%

42. All the drugs increase incidence of myelocele and myelomeningocele except
a. Phenobarbital
b. folate
c. phenytoin
d. carbamazepine
e. valproic acid

43. All are true regarding diastematomyelia except
a. frequently decreased the sagittal dimension of the vertebral bodies
b. norrowed the interpediculate distance at the level of diastematomyelia.
c. spina bifida
d. intersegmental fusion of laminae
e. segmentation abnormalities in 85% of cases

44. All are true regarding pituitary adenoma except
a. lengthening of both T1 and T2 relaxation in comparison to normal pituitary tissue.
b. microadenomas show a focal hypointense lesion on T1W in 80-95% of cases
c. Small isointense adenomas constitute the majority of false-negative MR examinations
d. Hyperintensity in adenomas is accounted for by the presence of old blood in the tumor
e. About two third to one half of microadenomas are hyperintense with T2 weighting

45. All are true regarding epidermoid except
a. result from inclusions of epithelium during the time of neural tube closure
b. the most frequent site of occurrence --the cerebellopontine angle followed by the parasellar region
c. The interior of the cyst is composed of a waxy material
d. lesions of adulthood,
e. predominantly located in the basal cisterns and are midline in position.

46. All are true regarding intracranial pathology except
a. Almost all cranial chordomas are found in relation to the clivus
b. Ecchordosis refers to a nodule of benign cells of notochordal origin
c. Pituicytoma and Granular Cell Tumors is situated anteriorly within the gland
d. Pituicytoma and Granular Cell Tumors are extremely vascular
e. chordomas are histologically benign but locally invasive and destructive

47. All are true regarding MR imaging of fetal brain except
a. avoid MR in the first trimester whenever feasible.
b. Isolated mild ventriculomegaly is defined as a transverse atrial measurement of 08 to 10 mm
c. MR has been found to be beneficial in callosal dysgenesis and heterotopias and polymirogyria
d. A cisterna magna measuring

greater than 10 mm raises the possibility of an anomaly in the Dandy-Walker spectrum
e. In arachnoid cyst the cerebellar structures are present but displaced.

48. The only clue of the hemorrhagic episode after several months or years may be
a. the collapsed cleft of hemosiderin and ferritin in the adjacent brain
b. the collapsed cleft of methemoglobin in the adjacent brain
c. No residue
d. hyperintense cleft
e. None

49. All are true regarding brainstem except
a. Brainstem DAI lesions are located in the dorsolateral quadrants of the rostral brainstem
b. intrinsic secondary lesions typically (87%) found in the ventral and ventrolateral aspects
C. multiple petechial hemorrhages is associated with grim prognosis
d. Duret hemorrhages are usually located in the dorsolateral aspects of the brainstem
e. brainstem infarcts occurs in the central tegmentum of the pons and midbrain

50. All are true regarding supratentorial pilocytic astrocytoma of children except
a. the most common glial origin tumors in the pediatric population
b. commonly occur in the optic chiasm, hypothalamus, and optic nerves
c. most often are associated with the predisposing syndrome of NF1
d. Tumor response to treatment is measured by a change in enhancement
e. cysts on the surface of the tumor

51. All are true regarding MR diffusion imaging except
a. exploits the presence of Brownian motion of water molecules to produce image contrast
b. a pair of diffusion sensitizing gradients applied symmetrically around a 180 refocusing RF pulse of a T2W
c. loss of signal is proportional to the degree of microscopic motion that occurs during the pulse sequence
d. regions of relatively stationary water molecules appear much brighter than areas with a higher molecular diffusion
e. signal loss is independent of the strength and duration of the diffusion sensitizing gradient (the 'b-value'.)

52. All are true regarding MR perfusion imaging except
a. Dynamic susceptibility-weighted contrast-enhanced MR imaging provides an indirect measure of tumour neovascularity
b. contrast enhancement is an indicator of vascular endothelial (blood–brain barrier) integrity
c. rCBV derived from PWI correlate poorly with angiographic and histological markers of tumour vascularity
d. PWI significantly increases the specificity and sensitivity of conventional MRI in the classification of gliomas

e. Maps of rCBV may be a useful adjunct for stereotactic tumour biopsies

53. All are true regarding brain metastases except
a. deposits from malignant melanoma hyperdendse on CT
b. Increasing relaxivity of gadolinium compounds improve detection of metastases
c. Well-differentiated adenocarcinoma metastases are hypointense on trace-weighted DWI,
d. PWI and MRS of intratumoural region useful in differentiating single metastasis from a glioma
e. DWI is helpful to differentiate cystic metastasis from cerebral abscesses

54. All are true regarding Alberta Stroke Program Early CT Score (ASPECTS) except
a. the affected middle cerebral artery territory is divided into ten segments
b. six segments for cortical areas are scored
c. One point is lost for each area that shows early ischaemic changes (swelling or reduced attenuation)
d. ASPECTS can be used to predict outcome and risk of post-thrombolysis haemorrhage
e. score correlates well with DWI findings at presentation

55. All are true regarding aneurysm except
a. a 'four vessel' catheter angiogram performed because of multiplicity of up to 20% of aneurysm
b. Angiography should be performed after 48 hrs of SAH
c. Three-dimensional angiography reduces the need for multiple angiographic runs
d. electrically detachable platinum coils are used in endovascular coiling
e. superior outcomes at 1 year for coiling over clipping noted

56. Features that favour a diagnosis of lymphoma over toxoplasmosis in HIV-related CNS disease
a. A single enhancing mass lesion
b. larger lesions
c. central low intensity on T2W images
d.. Subependymal spread
e. lesser uptake on Thallium-201 SPECT and FDG-PET

57. All are true regarding syringomyelia except
a. the cervical cord is involved most often
b. the spinal cord is enlarged in about 80 per cent
c. 70-90 % of cases of syringomyelia are associated with cerebellar ectopia
d. more than about 25 per cent of cysts extend cranial to C2
e. fusiform syrinx is found confined to only a few spinal segments

58. All are true regarding cerebral malformations except
a. The holoprosencephalies are abnormalities of dorsal induction.
b. Neurones form and proliferate in the germinal matrix from around 7 weeks gestation
c. the layers of the cerebral cortex from 2 to 5 months' gestation

d. the deeper layers of the cerebral cortex forms first
e. Anencephaly is the most common cerebral malformation in the fetus

59. All are true regarding inborn metabolic brain disorders except
a. Alexander's disease shows extensive white matter abnormality beginning in the frontal and periventricular white matter
b. L-2 hydroxyglutaricaciduria involve the periventricular white matter and corpus callosum
c. bilateral symmetrical involvement of the globus pallidus with sparing of the thalami is seen in methylmalonic acidaemia
d. Bilateral pallidal involvement is seen as T2 hyperintensity in Kearns–Sayer syndrome
e. Lorenzo's oil may delay disease progression of ALD

60. All are true regarding intracranial infections except
a. in utero infections acquired before 16–18 weeks produce lissencephaly and a small cerebellum
b. branching curvilinear hyperechogenicity in the basal ganglia is seen in congenitaql CMV
c. Toxoplasmosis cause cerebellar hypoplasia and polymicrogyria
d. congenital HSV cause rapidly disseminating diffuse encephalitis
e. Global atrophy and bilateral basal ganglia calcification are the m/c imaging findings in congenitally AIDS

TEST PAPER 14(ANSWER)

1.----b
The Dutch physicist C. J. Gorter first proposed the NMR concept in 1936

2.---b
Typically, venous infarctions are accompanied by hemorrhage within the affected tissue, which is particularly frequent in the white matter or near the gray–white junction. This stands in contrast to the cortical location of hemorrhage associated with most arterial infarctions. The most commonly involved sinus is the superior sagittal sinus, followed by the transverse sinus and then the straight sinus.

3.---e
Intravascular contrast enhancement is noted in acute infarction.(Chapter 15,,Atlas)

4.---e

5.---c
MR imaging is the most specific and sensitive noninvasive modality for the detection of intracranial vascular malformations of all types, whether angiographically demonstrable or angiographically occult

6.---a

7.---e

8.—b
Developmental venous anomalies (DVAs) /venous angiomas / venous malformations is an incidental malformations of venous drainage patterns. There is no arterial component in this entity. Intervening brain tissue is present between the veins comprising the lesion, and this brain tissue is usually normal without evidence of hemosiderin staining or gliosis.

9.---a
More than half of DAVMs are in the posterior fossa.

10.—b
The actual site of the fistulous communication in DAVM is virtually never seen on MR. The failure to visualize the site of shunting is ascribed to the small size of the area of AV communication, the location within the leaves of dura, and the lack of contrast between the signal void of rapidly flowing blood and that of adjacent bone. MR is usually unable to delineate the arterial supply to DAVMs ,again because of the relatively small size of meningeal feeding arteries. Nevertheless, MR is extremely useful in the evaluation of patients with DAVM particularly those with the potential for an aggressive course because of pial venous drainage. DAVM should be suspected when large draining veins and feeding vessels are found exclusively in superficial dural-based locations .Dilation of cortical veins in the absence of visualization of a parenchymal vascular nidus should suggest the diagnosis of DAVM.

A highly suggestive, if not specific, MR sign of DAVM with venoocclusive disease is the finding of prominent medullary veins.
We believe that the demonstration of medullary vein enlargement on MR is a specific sign of venous hypertension due to DAVM with venous outflow obstruction

11.---a
Populations that May be at Higher Risk for Intracranial Aneurysms—
Polycystic kidney disease
Coarctation of the aorta
Fibromuscular dysplasia
Family history of saccular aneurysm
Marfan syndrome
Ehlers-Danlos syndrome

12---b
Before FLAIR imaging, MR was notoriously poor for documenting acute SAH unless the SAH is massive. It has been proposed that the lack of visualization of diffuse subarachnoid blood on SE MR images is related to the relatively high Po$_2$ in the cerebrospinal fluid (CSF), which thereby prevents paramagnetic deoxyhemoglobin from forming. With FLAIR imaging, acute subarachnoid hemorrhage is clearly seen as high intensity compared to the normal low intensity of normal CSF.

13.---b
The Barkhof and Tintore criteria require three of four of the following findings (a) One gadolinium- enhancing lesion, or nine T2-hyperintense lesions if there is no gadolinium-enhancing lesion. (b) At least one infratentorial lesion. (c) At least one juxtacortical lesion (involving the subcortical U-fibers). (d) At least three periventricular lesions.

14.----a
15.---b
16.---a
CT is an appropriate choice in emergency setting for evaluation of new-onset seizure patients with symptomatic causes (i.e., focal deficits, persistent altered mental status, fever, trauma, persistent headaches, history of cancer, anticoagulation, ventriculoperitoneal shunts, or acquired immunodeficiency syndrome) and in the elderly, in whom acute stroke and tumors are the most likely causes.

17.---d
Hippocampal sclerosis include ipsilateral loss of hippocampal head digitations, dilation of temporal horn of lateral ventricle, and atrophy of the white matter in parahippocampal gyrus between the hippocampus and collateral sulcus. Increased T2 signal in the anterior temporal lobe white matter and atrophy of fornix and mammillary bodies from degeneration of hippocampal tracts can also be seen. Actual quantitative measurements of T2 signal (T2 relaxometry) obtained on a single-slice multiecho sequence through the hippocampal body have also been shown to be abnormally elevated in approximately 70% of cases with

hippocampal sclerosis
18.---b
19.---c
Extraaxial masses are most frequently benign in nature
20.----c
Tumour cysts are hyperintense to normal CSF on FLAIR.
21.-----c
22.---e
Localized (noninfiltrative) astrocytic tumors are pilocytic astrocytoma, pleomorphic xanthoastrocytoma (PXA), and subependymal giant cell astrocytoma. The better outlook for patients harboring these lesions is due to a limited capacity for invasion and spread and a limited tendency to progress into more malignant forms.
23.---d
The mass in subependymal giant cell astrocytoma is truly a parenchymal astrocytic neoplasm that projects into the ventricle from a subependymal location—it is not a tumor of the ependyma itself.
24.----d
Pineal cell tumour do not exhibit a striking gender predilection.
25.---c
Contrast enhancement on MR is almost always identifiable, even when meningiomas are densely calcified
The most striking finding of contrast-enhanced MR in meningiomas is dural enhancement adjacent to the lesion. En plaque meningiomas and globular convexity and basal meningiomas may infiltrate adjacent dural surfaces for several centimeters
Dural enhancement is not specific for meningioma; rather, it indicates dural involvement by any adjacent mass, whether the mass is meningioma, metastases, or invasive primary brain tumor
Regardless of the precise etiology of the dural thickening and enhancement, its determination in continuity with the margins of an intracranial tumor adds another valuable MR diagnostic feature of extraaxial dural-based tumors
26.---a
27.----d
DWI: patchy restricted diffusion (even with normal MRI) is seen . Restricted diffusion in the face of elevated perfusion would point to encephalitis over any other entity
MR imaging techniques are far more sensitive than CT in demonstrating parenchymal involvement.
Hyperintense signal involves both cortex and white matter and may be seen within hours after the onset of signs and symptoms compared with the reported delay of up to 3 to 5 days on CT and 4 to 11 days for single photon emission computed tomography (SPECT) brain scans using either ^{123}I-iodoamphetamine or ^{99m}Tc-hexamethylpropyleneamine oxime.
MR has been used to monitor response to treatment with acyclovir
28.----a
29.---d

HIV encephalitis has a pattern of diffuse centrum semiovale and periventricular white matter hyperintensity in contrast to the unifocal or asymmetric multifocal pattern typically produced by PML The demyelination lesions of HIV encephalitis tend to be more symmetric and central than those of PML
The lesions of HIV demyelination are usually unapparent on T1-weighted images, whereas those of PML are often clearly hypointense and well-demarcated on T1-weighted images.In PML, lesions often involve the posterior fossa and tend to be located in the posterior portion of the brain. The frontal lobes are the most common sites of involvement in HIV encephalitis. HIV encephalitis often manifests as a global encephalopathy, whereas PML is usually associated with a focal neurologic deficit.

Differential Diagnosis: Human Immunodeficiency Virus (HIV) Versus Progressive Multifocal Leukoencephalopathy (PML)------
HIV
  Diffuse periventricular white matter hyperintensity
  More symmetric and central
  Usually unapparent on T1-weighted imaging, no enhancement
  Frontal lobes most commonly involved
  Global encephalopathy
  Magnetic resonance spectroscopy: ↑ choline, ↓ NAA, ↑ mI
PML
  Multifocal (or unifocal) pattern
  More asymmetric and peripheral
  Hypointense and well-demarcated on T1-weighted imaging
  Occasional enhancement at periphery of lesion
  Posterior fossa and posterior lobes most commonly involved
  Focal neurologic deficit
Magnetic resonance spectroscopy: ↑ lactate/lipids; ↓ NAA

mI, myo-inositol; NAA, *N*-acetylaspartate.

30.-----a
JC polyomavirus causes infection of oligodendrocytes
MR demonstrates far greater sensitivity than CT in the imaging of PML for defining both the extent and the number of lesions and is always the procedure of choice in imaging any patient with suspected PML.

31.----d
Hemorrhage in Toxoplasma lesions is rare.
On CT, Toxoplasma encephalitis characteristically appears as multiple areas of isointensity or hypodensity that demonstrate a ring or, in fewer cases, a nodular enhancement.
Double-dose delayed technique (using 200 mL of intravenous contrast by bolus/drip infusion with delayed scanning at 1 hour) has been extremely effective in detecting lesions .
Lesions have a predilection for the basal ganglia (in 75% to 88% of cases), the thalamus, and the

corticomedullary junction of cerebral hemispheres, primarily in the frontal and parietal lobes
There is surrounding mass effect and edema of variable degree.
The asymmetric target sign was described as suggestive of a toxoplasmosis abscess and is characterized by a small, eccentric, enhancing nodule within the ring-enhancing lesion.
Toxoplasma encephalitis is the most common cause of brain space-occupying lesions in AIDS patients, and it occurs when CD4 counts fall below 100 cell/mm.
Chorea, an extremely rare sign, is thought to be a pathognomonic feature of CNS toxoplasmosis
Pathologically, three different morphologic types of focal lesions can be found: necrotizing abscesses, organizing abscesses, and chronic abscesses
Toxoplasma lesions do not have capsules.
Although small-vessel thrombosis and necrosis are characteristically associated with the lesions, arteritis of large vessels is absent.
MR has greater sensitivity than CT, particularly for small lesions at the corticomedullary junction, and detects a greater number of lesions.
The lack of multiplicity on a high-quality MR study should prompt suspicion of other possible pathologic conditions.

32.---c

As the cyst fluid content becomes turbid and gelatinous due to the proteinaceous fluid and debris accumulated, it appears slightly hyperintense to CSF on T1- and T2-weighted images and FLAIR images.
In the granular nodular stage, the cyst retracts and forms a granulomatous nodule that may show ring or solid enhancement

33.---d

Cerebral lesions are hypodense on CT but show variable signal on MRI. Lesions are hyperintense, hypointense, or both on long-TR sequences.
Gray matter nuclei involvement is more common and is usually bilateral and symmetric; white matter lesions usually are asymmetric. In a recent investigation of 100 patients with WD, signal abnormalities were present in the putamen in 72%, caudate nuclei in 61%, thalami in 58%, midbrain in 49%, cerebral white matter in 25%, pons in 20%, medulla in 12%, cerebellum in 10%, and cerebral cortex in 9%.

34.---d

Bilateral and usually symmetric involvement of the perimidline structures may permit a specific diagnosis of WE.
Less common sites of involvement include the perilateral ventricular caudate nuclei, the retroaqueductal quadrigeminal plate, and, in more clinically advanced cases, the cerebral cortex Involvement of the cerebral cortex appears to be associated with a very advanced presentation (deep coma) and a poor prognosis.

35---c

The TSC1 gene is located on

chromosome 9q34, and the TSC2 gene represents a locus on 16p13

36.---e
PHACES is a rare and recently described neurovascular syndrome with posterior fossa malformations, hemangiomas, arterial anomalies, coarctation of the aorta, cardiac defects, eye abnormalities, defects of the sternum, and abdominal raphe

37.---e
Band heterotopia is found most often in females.

38-.—e
Fat suppression sequences may be useful . . Chemical shift artifact is useful in the diagnosis
Dermoids may be show fat droplets "floating" within the frontal horns on axial or sagittal images of supine patients. These findings indicate rupture of the dermoid into the ventricular or subarachnoid space.The primary differential diagnosis is teratoma or lipoma
Associated midline anomalies such as callosal hypogenesis are common and may be a clue to the diagnosis.

39.—a
The most common sites of DVA are the frontal lobes and the posterior fossa
The final periods of intracranial venous development described by Padgett are stages 7 and 7a, referring to the "threshold of fetal period" and "fetus at the third month" . These periods are of particular interest because it is at this time that much of the definitive cerebral venous system appears

40.----c
Superficial siderosis is seen as marked hypointensity along the periphery of the cord on T2W

41---c
Particular susceptibility of the thoracic and lumbar cord regions to ischemia results from the poor collateral flow via adjacent segments of the ASA in the event of compromise of a major radiculomedullary artery. In contrast, the multiple collateral routes to the cervical ASA seem to provide some protection from infarction at these levels, at least in cases of proximal or radiculomedullary artery obstruction.

42.---b
Before 1980, myelocele and myelomeningocele occurred in 1 to 2 per 1,000 live births, up to 8 per 1,000 live births in specific populations . Since then, the incidence of these malformations has been reduced sharply (70% to 90%) simply by adding folate supplements to the diet of pregnant mothers in the period from before conception to 6 weeks after conception.
Neural tube defects are known to be associated with disorders of maternal methionine metabolism and with elevated maternal levels of homocysteine.
Neural tube defects have also been related to derangements in the paired box gene Pax3(Waardenburg syndrome I on chromosome 2q35-q37.3)
Myelomeningocele may also be

related to fragile X syndrome
43.---b
The sagittal dimension of the vertebral bodies is frequently decreased, and the interpediculate distance is characteristically widened at the level of diastematomyelia. The laminae are abnormal in nearly all patients and exhibit spina bifida, thickening of the laminae, and fusion between laminae of adjacent segments. The combination of spina bifida and intersegmental fusion of laminae is present in 60% of patients and is highly suggestive of the diagnosis

Eight-five percent of patients with diastematomyelia show segmentation anomalies such as hemivertebrae, butterfly vertebrae, and block vertebrae. Scoliosis and kyphosis are present in 50% to 60% of cases of diastematomyelia and are usually directly related to the segmentation anomalies.
Concurrent lesions seen with diastematomyelia include Klippel-Feil syndrome (2% to 7%) Sprengel deformity (7%), Chiari I malformation (3%) , dermal sinus (3%) , lipomyelomeningocele (3%), and teratomas (3%) .
44.---e
Hyperintensity in adenomas is accounted for by the presence of old blood in the tumor . About one third to one half of microadenomas are hyperintense with T2 weighting; most of the remainder are isointense.
45.---e

They are predominantly located in the basal cisterns and are lateral in position. The cerebellopontine angle is the most frequent site of occurrence, followed by the parasellar region.
Dermoids are more likely to be discovered in the pediatric age group and are more commonly located in the midline, most frequently in the fourth ventricle or vermis. The cyst wall contains various dermal appendages such as hair follicles and sebaceous and sweat glands, in addition to stratified squamous epithelium
46.---c
The specific anatomic site of the mass is the most telling feature of Pituicytoma and Granular Cell Tumors ,in fact, the diagnosis should be suspected when the pituitary mass is situated posteriorly within the gland and the normal posterior lobe hyperintensity cannot be identified. Of course, the most common posteriorly situated pituitary tumor is still the adenoma.
47.---b
Isolated mild ventriculomegaly is defined as a transverse atrial measurement of 10 to 15 mm
MR has been found to be beneficial in callosal dysgenesis and heterotopias and polymirogyria
48.---e
49.---d
Secondary (Duret) hemorrhages are usually located in the ventral and paramedian aspects of the midbrain and upper pons with

relative sparing of the dorsolateral aspects of the brainstem. The location of brainstem infarcts is typically in the central tegmentum of the pons and midbrain, whereas DAI usually involves the dorsolateral midbrain

50.---e
The WHO classifies pilocytic astrocytoma as a grade 1 tumor. There is virtually no evidence of malignant degeneration.
The tumour may or may not show contrast enhancement. A tumor that contrast-enhances on one examination may not do so on the next, and vice versa. The change in contrast enhancement from examination to examination does not necessarily indicate a change in aggressiveness or response to treatment. Tumor response is measured by a change in tumor size.
These tumors exude proteinaceous fluid from their surface, often producing locules of fluid, giving rise to cysts on the surface of the tumor.

51.—e
On diffusion-weighted images, regions of relatively stationary water molecules appear much brighter than areas with a higher molecular diffusion. The degree of phase shift and signal loss depends also on the strength and duration of the diffusion sensitizing gradient, which is expressed by the 'b-value'. B-values used for imaging of acute stroke lie typically around 1000s mm

52.---c
rCBV measurements derived from PWI correlate closely with angiographic and histological markers of tumour vascularity, and also with the expression of vascular endothelial growth factor (VGEF) in tumours, an important determinant of angiogenesis. High-grade glial tumours tend to have higher rCBV values than low-grade tumours and PWI significantly increases the specificity and sensitivity of conventional MRI in the classification of gliomas.

53.-------d
Metastases are characterized by oedema in the surrounding white matter, which appears dark on trace-weighted DWI and is often disproportionate to the size of the tumour itself.
Increasing the contrast dose or relaxivity of gadolinium compounds can improve the sensitivity for detection of metastases on MRI
Well-differentiated adenocarcinoma metastases are hypointense on trace-weighted DWI, whereas small cell and neuroendocrine metastases are hyperintense, due to their higher cellularity. On standard MRI it may occasionally be difficult to distinguish a single metastasis from a glioma. PWI and MRS of the peritumoural rather than intratumoural region were shown to be useful in differentiating the two.

54.----e
In simple rating scale of ASPECTS

the affected middle cerebral artery territory is divided into ten segments, namely: internal capsule, caudate nucleus, lentiform nucleus, insula and six segments for cortical areas. M1=anterior middle cerebral artery (MCA) cortex; M2=MCA cortex lateral to insular ribbon; M3=posterior MCA cortex; M4, M5 and M6 are anterior, lateral and posterior MCA territories immediately superior to M1, M2 and M3, rostral to basal ganglia. Subcortical structures are alotted 3 points (C, L and IC), MCA cortex is alotted 7 points (insular cortex, M1, M2, M3, M4, M5 and M6). A point is lost for each area that shows early ischaemic change (low density or swelling). The range of scores is 0–10, representing an infarct of the entire territory and normal findings, respectively.
It correlates well with DWI findings at presentation and facilitates more accurate interpretation of emergency CT by nonexperts.

55.----b
Angiography should be performed as soon as possible following SAH since the aneurysm re-bleed rate is greatest during the first 48 h and vasospasm can adversely affect the quality of angiograms performed several days after the haemorrhage. If a negative angiogram is marred by vasospasm, a repeat study is indicated

56.---e
Thallium-201 SPECT and FDG-PET show greater uptake in lymphoma than toxoplasmosis though this is unreliable in lesions smaller than 2 cm

57.---d
The cervical cord is involved most often.. Only about 10 per cent of cysts extend cranial to C2, where they split into two or deviate to right or left in a plane ventral to the floor of the fourth ventricle

58.---a
The earliest cerebral malformations to appear relate to the formation of the neural tube, i.e. abnormalities of dorsal induction or cranial dysraphism (3–4 weeks gestation). Anencephaly, cephalocele and Chiari II (Arnold–Chiari) malformation are consequences of abnormalities of dorsal induction. The events following the formation of the neural tube are termed ventral induction, when the two separate cerebral hemispheres are formed (5–8 weeks). The holoprosencephalies are all abnormalities of ventral induction.

59.---b
The MRI findings of L-2 hydroxyglutaricaciduria show white matter involvement with peripheral involvement, particularly of the subcortical U fibres, internal, external and extreme capsules, sparing of the periventricular white matter and corpus callosum, and with a slight frontal predominance. There is macrocephaly
Bilateral pallidal involvement is

seen as T2 hyperintensity in methylmalonic acidaemia ,GAMT (guanidinoacetate methyltransferase deficiency), Kearns–Sayer syndrome ,kernicterus and carbon monoxide poisoning

60.----c

Imaging features of of congenital toxoplasmosis microcephaly and parenchymal calcification are similar to CMV infection although cerebellar hypoplasia and polymicrogyria are not seen, and the ventriculomegaly may be due to an active ependymitis causing obstructive hydrocephalus rather than diffuse cerebral damage . The severity of brain involvement correlates with earlier maternal infection.

CMV is the most common cause of serious viral infection in fetuses and neonates in the West

TEST PAPER 15

1. All are correctly matched except
a) Experimental observation of NMR in solids and liquids-- Bloch and Purcell (1946)
b) Theory of nuclear spin relaxation/introduction of T1 and T2---Bloch(1946)
c) Spin echoes---- Damadian (1972),
d) Magnetic resonance imaging (MRI) using gradient fields--- Lauterbur (1973)
e) Human MRI using gradient fields---- Aberdeen, Nottingham, EMI (1976–1979)

2. The only approved therapy for acute ischemic arterial stroke in first 3 hours of stroke is
a. intravenous (i.v.) tissue plasminogen activator (tPA)
b. intraarterial thrombolytic therapy
c. the MERCI (Mechanical Embolus Removal in Cerebral Ischemia) retrieval device
d. Anticoagulation therapy
e. Endovascular therapy

3. All are chronic findings of periventricular infarction in preterm infant except
a. increased T1 signal in the periventricular white matter
b. thinning of the periventricular white matter volume
c. thinning of the corpus callosum
d. the development of porencephalic cysts
e. ventriculomegaly

4. All are possible etiologies of arterial infarction in Older Children and Young Adults except
a. cyanotic congenital heart disease
b. mitochondrial disorders
c. lysosomal disorders
d. organic acidurias
e. all

5. Intracerebral metastases most prone to hemorrhage include all except
a. melanoma
b. renal cell carcinoma
c. pancreatic carcinoma
d. bronchogenic carcinoma
e. thyroid carcinoma

6. The screening modality of choice for intracranial vascular malformations and most of their complications in almost all clinical settings is
a. CT scan
b. Catheter angiography
c. MRI
d. USG
e. X RAY

7. All are true regarding optic nerve glioma(OPG) except
a. primarily tumors of childhood
b. usually pilocytic astrocytoma
c. MR superior to CT for evaluating optic pathway gliomas
d. tram track appearance along the optic nerve/sheath complex
e. OPG in the setting of NF1 often behaves as a hamartoma

8. All are true regarding epidermoids except

a. may cause a chemical granulomatous meningitis
b. hyperintense to brain and CSF on FLAIR
c. show diffusion characteristics of solids
d. Calcification is very rare.
e. Enhancement occurs infrequently

9. Associated finding of AVMs on MRI are all except
a. intraparenchymal hemorrhage and SAHs
b. gliosis and/or secondary demyelination in adjacent area
c. Intraventricular /superficial cortical hemosiderosis
d. extraventricular obstructive hydrocephalus
e. massively dilated vessels (nearly always artery)

10. Causes of cryptic AVMs(angiographically occult small AVMs) are all except
a. compression of the lesion by adjacent hematoma
b. vasospasm
c. extremely slow flow
d. thrombosis
e. all

11. A young patient undergoes MRI of brain which show no abnormality on unenhanced SE images. The pons reveals lacelike region of stippled contrast enhancement on contrast study. The patient is asymptomatic. The most likely diagnosis is
a. lymphoma
b. cavernous angioma
c. capillary telangiectasia
d. venous angioma
e. developmental venous anomaly

12. All are true regarding normal embryogenesis of the vertebrae except
a. paraxial mesoderm forms somites
b. somites first form at about days 19 to 21 in the future cervical region
c. ventromedial portion of each somite express the markers Pax1 and Pax9
d. The perichordal mesenchyme differentiate into the pedicles, the neural arches, and the lateral ribs
e. dorsolateral portion of each somite to express Pax3, Pax7, and Myo-D

13. All are true regarding pituitary microadenoma except
a. The T1W sequence is the more reliable than the T2-weighted sequence for microadenoma detection
b. examine the gland at narrow display windows
c. the adenomatous tissue is isointense to adjacent temporal lobe gray matter on T1W
d. normal pituitary tissue is isointense with temporal lobe white matter on T1W
e. As a general rule, the contrast between adenoma and normal tissue is equal to that between gray and white matter

14. All are true regarding developmental venous anomalies except
a. no arterial component
b. intervening brain tissue is usually abnormal
c. may be the most common cerebrovascular malformation
d. clinically silent

e. may be associated with cortical dysplasias

15. All are true regarding venous angioma except
a. a tuft of abnormally enlarged medullary venous channels
b. parallel arrangement
c. drain into a central venous trunk
d. the common trunk drains intracerebrally into the deep or superficial venous system
e. anatomically variant but physiologically competent venous drainage pathways

16. All are true regarding dural arteriovenous malformations (DAVMs) except
a. acquired lesions
b. Cranial bruit, tinnitus, and headache are frequent
c. Spontaneous regression of the lesions seen
d. source of hemorrhage--- the nidus
e. Hemorrhage reported only in lesions with reflux into leptomeningeal veins

17. All are true regarding role of MR in DAVMs except
a. direct visualization of the shunt in DAVMs is generally not possible on MR
b. MRA demonstrates AV shunting in DAVMs
c. MRA may be useful in DAVMs near the skull base
d. MR exquisitely depict thrombosis of cavernous sinus or superior ophthalmic vein
e. MR study can definitively exclude DAVMs

18. The most frequent presenting manifestation of intracranial aneurysm
a. SAH
b. intraparenchymal hemorrhage
c. SDH
d. EDH
e. mixed

19. An isolated and complete third nerve palsy is a classic finding in patients with aneurysm of
a. The junction of the anterior cerebral and anterior communicating arteries
b. the ICA at the origin of the posterior communicating artery
c. the bifurcation of the MCA
d. the posterior cerebral artery
e. the bifurcation of the ICA

20. All are indirect signs of secondary brainstem injury except
a. Rotation, angulation and ovoid compression
b. craniocaudal shortening
c. dilatation of the fourth ventricle and basal cisterns
d. herniation of the parahippocampal gyrus into the tentorial incisura
e. posterior cerebral artery distribution infarcts

21. Multiple sclerosis shows a distinct propensity for involvement of certain regions of white matter. Such locations are all except
a. the periventricular white matter
b. optic nerves
c. brainstem
d. spinal cord
e. thalamus

22. All features are suggestive of PML except
a. more frequent involvement of parietal white matter
b. usually no enhancement on MR
c. posterior fossa involment
d. no optic nerve involvement
e. spinal cord involvement common

23. Extensive symmetric CSF-isointense white matter changes and radiating cystic degeneration is seen in which Vacuolating Leukoencephalopathies
a. Canavan disease
b. Cystic leukoencephalopathy without megalencephaly
c. Vanishing white matter disease
d. Megalencephalic leukoencephalopathy with subcortical cysts
e. Progressive cavitatory leukoencephalopathy

24. An appropriate choice in emergency setting for evaluation of new-onset seizure in the elderly is
a. CT
b. MRI
c. PET
d. USG
e. SPECT

25. All are true regarding myelocele and myelomeningocele except
a. The dorsal surface is exposed to the exterior
b. The dorsal roots arise from the ventral surface of the neural plate
c. dura forms dorsal to the neural placode.
d. The laminae are widely everted
e. the neural placode elevated well above the surface of the surrounding back in myelomeningocele

26. All are true regarding hippocampal sclerosis except
a. Hippocampal volumetry significantly increase the sensitivity over visual analysis in detection of hippocampal sclerosis
b. Hippocampal volumetry and T2 relaxometry routinely useful in diagnosis of bilateral hippocampal atrophy without visually appreciable signal changes
c. Bilateral hippocampal atrophy occurs in about 10% to 20% of cases
d. Bilateral hippocampal atrophy is frequently associated with developmental anomalies of temporal lobe
e. T2 relaxometry and FLAIR techniques are useful in detecting associated abnormalities of amygdala not seen on routine MR

27. The most frequent neoplastic lesion associated with late-onset seizures in the elderly patient is
a. glioblastoma multiforme
b. ganglioglioma
c. DNET
d. low grade glioma
e. cerebral metastases

28. Findings specific for extraaxial localization of brain tumour is
a. peripheral location along the inner table of the skull
b. associated bone change in overlying calvarium
c. enhancement of adjacent meninges
d. Cerebrospinal fluid cleft between brain and lesion

e. Displacement of brain from the skull

29. Causes of low Intensity in tumors on T2W MRI are all except
a. Ferritin/hemosiderin from prior hemorrhage
b. Scant cytoplasm (high nucleus:cytoplasm ratio)
c. Dense cellularity
d. Fibrocollagenous stroma
e. Very low (nonparamagnetic) protein concentration

30. All are true regarding perfusion imaging in MRI except
a. dynamic susceptibility contrast (DSC) MRI is most conventionally used to measure cerebral blood volume in brain.
b. dynamic contrast-enhanced (DCE) MRI is used to measure vascular permeability in brain
c. MTT has been the most widely used parameter derived from DSC PWI
d. the k_{trans} value is putatively a measure of the vascular permeability to contrast agent
e. the k_{trans} correlates with glioma grade

31. The most common astrocytoma in childhood
a. Pilocytic Astrocytoma
b. Tectal Glioma
c. pleomorphic xanthoastrocytoma (PXA)
d. subependymal giant cell astrocytoma
e. Gangliocytoma

32. All are true regarding subependymal giant cell astrocytoma except
a. WHO grade I
b. a well-circumscribed mass in the region of the foramen of Monro
c. in a young adult
d. tumor of the ependyma
e. present in up to 10% of patients with tuberous sclerosis

33. All are true regarding pineal germinoma except
a. peak incidence at puberty
b. striking female predominance in 90%
c. marked and homogeneous enhancement
d. highly prone to seed the subarachnoid space
e. isointense to gray matter on T2-W

34. CT is superior to MRI to reveal which feature of meningioma
a. Internal tumor vascularity
b. Venous sinus invasion
c. Transdural invasion
d. Bony hyperostosis
e. calcification

35. All are true regarding brain tumour except
a. metastases, meningiomas, and malignant gliomas are the most frequent tumors in adult
b. tumors of astrocytic origin comprise 40% to 55% of the total paediatric tumour
c. optic gliomas affect 5% to 15% of patients by age 20 years in case of NF1
d. tuberous sclerosis is frequently associated with medulloblastoma
e. Gorland syndrome is associated with intracranial neoplasm

36. All are true regarding cerebellar astocytoma in paediatric age group except
a. the most common cerebellar hemispheric tumor of glial origin

b. The most frequent astrocytoma is the pilocytic (85%) and fibrillary (15%)
c. The pilocytic astrocytoma belongs to grade II of WHO classification
d. The juvenile pilocytic astrocytomas (JPAs) are unencapsulated
e. Glioblastomas of the cerebellum may be radiation induced

37. All are true regarding supratentorial pilocytic astrocytoma of children except
a. optic gliomas found in 5% to 15% of NF1 patients by the age of 20yrs
b. the cysts in tumour can dissect into the surrounding brain tissue
c. can seed subarachnoid space /the intraventricular space
d. low ADC values
e. a mild elevation of choline relative to NAA and relative preservation of creatinine

38. HSV-2 is a major cause of neonatal encephalitis along with other TORCH. All are imaging features of HSV-2 except
a. T2WI and FLAIR: hyperintense cortex/subcortical white matter
b. Leptomeningeal involvement
c. Focal hemorrhagic necrosis
d. Cystic encephalomalacia
e. central gray matter involvement characteristic

39. All are true regarding CNS infection of AIDS except
a. Inflammatory changes occur in the subcortical regions
b. the most common neurologic manifestation ---AIDS dementia complex (ADC)
c. neurologic dysfunction is related to direct viral invasion of neurons
d. subacute encephalitis with microglial nodules is primary pathologic substrate of ADC
e. Diffuse atrophy is usually present in ADC

40. Proton MR spectroscopy is a valuable tool in the assessment of patients with HIV infection. Proton MR spectroscopy is able to depict brain metabolite changes in asymptomatic HIV-infected patients with no abnormalities on conventional MR imaging sequences. All are true in CNS infection of AIDS except
a. reduction in the levels of N-acetylaspartate
b. reduced N-acetylaspartate/creatine (NAA/Cr)
c. reduced N-acetylaspartate/choline (NAA/Cho)
d. reduced choline compounds
e. an increase in Myo-inositol

41. All are true regarding progressive multifocal leukoencephalopathy except
a. multifocal /unifocal pattern
b. more asymmetric and peripheral
c. hyperintense and well-demarcated on T1W
d. posterior fossa and posterior lobes most commonly involved
e. magnetic resonance spectroscopy: ↑ lactate/lipids; ↓ NAA

42. False regarding CNS lymphoma and toxoplasmosis in AIDS is

a. lymphoma---- is often solitary
b. lymphoma--- increased uptake on Thallium-201 brain SPECT
c. toxoplasmosis---an absence of radionuclide uptake on The ^{18}F-fluorodeoxyglucose–PET
d. lymphoma----hyperperfusion on CBV maps on Dynamic perfusion MR imaging
e. toxoplasmosis---lower Apparent diffusion coefficient values than in lymphomas.

43. All are true regarding neurocysticercosis except
a. different stages of the disease may be seen within an individual patient
b. the entire process of resolution of a single lesion can take 2 to 10 years in untreated host
c. the most common CT finding in intraventricular cysticercosis is hydrocephalus
d. the lateral ventricule is the most common site for intraventricular cysticercosis
e. cysticercosis lesions do not have hyperperfusion.

44. All are true regarding neuroimaging of Wilson disease except
a. "face of the giant panda" sign in medulla
b. the "bright claustral" sign
c. variable findings on DWI
d. significant decrease in the NAA/Cr ratio in the parietal-occipital cortex, frontal white matter, and basal ganglia
e. may improve and/or resolve after effective treatment

45. All are true regarding intracranial meningioma in NF 2 except
a. multiple
b. noted in the lateral ventricle more commonly than sporadic meningiomas
c. younger age at presentation
d. similar to sporadic tumors in their histology and radiologic appearance
e. a better prognosis than sporadic

46. All are associated with VHL except
a. Renal cyst
b. pancreatic cyst
c. hepatic cyst
d. testicular cyst
e. Renal cancer

47. All are true regarding genetic cause except
a. The isolated lissencephaly sequence (ILS) may result from mutations of the DCX
b. LIS1 gene mutations may result subcortical band heterotopia (SBH)
c. DCX mutations can result in SBH
d. bilateral perisylvian polymicrogyria may result from mutations at locus Xq28
e. DiGeorge syndrome may result from mutations of the DCX

48. The lissencephaly band heterotopia spectrum is associated with all the following genes except
a. LIS1 mutations.
b. DCX (doublecortin) mutations.
c. PROKR2
d. ARX mutations.
e. RELN mutations

49. All are true regarding epidermoid cyst except
a. epidermoids are of entirely

ectodermal origin
b. the majority involve the basal surface of the brain
c. tend to lie laterally
d. The most common cranial sites --- subfrontal and interhemispheric regions
e. typically insinuate into the subarachnoid cisterns and sulci

50. All are true regarding Meningiomas of the spinal canal except
a. primarily intradural extramedullary
b. 80% found in the cervical region in general population
c. Calcifications are present in up to 72% of the cases
d. hypointense to isointense to the spinal cord on T2W.
e. usually enhance immediately, intensely, and homogeneously

51. All are true regarding astrocytoma of spinal cord except
a. represent more than 50% of intramedullary mass lesions in children
b. most often are located in the cervical cord
c. decreases in prevalence in the lower thoracic and lumbar regions
d. eccentric in location, usually posteriorly located by the posterior columns
e. frequently involve the spinal cord over multiple segments

52. All are true regarding pyogenic Spondylitis except
a. The most common sources of septic emboli is infections from genitourinary tract
b. Staphylococcus aureus is the most common organism (up to 60%)
c. The lumbar spine is most frequently involved.
d. changes on plain radiographs occur at 2 to 8 weeks after the beginning of the process
e. Sensitivity of MRI is 100%

53. All are true regarding Xenon computed tomography except
a. xenon is freely diffusable and penetrates the blood–brain barrier
b. Xenon computed tomography can be used to assess cerebral blood perfusion
c. The washout of xenon occurs relatively slowly
d. patient movement during period of imaging causes misregistration of data
e. patient inhale of a gas containing 28 per cent xenon

54. All are PHYSIOLOGY-BASED MR IMAGING except
a. DWI
b. PWI
c. MRS
d. BOLD –functional MRI
e. proton-density MRI

55. All are true regarding Primary cerebral lymphoma (PCL) except
a. hyperdense on CT and hypointense on T2W images
b. often abutting an ependymal / meningeal surface
c. uniform enhancement in immunocompromised patients
d. The ADC value is lower than in gliomas / toxoplasmosis
e. a modest increase in rCBV--- much less marked than in high-grade gliomas

56. All are true regarding infarction except

a. swelling with obvious low density on CT indicates of infarction
b. Hypodensity affecting more than 50 per cent of the MCA territory is associated with a high mortality rate
c. involvement of MCA territory of greater than two-third is commonly a contraindication to thrombolysis
d. The sensitivity of CT for infarcts has been reported to be 30 per cent at 3 h
e. lower total score on ASPECTS carry a worse prognosis

57. All are true regarding aneurysm except
a. CTA is at least the equalvalent to of 2D- DSA for the diagnosis and anatomical assessment of aneurysms
b. The sensitivity of MRA is 77–94 per cent for aneurysm > 5mm
c. CTA outperforms DSA for aneurysm less than 3mm
d. Giant aneurysms are rarely visualized in their full extent on 3D TOF MRA
e. CTA is a reasonable first-line option for elective imaging of aneurysms

58. the commonest cause of a cerebral mass lesion in AIDS is
a. Cryptococcomas
b. Lymphoma
c. Tuberculosis
d. Candida
e. Toxoplasmosis

59. All are true regarding following diseases except
a. intradural arachnoid cysts arise from arachnoidal duplications or spinal arachnoiditis
b. Perineural arachnoid cysts (Tarlov cysts) occur commonly in the lumber region
c. the type I NF form is usually associated with skeletal dysplasia
d. marked and extensive thickening of the dura and extradural tissues noted Maroteaux-Lamy diseases.
e. retromedullary subarachnoid space in the thoracic spine is commonly wide

60. All are true regarding malformations except
a. The posterior fossa is of normal size in cerebellar hypoplasia
b. Torcular–lambdoid inversion is seen in Dandy –Walker syndrome
c. 'batwing appearance' of the fourth ventricle is seen in Joubert's syndrome
d. The 'Molar tooth' appearance is noted in rhombencephalosynapsis
e. a nonenhancing mass with diffusely enlarged cerebellar folia is feature of L'Hermitte-Duclos

TEST PAPER 15(ANSWER)

1.---c
Spin echoes----Hahn(1950), Whole-body NMR for medical diagnosis--- Jackson (1968), Damadian (1972), Abe (1973)

2.----a
Currently, intravenous (i.v.) tissue plasminogen activator (tPA) administered in the first 3 hours after stroke is the only approved therapy for acute ischemic stroke (FDA)
Endovascular therapy is playing a much more prominent role in the time window extending beyond 3 hours. The Prolyse in Acute Cerebral Thromboembolism (PROACT II) study showed a benefit to intraarterial thrombolytic therapy up to 6 hours after ischemic stroke onset
The U.S. Food and Drug Administration has approved the MERCI (Mechanical Embolus Removal in Cerebral Ischemia) retrieval device for removal of thrombus in patients with ischemic stroke.

3.---a
There is increased T2 signal in the periventricular white matter due to gliosis. .

4.---e

5.---c
Intracerebral metastases most prone to hemorrhage include melanoma, chordocarcinoma, renal cell carcinoma, bronchogenic carcinoma, and thyroid carcinoma.Of primary gliomas, glioblastoma multiforme, oligodendroglioma, and ependymoma are most likely to demonstrate significant hemorrhage pathologically. .

6.—c
As a general rule, MR has replaced CT as the screening modality of choice for intracranial vascular malformations and their complications in all clinical settings, except in the search for acute subarachnoid blood , where the clinical data on FLAIR are incomplete.

7.---d
The differential diagnosis of OPG involving the optic nerve is mainly with perioptic meningioma which may have a tram track appearance along the optic nerve/sheath complex, creating a fusiform appearance.

8.---a
Slow expansile growth is characteristic of dermoid, and they tend to insinuate within and around adjacent neural structures, conforming to the space within which they are situated. Rarely, the cyst ruptures and produces a chemical granulomatous meningitis. Epidermoids are characteristically hyperintense to brain and CSF on these sequences compared with arachnoid cysts, which remain isointense to CSF . Diffusion-weighted images may also be used because they demonstrate

diffusion characteristics of solids in epidermoids, whereas arachnoid cysts possess diffusion characteristics similar to CSF . Other features include a slightly inhomogeneous internal architecture and scalloped margins . Calcification is very rare. Enhancement occurs infrequently and, when present, occurs only along the periphery. Dermoids are more heterogeneous in a signal pattern . Most have evidence of a fatty component (hyperintense on T1-weighted images) and small areas of dense calcification , but on those occasions when fat or calcium is not in the tumor, dermoids may mimic the appearance of epidermoids or even arachnoid cysts.

9.---e

Venous occlusive disease is probably an important pathophysiologic feature of many AVMs, and should be sought on MR. This can be suggested by massively dilated vessels (nearly always representing veins) of either the deep or superficial venous system. Enlargement of the medullary veins, even in the contralateral hemisphere from the site of the AVM, is an important clue to venous occlusive disease (particularly in dural AV fistulas)

10.---e

11.---c

The key to distinguishing the enhancement of capillary telangiectasia from other, similar enhancing lesions, notably lymphoma when periventricular, is the absence of any signal abnormality on the unenhanced images.

12.---d

The sclerotome form the cartilage, bone, and ligament of the vertebral column and the ribs. The medial and the lateral portions of the sclerotome have divergent fates.Perichordal mesenchyme differentiate into the vertebral bodies and intervertebral disks. The perineural mesenchyme differentiate into the pedicles, the neural arches, and the lateral ribs

13.—a

The T1-weighted sequence is the more reliable for microadenoma detection than the T2-weighted sequence.

14.—b

Developmental venous anomalies (DVAs) **/venous angiomas / venous malformations** is an incidental malformations of venous drainage patterns. There is no arterial component in this entity. Intervening brain tissue is present between the veins comprising the lesion, and this brain tissue is usually normal without evidence of hemosiderin staining or gliosis .**15.—b**

Venous angioma consists of a tuft of abnormally enlarged medullary venous channels that are radially arranged around, and drain into, a central venous trunk . The common trunk drains intracerebrally into the deep or superficial venous system.

16.---d

Hemorrhage from DAVMs has been demonstrated to occur through leptomeningeal venous connections rather than through the nidus itself. Hemorrhage has been reported only in lesions with reflux into leptomeningeal veins and not in those cases in which drainage is confined to the dural sinuses. Consequently, the risk of hemorrhage in DAVM is related to the presence of leptomeningeal venous drainage, which in turn is a factor of the location of the lesion

17.---e

Because direct visualization of the shunt in DAVMs is generally not possible on MR, the technique cannot definitively exclude DAVMs, particularly those without cortical venous drainage.

18.---a

19.---b

Any adult with a painful complete third nerve palsy must be given the diagnosis of aneurysm until proven otherwise because in such patients a high percentage have unruptured posterior communicating-ICA aneurysm. Isolated third nerve palsy can also be a sign of microvascular disease, particularly common in diabetes. The third nerve palsy of diabetes (or any etiology of infarction) characteristically spares the pupil (pupillary fibers run in the peripheral portion of the nerve, and infarctions characteristically involve the central nerve) and often recovers completely over several weeks. **20.---c**

Rotation, angulation, ovoid compression, and craniocaudal shortening of the upper brainstem are some of the more commonly observed indirect signs of secondary BSI. Other common but less specific indirect signs include compression of the fourth ventricle and basal cisterns, herniation of the parahippocampal gyrus into the tentorial incisura, and posterior cerebral artery distribution infarcts.

21.---e

22----e

Spinal cord involvement is extremely rare in PML. Mass effect is more common with lymphoma and toxoplasmosis but can occasionally be present in PML. Encephalitides, including cytomegalovirus, toxoplasmosis, or HIV-1 encephalopathy may mimic PML in case of AIDS patients.

23.----c

24----a

25.---c

The dura encloses the cerebrospinal fluid ventrally and laterally and then becomes lost in the tissue lateral to the neural placode. No dura forms dorsal to the neural placode.

26.—a

Quantitative evaluation of hippocampal volume has been found to marginally increase the sensitivity over visual analysis in detection of hippocampal sclerosis. Qualitative assessment of hippocampal atrophy by an experienced observer achieves a

sensitivity of 80% to 90%, whereas quantitative methods are about 90% to 95% accurate.
27.---e
28.----d
29----e
Causes of Low Intensity in Tumors on T2-Weighted Magnetic Resonance Images----
Paramagnetic effects
  Iron within dystrophic calcification or necrosis
  Ferritin/hemosiderin from prior hemorrhage
Deoxyhemoglobin in acute hemorrhage
  Intracellular methemoglobin in early subacute hemorrhage
  Melanin (or other free radicals)
Low spin density
  Calcification
  Scant cytoplasm (high nucleus:cytoplasm ratio)
  Dense cellularity
Fibrocollagenous stroma
Macromolecule content
Very high (nonparamagnetic) protein concentration
Intratumoral vessels
  Signal void from rapid flow
30.---c
rCBV has been the most widely used parameter derived from DSC PWI
31.---a
Pilocytic Astrocytoma represents one of the most benign forms of glial neoplasm and is the most common astrocytoma in childhood
32.---d
The mass in subependymal giant cell astrocytoma is truly a parenchymal astrocytic neoplasm that projects into the ventricle from a subependymal location—it is not a tumor of the ependyma itself.
33.---b
Pineal germinoma shows striking female predominance in 90%.
34.----e
With MR, tumor vascularity and encased arteries with rapid flow remain hypointense on all imaging sequences even after the administration of contrast.

Meningioma calcification is less well defined with MR than with CT. Gradient echo imaging markedly improves the sensitivity for the detection of calcifications but specificity for this alteration will not be as great as with CT because other tissue substances such as acute or old blood products can cause a similar signal loss on gradient echo sequences.

35.---d
In tuberous sclerosis, giant cell tumors arise with significant frequency . Other genetic conditions that predispose to intracranial neoplasms include Gorland syndrome, basal cell nevus syndrome, Turcot syndrome (in which one fourth of all cerebral neoplasms are PNETs), and tumors associated with neurofibromatosis type II.
36.---c
The pilocytic astrocytoma falls under the World Health Organization (WHO) classification as grade I, meaning extremely benign and generally curable if it

can be completely resected. Although unencapsulated, they remain remarkably circumscribed and do not undergo malignant differentiation with time.

37.---d
Diffusion imaging shows increased motion of water throughout the tumor with elevated ADC values.

38.---e
Neuroimaging reflects various degrees of parenchymal inflammation and leptomeningeal involvement, evolving to necrosis. CT may reveal only subtle hypodensity of the periventricular white matter with relative sparing of the central gray matter, including basal ganglia and thalami, and the posterior fossa. Varicella CNS infection may result in transverse myelitis, meningoencephalitis, cerebellar ataxia
In immunocompetent patients, cranial and peripheral nerve palsies are the most common neurologic disorders seen in zoster infections whereas diffuse encephalitis is the most frequent manifestation seen in AIDS patients and other immunosuppressed patients. Five different patterns of CNS involvement in AIDS patients have been proposed: multifocal leukoencephalitis, ventriculitis, acute meningomyeloradiculitis, focal necrotizing myelitis, and necrotizing angiitis involving leptomeningeal arteries with cerebral infarction.

39.---c
ADC is not related to direct viral invasion of neurons. Clinicopathologic correlation in patients with ADC suggests that the primary pathologic substrate is subacute encephalitis with multinucleated giant cells rather than microglial nodules.

40.----d
A reduction in the levels of N-acetylaspartate, a neuronal functional marker, is evident in the early onset of infection, even in asymptomatic individuals. The decline is greater in symptomatic than asymptomatic patients. MR spectroscopy may reveal an increase in choline compounds earlier than the NAA reduction in patients with cerebral HIV infection. Thus, an elevated choline level appears to be a useful marker for early cerebral injury secondary to HIV and is high before the onset of clinical dementia. The increased choline is present in both early and late stages of HIV infection. Choline levels are not directly related to clinical status or CD4 counts. Myo-inositol seems to be elevated in the early course of cerebral HIV infection, it may be less prominent with advancing dementia. In summary, MR spectroscopy analysis in early stages of HIV dementia seems to be associated with an increase in both choline and mI levels.

41.---c
PML appears as multifocal hypodense white matter lesions involving the subcortical or periventricular regions without causing significant mass effect

and usually without enhancement on imaging. Occasional enhancement at periphery of lesion are noted.
PML lesions on MR images are hypointense on T1-weighted images and hyperintense on T2-weighted images involving the periventricular and/or subcortical white matter, producing a "scalloped" appearance . Lesions usually have a bilateral, multifocal, and asymmetric distribution pattern

42.---e
Apparent diffusion coefficient values are higher in toxoplasmosis than in lymphomas.
Although pyogenic abscesses have showed restricted diffusion on previous reports, toxoplasmosis lesions have revealed increased diffusibility. A possible cause for high apparent diffusion coefficient values within toxoplasmosis abscesses may be explained by the fact that the immune responses are impaired and viscosity is diminished within the lesion . Lymphoma is a highly cellular lesion, causing narrowing in the extracellular space and hampering mobility of free water molecules. A reduction in apparent diffusion coefficient values is not infrequently observed in these lesions. Thus, diffusion-weighted imaging can be of great use in distinguishing between these two conditions.
MR spectroscopy may also be helpful in differentiating toxoplasmosis from primary CNS lymphomamarkedly elevated lipid and lactate peaks, whereas all other normal brain metabolites are virtually absent or reduced. In contrast, primary CNS lymphoma shows a mild to moderate increase in lactate and lipids, a markedly elevated choline peak, and preservation of some normal metabolites with variably decreased levels of NAA and Cr
Toxoplasmosis and lymphoma are the most common brain enhancing mass effect lesions in AIDS patients
Toxoplasmosis is the second-most-common cause of congenital CNS infection. The most common cause is CMV.
A classic triad suggests the diagnosis of congenital toxoplasmosis: chorioretinitis, hydrocephalus, and cerebral calcifications.

43.----d
The fourth ventricule is the most common site for intraventricular cysticercosis

44.---a
Two specific MRI signs have been described in WD. The better known is the "face of the giant panda" sign , which describes hyperintense signal on long-TR sequences throughout the midbrain with sparing of the red nucleus, the lateral portion of the pars reticulata of the substantia nigra, and a portion of the superior colliculus.
The other sign, the "bright claustral" sign, correlates with focal hyperintense signal of the claustrum on long-TR sequences . In a recent investigation, the "face

of the giant panda" sign was found in 12% and the "bright claustral" sign in 4% of patients with WD.

45.---e

Any meningioma presenting in childhood or young adulthood should alert the physician to be particularly suspicious for NF2. Meningiomas are usually slowly growing, benign tumors that can be resected for cure. However, some researchers have suggested that the meningiomas occurring in NF2 may have a worse prognosis

46.---d

Epididymal cyst is seen

47.----e

DiGeorge syndrome may result from mutations of the GPR56 gene

48.---c

PROKR2 gene is associated with Kallman syndrome.
Kallmann syndrome may be of X-linked, autosomal dominant, or autosomal recessive inheritance. It can be divided by genotype into four different types: KAL1 (X-linked) and the autosomal types KAL2, KAL3, and KAL4.
VLDLR mutations is associated with the lissencephaly band heterotopia spectrum.
LIS1 mutations may result in the phenotypes of the Miller-Dieker syndrome, isolated lissencephaly sequence (ILS), or subcortical band heterotopia (SBH)
The DCX gene, or XLIS located on Xq22.3-q23, encodes a protein named doublecortin, which, similar to LIS1, depending on the type of mutation, may result in the phenotype of ILS, SBH or central pachygyria

49.---d

The most common cranial sites include the cerebellopontine angle and parasellar regions. Following these sites are the rhomboid fossa (ventral to the brainstem), ventricles and choroidal fissures, and subfrontal and interhemispheric regions. Epidermoids typically insinuate themselves into the subarachnoid cisterns and sulci enveloping cranial nerves and vessels.
The epidermoid tend to lie laterally, as opposed to dermoids, which tend to be midline

50.---b

In females, 83% of spinal meningiomas are in a thoracic location, with a 7:1 ratio of thoracic to cervical meningiomas. In males, approximately 47% of meningiomas are found in a thoracic location and 41% at the cervical level. Considering the population as a whole, approximately 80% of meningiomas are found in the thoracic region, 16% are cervical, and 3% are lumbar. Within the cervical spine, excluding the foramen magnum, the segments most often affected are C3 and C4.

51.----b

Astrocytomas most often are located in the thoracic cord. Prevalence of astrocytomas decreases in the lower thoracic and lumbar regions, unlike the prevalence of ependymomas, which increases in the caudal

spinal canal .
52.---e
Diagnostic Studies in Spinal Osteomyelitis

	Magnetic resonance	Gallium and bone scanning	Bone scans
Sensitivity	96%	90%	90%
Specificity	92%	100%	78%
Accuracy	94%	94%	86%

MR is as accurate as and more sensitive than radionuclide scanning in the characterization of osteomyelitis . MR is the most sensitive technique for diagnosing spondylodiscitis.
53.---c
The washout of xenon occurs relatively rapidly, allowing a repeat examination after 15–20 min.
54.----e
55.---c
Primary cerebral lymphoma (PCL) has tripled in incidence over the past 2 decades. This is partly due to a rise in patients with AIDS but PCL has also increased in immunocompetent patients. Enhancement is uniform in immunocompetent patients and ring-like in immunocompromised patients, in whom PCL frequently contains areas of central necrosis. The high cellular density and nucleus-to-cytoplasm ratio make PCL appear hyperdense on CT and hypointense on T2W images. PCL grows in an angiocentric fashion around existing blood vessels without extensive new vessel formation. Perfusion-weighted MRI therefore shows only a modest increase in rCBV, much less marked than in high-grade gliomas, where angiogenesis is a prominent feature
A characteristic finding is rapid resolution of the tumour following administration of steroids and/or radiotherapy.
56.---c
Greater than one-third involvement of MCA territory is commonly a contraindication to thrombolysis.
57.---e
Giant aneurysms are rarely visualized in their full extent on 3D TOF MRA because of slow and turbulent flow in their fundus. The lumen is properly opacified on CTA, which also shows mural thrombus and the aneurysm wall. MRA is a reasonable first-line option for elective imaging of aneurysms. It is also used for following coiled aneurysms. CTA is now preferable in acute SAH.
58.----e
59.----b
Perineural arachnoid cysts (Tarlov cysts) occur commonly in the sacrum, especially on the second sacral root. They can be large, multiple and are often associated with eccentric pressure erosion of the sacral canal and are well shown by MRI.
60.---d
Joubert's syndrome is considered as generalized developmental disorder of the midbrain and

hindbrain. The imaging findings reflect a failure of formation of the decussation of the superior cerebellar peduncles, lack of the pyramidal decussations and other anomalies of the midbrain crossing tracts and their nuclei. On cross-sectional imaging the fourth ventricle is enlarged with a 'batwing appearance' and there is a cleft in the vermis. The midbrain is small. The 'molar tooth' appearance seen on axial images arises from the lack of the superior cerebellar decussation and the superior peduncles also appear enlarged.

TEST PAPER 16

1. **Who were jointly awarded the Nobel Prize in Physiology or Medicine (2003) "for their discoveries concerning magnetic resonance imaging"**
a) Lauterbur and Sir Peter Mansfield
b) Bloch and Purcell
c) Ernst and Anderson
d) Jackson and Damadian
e) Aberdeen and Nottingham

2. **All are true regarding conventional magnetic resonance imaging of infarction except**
a. T2-weighted imaging --- repetition time, 400 to 600 ms; echo time, 20 to 35 ms,
b. T1-weighted imaging is generally done to provide anatomic definition
c. T1-weighted imaging is done for detection of methemoglobin in subacute hemorrhage.
d. T2-weighted imaging is used to demonstrate sites of parenchymal insult
e. T2-weighted imaging is used for detection of acute or remote hemorrhage

3. **All are true of pattern of ischemic injury except**
a. periventricular white matter in pre-term
b. the thalami, basal ganglia, and brainstem in premature
c. cortical and subcortical injury in a watershed distribution in term-infant
d. the thalami and basal ganglia with relative sparing of the cortex in term infant with profound hypotension
e. Bilateral frontal lobe infarction in the neonate with severe symptomatic hypoglycemia

4. **All are true of remote haematoma except**
a. Ferritin is a water-soluble protein with a crystalline core of ferric oxyhydroxide
b. Hemosiderin is insoluble aggregation of ferric oxyhydroxide with less protein than ferritin.
c. Ferritin and hemosiderin are antiferromagnetic in nature at biological temperatures
d. The iron in ferritin and hemosiderin show no relaxivity effects
e. Magnetic susceptibility variations are present in tissues containing ferritin and hemosiderin (observed on T2*)

5. **Specific pattern of hemorrhage on magnetic resonance imaging of Hemorrhagic neoplasm are all except**
a. Multiple stages of hematoma in same lesion
b. Debris–fluid levels
c. Persistent deoxyhemoglobin, absent hemosiderin
d. Identification of nonneoplastic tissue
e. all

6. **The gold standard for aneurysm diagnosis is**
a. CT angiography
b. Catheter angiography
c. MR angiography

d. USG
e. X RAY

7. All disorders are correctly matched except
a. Dandy-Walker malformation – ventral induction
b. callosal agenesis---cellular migration
c. Lhermitte-Duclos disease---cellular migration
d. myelocystocoele---secondary neurulation
e. septo-optic dysplasia---secondary neurulation

8. A young patient undergoes MRI of brain which show no abnormality on unenhanced SE images. The pons reveals lacelike region of stippled contrast enhancement on contrast study .The patient is asymptomatic. The most likely diagnosis is
a. lymphoma
b. cavernous angioma
c. capillary telangiectasia
d. venous angioma
e. developmental venous anomaly

9. All are true regarding venous angioma except
a. a spoke wheel–appearing collection of small, tapering veins arranged in a radial pattern
b. normal arterial and capillary phases
c. opacification of the lesion usually remain opacified through the late venous phase
d. intimately associated with the lateral ventricle and draining into a subependymal vein
e. MRA is necessary in most cases.

10. All are true regarding dural arteriovenous malformations (DAVMs) except
a. the most common DAVMs is that involving the sigmoid-transverse sinuses
b. the incidence of hemorrhage in sigmoid-transverse DAVMs is low
c. the second-most-common location of DAVMs is the cavernous sinus
d. intracranial hemorrhage from cavernous DAVM is very common
e. DAVMs of the tentorial-incisural region commonly present with intracranial hemorrhage

11. All are role of MR in DAVMs except
a. To document parenchymal complications of lesions
b. to suggest venoocclusive disease by defining abnormal cortical venous drainage
c. to indicate venous hypertension
d. to exclude other causes of venous dilation
e. for direct visualization of the shunt in DAVMs

12. Morbidity and mortality of SAH is
a. morbidity (20% to 25%) and mortality (50% to 60%)
b. morbidity (15% to 20%) and mortality (40 % to 50%)
c. morbidity (10% to 15%) and mortality (30% to 40%)
d. morbidity (5% to 10%) and mortality (20% to 30%)
e. morbidity (0% to 5%) and mortality (10% to 20%)

13. Probably the most useful noninvasive imaging modality in the postoperative assessment of aneurysmal clipping is
a. CT
b. MRI

c. PET
d. USG
e. none

14. All criteria are related to Multiple sclerosis except
a. the Poser criteria
b. the McDonald criteria
c. the Barkhof and Tintore criteria
d. the rose criteria
e. Bartel criteria

15. All are true regarding HIV encephalopathy except
a. occurs in patients with advanced immunosuppression
b. the cortex is preferentially affected
c. the most distinctive microscopic feature of HIV encephalopathy--- Multinucleated giant cells, often associated with microglial nodules
d. the most common finding on imaging ---- atrophy of the brain
e. multifocal confluent lesions / diffuse symmetric high signal intensity in the periventricular and deep white matter.

16-. Sudanophilic Leukodystrophies are
a. Canavan disease and Alexander disease
b. Pelizaeus-Merzbacher disease and Cockayne syndrome
c. Canavan disease and Cockayne syndrome
d. Alexander disease and Pelizaeus-Merzbacher disease
e. Vanishing white matter disease and Canavan disease

17. The appropriate neuroimaging study of choice of children with new-onset seizures who have no detectable symptomatic cause is
a. CT
b. MRI
c. PET
d. USG
e. SPECT

18. All are true regarding dual pathology in epilepsy patient except
a. hippocampal sclerosis with another potentially epileptogenic extrahippocampal abnormality
b. observed in 15% of surgical epilepsy cases with MR imaging
c. associated with less favorable surgical outcome
d. the most often encountered associated abnormality is DNET
e. both pathology must be resected for successful control of seizures

19. All are specific findings for extraaxial localization of brain tumour except
a. Cerebrospinal fluid cleft between brain and lesion
b. Vessels interposed between brain and lesion
c. Cortex between mass and edematous white matter
d. Dura between epidural mass and brain
e. Enhancement of adjacent meninges

20. All shows restricted diffusion except
a. lymphoma
b meningioma
c. glioblastoma multiforme
d. pyogenic abscesses
e. arachnoid cyst

21. All are true regarding chordoid glioma except
a. typical location in frontal lobe
b. thought to arise from the

region of the lamina terminalis
c. signal abnormalities extending into the proximal optic tracts bilaterally
d. appear to be benign
e. the strong staining for glial fibrillary acidic protein

22. The most frequent neuroanatomic location of the pilocytic astrocytoma is
a. the cerebellar hemisphere
b. the optic nerve
c. diencephalon
d. floor of the third ventricle
e. cerebral hemisphere

23. All are true regarding pineal germ-cell tumour except
a. The second-most-common pineal germ cell tumor is a teratoma
b. teratoma contain hair, teeth, bone, and fat on pathologic examination
c. teratoma are virtually always solid and commonly hemorrhagic
d. teratoma has strikingly heterogeneous appearance on MRI
e. Rhabdoid tumour is DD of pineal teratoma

24. All are true regarding intraventricular meningioma except
a. arise from arachnoid cells of the tela choroidea
b. most commonly occur in the lateral ventricles
c. usually appearing in the middle-aged and elderly population
d. have a smooth margin and are generally oval in configuration
e. difffuse hydrocephalus

25. All are true regarding protocol of MR in paediatric brain tumour except
a. a T2 gradient echo susceptibility scan can be done in case of suspicion of calcification /hemorrhage
b. Diffusion imaging is included in evaluations of all cases of brain tumors
c. The navigational study is obtained through the entire head at 20-degree angulation to the orbitomeatal line
d. task activation functional MRI is done when the tumor is in or near a sensitive region
e. Diffusion tensor imaging with fiber tracking provide specific information about the effect of the tumor on tracts

26. All are true regarding brainstem glioma except
a. pontine glioma occurs most often between 5 and 6 years of age
b. pontine glioma is diffusely infiltrating and tends to run a malignant course
c. In general, midbrain tumours have a tendency to be indolent and of low-grade astrocytic nature
d. Contrast enhancement of a medullary tumor does not necessarily mean an aggressive tumor
e. Hydrocephalus is relatively infrequent in midbrain tumour tumors

27. An adult patient present acutely with a lowered level of consciousness, together with focal neurologic deficit, seizures, and fever . The most radiological finding suggestive of herpes encephalitis (type 1) is

a. unilateral / bilateral involvement of the insula in association with other frontal and temporal cortex
b. lone involvement of the hippocampus without any insular and temporal cortex changes.
c. bilateral involvement from beginning
d. involvement of the basal ganglia
e. involvement of posterior occipital cortex

28. All are true regarding MR imaging of congenital cytomegalovirus infection except
a. Macrocephaly
b. porencephaly
c. atrophy and encephalomalacia
d. ventricular enlargement and periventricular calcification
e. the lissencephaly–pachygyria spectrum

29. All are true regarding HIV encephalitis except
a. Cortical atrophy ----the most frequent MR finding
b. ventricular ex vacuo dilation
c. hyperintense lesions in the periventricular white matter and centrum semiovale on T2W and FLAIR
d. non-enhancemrnt of lesions
e. significant mass effect

30. All are true regarding paediatric CNS infection of AIDS except
a. Brain atrophy ---the most common imaging finding
b. extensive calcific vasopathy
c. No calcification i in the basal ganglia
d. the most common intracranial mass lesion ----CNS lymphoma

e. reduced NAA/Cr ratio

31. All are true regading brain abscess except
a. an abscess often exhibit mesial thinning of the ring
b. Abscesses tend to demonstrate high signal intensity on DWI
c. lactate (1.3 ppm), and pyruvate are fairly specific markers for pyogenic abscesses
d. an amino acid peak (valine, leucine, and isoleucine) at 0.9 ppm are seen in necrotic/cystic tumour
e. The spectra of S. aureus abscesses donot demonstrate increased peaks of succinate and acetate or amino acid resonance

32. All are true regarding vesicular stage of neuro-cysticercosis except
a. A small cyst with eccentric scolex
b. little or no contrast enhancement
c. the mural nodule is best seen T2W image
d. The cysts are isointense to CSF on all MR sequences
e. MR often reveals a greater number of viable lesions compared to CT

33. All are true regarding Alzheimer disease except
a. beta amyloid is a component of the microtubule system
b. Neurofibrillary tangles consist of pathologic aggregates of tau protein
c. Neuritic plaque consists of a dense central β-amyloid core
d. The most promising biomarker appear to be CSF Aβ$_{1-42}$ protein levels

e. the neurofibrillary pathology of AD begins in the transentorhinal area

34. All are true regarding Wernicke encephalopathy (WE) except
a. acute neurologic emergency due to thiamine (vitamin B_1) deficiency
b. the classic triad of ophthalmoplegia, ataxia, and confusion
c. perimidline focal cerebral lesions characteristic
d. hyperintense signal on T2-weighted and FLAIR sequences
e., enhancement always noted

35. All are regarding features of NF1 and NF2
a. NF1 more common than NF2
b. NF2 are prone to develop neoplasia of the astrocyte and neuron
c. neurofibromas are relatively uncommon in NF2
d. NF2 patients develop multiple schwannomas meningiomas, and ependymomas
e. significant risk for various visceral and skeletal problems in NF1

36. All are true regarding hemangioblastoma except
a. "Cyst with nodule" appearance occurs in about one third of hemangioblastomas
b. presence of stromal cells distinguishes it from cavernous angiomas and arteriovenous malformations
c. The hyporvascular neoplastic nodule is usually located in a superficial subpial location
d. The solid portions of the tumor donot show intense enhancement after contrast infusion.
e. the cyst margin do not enhance.

37. All are true regarding lissencephaly except
a. a smooth brain
b. a figure-eight appearance.
c. agyria more pronounced frontally in XLIS mutations
d. separation of the the cortex from band heterotopia by white matter
e. horizontally-oriented sylvian fissures

38. All are true regarding imaging of epidermoid except
a. lobulated, extraaxial masses
b. low density, often similar to CSF
c. typically intense contrast enhancement
d.. insinuation of contrast into the interstices of the epidermoid on intrathecal contrast
e. restricted diffusion on DWI

39. All the features favour meningioma over neurofibroma in spine except
a. more posterior location within the spinal canal
b. multiplicity
c. not attached to the dura
d. more mobility
e. a central area of decreased signal on T2W

40. All the tumours seed the CSF space except
a. medulloblastoma
b. Glioblastoma and high-grade astrocytomas (grades III and IV)
c. Ependymoma
d. oligodendroglioma
e. neurofibroma

41. All are true regarding Spinal Cord Arteriovenous Fistula(

SCAVF) except
a. The intradural location of the shunt
b. constant involvement of arteries supplying the spinal cord
c., typical location ventral to the cord
d. lack of intervening nidus
e. no spinal subarachnoid hemorrhage

42. All are true regarding genetics of spine except
a. The homeotic genes define the specific identity of the individual spinal segments
b. Transforming growth factor β selectively activates anterior homeobox genes
c. Fibroblast growth factor selectively activates posterior homeobox genes
d. The concentration gradient of retinoic acid ----a major factor in determining the specific rostrocaudal fate of neuralized ectoderm
e. Activin β and activin receptor II are expressed only on the left of Hensen's node

43. All are true regarding Diastematomyelia except
a. single arachnoid/dural sheath in 50% to 60% cases
b. type I Diastematomyelia has dual dural-arachnoid tubes
c. fibrous partition of diastematoyelia refers to double layer of dura
d. bony spur appears to be more intimately associated with the laminae than the vertebral body
e. The spinal canal is nearly always markedly abnormal

44. All are true regarding pituitary adenoma except
a. Nelson syndrome is caused by TSH hypersecretion
b. The prolactin-growth hormone adenoma is the most common of the plurihormonal adenomas.
c. nonfunctional pituitary adenomas present because of adjacent compression/invasion .
d. pituitary apoplexy occurs due to intratumoral hemorrhage
e. lengthening of both T1 and T2 relaxation

45. .All are true regarding intracranial germinoma except

a. frequent cystic components
b. mildly hypointense on T1W and often isointense to gray matter on T2W
c. Marked contrast enhancement
d.. prominent lipid peaks
e. pineal lesion in conjunction with a suprasellar lesion in a young person

46. All are true regarding Chiasmatic and Hypothalamic Glioma except
a. 75% occur in the first decade of life
b. a definite association with neurofibromatosis
c. more aggressive than those originating from the optic nerves
d. Calcification and hemorrhage common features
e. Contrast enhancement in about half of all cases

47. All are features of optic nerve glioma(OPG) in NF-1 (in comparison to sporadic glioma) except
a. present in early childhood, usually by the age of 5 to 6 years

b. more frequently found along the orbital or intracranial portion of the optic nerve
c. greater number of T2 hyperintense lesions in the brain
d. more heterogeneous in signal intensity and exhibit greater T2 hyperintensity than OPGs
e. perineural tumor growth around the optic nerve within the dural sheath

48. Reid's or Frankfurt line refers to
a. line drawn from the upper margin of the orbit to the superior border of the external auditory meatus
b. line drawn from the lower margin of the orbit to the superior border of the external auditory meatus
c. line drawn through both pupils
d. line drawn vertically through the EAM
e. line from the outer canthus to the centre of the meatus: orbitomeatal (OM) line.

49. Commonly calcified brain tumours are all except
a. Oligodendrogliomas (90%)
b. Choroid plexus tumours
c. Ependymoma
d. Metastases
e. Central neurocytoma

50. All are true regarding pineal region tumours, germinoma except
a. often grey matter isointensity on standard MRI
b. poor contrast enhancement
c. virtually never calcify.
d. the hypothalamic region ----the second commonest site of germinoma
e. show diffuse subependymal and subarachnoid spread

51. All are true regading pathophysiology of stroke except
a. A CBF of around 23 ml 100 g^{-1} min^{-1} causes a reversible neurological deficit.
b. electrical activity ceases below about 18–20 ml 100 g^{-1} min^{-1} of CBF
c. cytotoxic edema develops at 10–15 ml 100 g^{-1} min
d. Most carotid territory infarcts involve the middle cerebral artery.
e. The commonest cause of ACA infarcts is embolism

52. All are true regarding aneurysm except
a. 30 per cent arise from vertebral or basilar arteries
b. Giant aneurysms account for approximately 5 per cent of all cerebral aneurysms
c. A clot in the septum pellucidumis is virtually diagnostic of an aneurysm of the anterior communicating artery
d. the basilar artery bifurcation aneurysm rupture ----- blood in the interpeduncular fossa, brainstem or thalamus
e. the posterior inferior cerebellar arteries aneurysm often haemorrhage into the ventricular system.

53. Cause white matter disease in HIV-related CNS disease is/are
a. Small nonspecific focal white-matter hyperintensities on T2W
b. HIV encephalopathy
c. PML
d. viral encephalitis—CMV
e. all

54. All are true regarding spinal cord supply except
a. supplied by the midline anterior spinal artery and two posterolateral spinal arteries
b. artery of Adamkiewicz is found in the thoracolumbar region
c. artery of Adamkiewicz is usually on the left side, between T8 and L1–2
d. The anterior spinal artery supplies the major portion of the cord substance
e. posterolateral spinal arteries supply the motor cells of the anterior horns

55. All are true regarding normal gyration except
a. the interhemispheric fissure and Sylvian fissures is formed by 16 weeks gestation
b. the callosal sulcus and parieto-occipital fissure are recognizable at 22 weeks gestation
c. The central sulcus is seen in most infants by 32 weeks
d. The slowest regions of gyration are the frontal and temporal poles
e.. By term the gyral pattern is nearly the same as the appearance in adults

56. All are true regarding spine except
a. The spinal cord termination ---- abnormal if seen at or below L3
b. myelomeningoceles are virtually always associated with Chiari II malformation
c. The filum terminale lipoma is considered to arise from a disturbance of caudal regression
d. The 'tight' filum terminaleis refers to short, thick filum greater than 2 mm in diameter
e. dermal sinus is typically seen in the thoracic lumbosacral region

57. Congenital cause of hydrocephalus is /are
a. aqueductal stenosis/gliosis
b. Chiari II malformation
c the Dandy–Walker malformation
d. vein of Galen malformation
e. all

58. All are true regarding ONYX except
a. non-adhesive liquid embolic agent
b cosists of ethyl-vinyl alcohol polymer (EVOH)
c. dimethyl sulfoxide (DMSO) used as solvent
d. tantalum used to make it radiopaque
e. it solidifies more rapidly than NBCA

59. All are true regarding calcification in brain tumour except
a. oligodendroglioma calcify in 50% cases
b. craniopharyngioma show calcification in over 75% of cases
c. calcification in craniopharyngioma is in midline and above the sella
d. calcification in meningioma is characteristically ball-like and amorphous
e. medulloblastoma calcify.frequently

60. All are causes of large head in infancy except
a. Pelizeazius –merzbacker disease
b. Lipidoses
b. Spongy degeneration
c. Alexander's disease
d. Tuberous sclerosis

61. All are true regarding azygous

ACA except
a. solitary unpaired vessel
b. arise as single trunk
c. arise from the confluence of the A1 segment of the right and left ACAs
d. very common anomaly
e. often associated with other intracranial anomalies

62. All the factors increase the hemorrhagic risk of AVM except
a. smaller size
b. central/deep venous drainage pattern
c. peri-or intraventricular location
d. presence of an intranidal aneurysm
e. presence of angiomatous changes

63. All are true regarding lateral ventricles except
a. septum is absent in corpus callosum dysgenesis
b. septum pellucidum thicker than 3mm is suspicious for neoplasm
c. the most common primary septal tumour is astrocytoma
d. dysplastic thickening of septum is seen in NF1
e. subependymoma show strong predilection for frontal horn

64. All are true regarding neurocysticercosis except
a. nodular or microring enhancement at nodular calcified stage
b. most common site ---brain parenchyma>ventricles>subarachnoid space
c. round CSF-like cyst with mural nodule in vesicular stage
d. edema and cyst wall enhancement in colloidal vesicular stage
e. isodense cyst with hyperdense calcified scloex in granular nodular stage

65. Which is a neuroepithelial cyst ?
a. choroid fissure cyst
b. arachnoid cyst
c. dermoid cyst
d. epidermoid cyst
e. posterior fossa cyst

66. All are true regarding fungal CNS infection except
a. aspergillosis may cause hemorrhagic infarcts
b. mucor tends to spread along perineural channel
c. cryptococcosis cause pseudocyst in basal ganglia
d. caseating granuloma is common in coccidiodomycosis
e. aspergillosis reach CNS by direct extension

67. All are true regarding following disoreder except
a. Leigh disease show high density areas in the putamina and caudate nuclei on NECT
b. Multiple infarcts seen in MERRF and MELAS
c. occipital lobes are most common site for MELAS
d. Neuronal migration discrder with general decrease in white matter volume is noted in Zellweger Syndrome
e. caudate nucleus volume is seen in Huntington disease

68. All are common causes of bilateral basal ganglia lucencies except
a. lacunar infarct
b. dilated perivascular spaces
c. HIE
d. toxic encephalopathy

e.Wilson disease

69.All are true regarding multiple sclerosis of spinal cord except
a.preferentially in the ventrolateral cord
b.donot respect boundaries between gray and white matter
c.predilection for cervical spinal cord in early stage
d.elongated hyperintense lesion on T2W
e.enhancing lesion in acute stage

70.All are true regarding detachable balloons except
a.mechanical devices for embolism
b.made of titanium
c.used to occlude carotico-cavernous fistula
d.the risks of the accidental detachmen in an unwanted position
e.non-detachable balloons used for temporary test occlusions.

71.All are true regarding endovascular treatment of cerebral AVMs except
a. aim is the prevention of cerebral haemorrhage or re-haemorrhage
b. The most commonly used approach is venous embolisation using a permanent fluid agent
c. may be used to reduce the size of the AVM prior to radiosurgery
d. partial AVM embolisation can be effective in improving the control of epileptic seizures
e. partial AVM embolisation bring relief of symptoms related to venous hypertension

72.All are true regarding tumour except
a.Dermoids are found most commonly just above the outer angle of the orbit
b. moth-eaten' appearance is seen in mets of carcinoma
c. Neurohlastorma involve suture margins
d. Histiocytosis produce non-sclerotic margin
e. 'double' floor is seen in pituitary microadenoma

73.All are features of r CBF in dementia except
a. The typical defect of Alzheimer's disease is a reduction of flow in the posterior parietal and temporal areas
b. The blood flow response to Diamox is relatively normal in AD.
c. perfusion abnormality in Lewy body disease (LBD) is broadly similar in distribution to AD
d. the basal ganglia blood flow are typically abnormal in LBD, but normal in AD
e. Pick's disease show asymmetrical reduction in rCBF in both frontal lobes initially

74.All are true regarding cerebral herniation except
a.subfalcine hernation leads to shift of the cingulate gryrus across the midline
b.PCA is displaced in descending transtentorial herniation
c.fourth ventricle is compressed and displced posteriorly in descending transtentorial herniation
d.frontal lobe is forced posteriorly over the greater sphenoid ala in descending transalar herniation
e.tonsillar herniation is best seen

on saggittal MR studies

75. The most common tumours in children less than 2yrs are
a. PNET
b. asrocytoma
c. teratoma
d. choroid plexus tumour
e. medulloblastoma

76. The most common cause of nontraumatic scalp masses in children is
a. cephalhematoma
b. eosinophilic granuloma
c. cephalocele
d. dermoid tumours
e. hamartoma

77. All are true regarding imaging of meningioma except
a. mother-in-law sign on angiography
b. 70% to 75% hyperdense
c. typically isodense with gray matter
d. dural tail in 95%
e. sunburst of enlarged dural feedres

78. All are common causes of ependymal enhancement except
a. ventriculitis/ependimitis
b. anaplastic astrocytoma/GBM
c. lymphoma
d. choroid plexus tumour
e. germinoma

79. All are true regarding x-linked adrenoleukodystrophy except
a. a bilaterally symmetric demyelination
b. cortex normal
c. demyelination occurs first in the occipital lobe and the corpus callosum splenium
d. outermost zone show enhancement on MRI
e. auditory pathway involvement common

80. All are common causes of multifocal white matter lesions except
a. perivascular spaces
b. myelin pallor
c. multiple sclerosis
d. metastases
e. vasculitis

81. All disorders are correctly matched except
a. Dandy-Walker malformation – ventral induction
b. callosal agenesis---cellular migration
c. Lhermitte-Duclos disease---cellular migration
d. myelocystocoele---secondary neurulation
e. septo-optic dysplasia---secondary neurulation

82. All are true regarding Chiari I malformation except
a. tosnsil displaced at least 6 mm in the first year of life
b. brrain usually normal
c. syringomyelia in 30 to 60% of symptomatic patients
d. basilat invagination -29% to 50%
e. Klippel-Feil syndrome 5% to 10%

83. All are true regarding inborn metabolic brain disorders except
a. bilateral and symmetrical
b. Macrocephaly seen in Canavan's and Alexander's leukoencephalopathies
c. frequent finding of delayed myelination /hypomyelination
d. T1W often shows more severe hypomyelination compared to T2W in in Pelizaeus Merzbacher disease
e. T2-weighted hyperintensity is noted specifically in the splenium

and peritrigonal white matter in ALD

84. All are true regarding hypoxic–ischaemic injury in term patterns
a. posterolateral putamina, ventrolateral thalami and adjacent capsular white matter most vulnerable
b. bilateral and symmetrical
c. parasagittal distribution in partial hypoxic ischaemia
d. ulegyria in partial hypoxic ischaemia
e. involvement of the cerebral hemipheres with the posterior fossa structures

85. All are true regarding angioplasty and stenting of exctracranial vessels except
a. primary stenting is the endovascular technique of choice for carotid artery stenosis,
b. most common cause of major strokes after carotid PTA is due to dissection of the carotid artery.
c. Carotid stenting is generally performed under general anaesthesia
d. filters and occlusion balloons are used to catch any embolic material released during stenting
e. The self-expandable stent adapts to the different diameters of the common and internal carotid arteries

86. All are true regarding management Galen aneurismal malformation except
a. deferred to allow for growth of the child
b. intervention in neonate technically easy
c. arterial approach using NBCA most often used
d. the initial aim --- to reduce the level of arteriovenous shunting to manage cardiac failure
e. staged treatment performed after maturation of the child

87. Geographic skull is seen in
a. multiple myeloma
b. histiocytosis
c. chordoma
d. epidermoid
e. metastases

88. All are true regarding r CBF imaging in crebrovascular disease except
a. 90% of patients show local blood flow abnormalities after 8hrs of acute storke on SPECT imaging.
b. help in monitoring thrombolytic therapy
c. The appearance of 'luxury perfusion' commonly occurs 2-28 days after the onset of a stroke
d. thalamic blood flow is usually used as a reference point for assessing cortical regional flow
e. Loss of cerebellar perfusion reserve carries a poor prognosis

89. All are true regarding location of diffuse axonal injury except
a. lobar white matter
b. corticomedullary junction
c. frontotemporal region
d. posterior body and splenium of corpus callosum
e. ventral aspect of the upper brainstem

90-. Pseudodelta sign is seen in
a. SAH
b. SSS thrombosis
c. oligodendrogioma
d. tuberous sclerosis
e. AVM

91. Common unilateral cavernous masses are all except
a. Schwannoma
b. meningioma
c. lymphoma
d. metastases
e. carotid cavernous fistula

92. All are true regarding location of meningioma except
a. prasaggittal—25%
b. cerebral convexity---20%
c. sphenoid ridge----15% to 20%
d. olfactory groove---5% to 10%
e. posterior fossa ---1%

93. All are true of congenital HIV except
a. maternally transmitted
b. diffuse cerebral atrophy
c. basal ganglia calcification
d. progressive encephalopathy in 30 to 50% cases
e. good prognosis

94. All are true regarding Krabbe disease except
a. symmetric demyelination
b. sparing of U fibres
c. high incidence in Sweden
d. the centrum semiovale –rarely affected
e. thalami and basal ganglia hperdense on NECT

95. All are true regarding toxic demyelination except
a. transeverse pontine fibres are spared in osmotic myelinolysis
b. pontine plus concomitant basal ganglia involvement is fairly specific for osmotic myelinolysis
c. Marchiafava-Bignami disease --- demyelination and necrosis of corpus callosum
d. Wernicke encephalopathy --- hyperintense areas surrounding the third ventricle and aqueduct
e. mammillary body atrophy is seen in chronic Wernicke encephalopathy

TEST PAPER 16(ANSWER)

1.----a
2. -----a
Routine evaluation of the ischemic stroke patient (particularly in the subacute and chronic stages of infarction) typically includes some form of T1-weighted and T2-weighted spin echo or fast spin echo imaging and supplemental gradient echo imaging for hemorrhage
T1-weighted imaging --- repetition time, 400 to 600 ms; echo time, 20 to 35 ms, T2-weighted imaging --- repetition time, greater than 2,500 ms; echo time, 80 to 120 ms.
3.---e
Hypoglycemia is associated with perinatal ischemic stroke and appears to be an independent risk factor for the development of stroke in this time period. Bilateral occipital lobe infarction has been noted in the neonate with severe symptomatic hypoglycemia.
4.---c
Storage forms with large aggregates of iron (ferrritin and hemosiderin) behave paramagnetically at biological temperatures, but at very low temperatures they behave antiferromagnetically and probably superparamagnetically.
An area of marked hypointensity on T2-weighted images and particularly on GRE images can remain at the site of an old hemorrhage indefinitely and is due to ferritin and hemosiderin accumulated within the lysosomes of macrophages and glial cells.
5.---e
Inappropriate enhancement with acute hematoma ,perihematoma "edema" and mass effect in late hemorrhage are other features of hemorrhagic neoplasm. There is marked heterogeneity, due to mixed stages of hemorrhage, debris fluid (intracellular-extracellular blood) levels, edema + tumor + necrosis with blood.There is delayed evolution of blood-breakdown products. Absent, diminished, or very irregular hypointense rim representing iron storage forms is noted
6.---b
Conventional intraarterial catheter angiography is the the gold standard for aneurysm diagnosis.
7.---e
Septo-optic dysplasia---Ventral induction
8.---c
The key to distinguishing the enhancement of capillary telangiectasia from other, similar enhancing lesions, notably lymphoma when periventricular, is the absence of any signal abnormality on the unenhanced images.
9.----e
MRA is unnecessary in most cases. GRE imaging can occasionally show marked hypointensity within venous angiomas. This should not be mistaken for hemorrhage; it is simply a reflection of the paramagnetic deoxyhemoglobin within venous blood.
10.---d
Leptomeningeal venous drainage is uncommon in the cavernous sinus DAVMs and consequently

intracranial hemorrhage from this lesion is rare.

DAVMs of the tentorial-incisural region, anterior fossa, convexity-sagittal sinus, and sylvian-middle fossa has very high incidence of leptomeningeal venous drainage ,Consequently, most lesions in these locations have a very aggressive course, and most commonly present with intracranial hemorrhage.

11.---e

Direct visualization of the shunt in DAVMs is generally not possible on MR.MR is useful in defining the relationship of the components of the DAVM to neuroanatomic structures ,particularly in lesions with both intracranial and extracranial involvement. MR is useful to indicate venous hypertension and thereby implicate DAVM with venous outflow obstruction by delineating enlarged deep medullary veins.

12.---a

13.---b

All aneurysm clips in use are composed primarily of nonferromagnetic material, which generally shows no movement in a magnetic field. Although Phynox and Sugita Elgiloy contain ferromagnetic material, they usually do not demonstrate movement when introduced into MR scanners at currently used field strengths.

14.----d

15.---b

The central cerebral white matter and deep gray matter are preferentially affected, whereas the cortex is relatively spared

16.---b

17.—b

18.----d

The most often encountered associated abnormality is cortical dysgenesis

Dual pathology is associated with less favorable surgical outcome. For successful control of seizures, both abnormalities must be resected .

19.----d

20.---e

21.---a

Chordoid glioma is a recently recognized tumor that has a typical location in the anterior third ventricle and hypothalamic region, with histologic features distinct from those of other glial tumors . This lesion has shown cords and clusters of epithelioid cells with mucinous background, with low-grade lymphoplasmacytic infiltrate, similar to chordoma or chordoid meningioma.

22.---a

The most frequent neuroanatomic location of the pilocytic astrocytoma is the cerebellar hemisphere.

23.---c

Teratoma are virtually always partially cystic and commonly hemorrhagic.

24.---e

Intraventricular meningiomas can usually be differentiated from choroid plexus papillomas both clinically and with MR. Lateral ventricular choroid plexus papillomas develop mainly in young children, with meningiomas usually appearing in the middle-aged and elderly population. Meningiomas have a smooth margin and are generally oval in configuration whereas papillomas frequently demonstrate very nodular, heterogeneous, irregular surfaces. Papillomas also usually present with diffuse hydrocephalus and not just dilation of the trapped ventricular segment. This occurs either because of their overproduction of CSF or their frequent bleeding, which may cause obstructing basal arachnoiditis and/or intraventricular ependymitis. Although papillomas are more frequently very heterogeneous, intraventricular meningiomas can also show significant heterogeneity and extensive edema . Therefore, the location of the lesion and the age of the patient are the two most valuable clues to the diagnosis

25.---c
The navigational study includes axial post–contrast enhanced T1 and T2 1-mm-thick slices obtained through the entire head at zero-degree angulation to the orbitomeatal line.

26.----e
Hydrocephalus is relatively infrequent in pontine tumors .In contrast to pontine and medullary tumors, hydrocephalus is the common presenting finding in patients with midbrain tumors. On a nonenhanced CT, one third of the pontine tumors are hypodense, one third are isodense, and one fourth are mixed density, both decreased and isodense. Only 5% of tumors are of increased density, with the increased density representing either calcification or blood, and the hemorrhagic focus usually indicating a malignant zone within the tumor

Masses that are predominately hyperdense in pons, with or without surrounding focal edema, should be considered as possible cavernomas . The mass that shows a rim of hemosiderin hypointensity on T2 or T2* should be thought of as a cavernoma of the brainstem and followed with imaging.

27.---a
Herpes encephalitis is often but not always hemorrhagic, affecting primarily the medial temporal and inferior frontal lobes. In most cases, herpes encephalitis is initially unilateral, with asymmetric contralateral involvement seen in later stages. The most suggestive finding to be sought by the radiologist is unilateral or bilateral involvement of the insula in association with other frontal and temporal cortex. Despite the fact that this is a limbic inflammation, commonly affecting cingulate and parahippocampal gyri, the diagnostic radiologist should note that it would be highly atypical for herpes encephalitis to involve the hippocampus alone, that is, without any insular and temporal cortex changes. This stands in contrast to other disease states affecting hippocampi (including limbic encephalitis, a paraneoplastic noninfectious process, and status epilepticus),

which can be isolated to unilateral or bilateral hippocampus.
Extension from the temporal lobes across the sylvian fissure to the isle of Reil is frequently seen, sparing the putamen. The disease often spares the basal ganglia
In immunocompetent individuals, HSV-1 encephalitis may result in necrotizing encephalitis involving mostly the temporal lobes and orbital surfaces of the frontal lobes.

28.---a
Microcephaly is found in congenital CMV .
Owl's-eye appearance is a pathologic hallmark of CMV.
CT is virtually always less sensitive than MR in detecting CMV encephalitis abnormalities . CT grossly underestimates the degree of involvement by CMV . Typically, CT may reveal atrophy, the most common finding , and, less commonly, white matter hypodensity and ring-enhancing lesions.
MR imaging depicts patchy and, less often, confluent periventricular white matter lesions with hypointense signal on T1-weighted images, as well as a hyperintense signal on T2-weighted images . Infrequently, subependymal enhancement is evident and, if present, is a valuable diagnostic clue.

29----e
There is little edema and a paucity of inflammatory cells in ADC, correlating with the lack of any mass effect on imaging studies.

30.----c
Calcification is often present in the basal ganglia and is usually bilateral, so CT can suggest this entity with more accuracy than MR. On MR, basal ganglia calcifications are often invisible but can be seen as hypointense areas on T2-weighted images or even hyperintensity on T1-weighted images. This is a unique finding related to vertical transmission.

31.---d
Acetate and succinate are not seen in association with necrotic tumors and are therefore fairly specific markers for pyogenic abscesses
The differential diagnosis for a ring-enhancing lesion includes primary brain tumor (high-grade astrocytoma), metastasis, infarction (bland or septic), resolving hematoma, thrombosed aneurysm, arteriovenous malformation, radiation necrosis, AIDS-related lymphoma, and other inflammatory conditions (e.g., demyelinating disease, granulomata, etc.)
Abscesses tend to demonstrate high signal intensity on DWI, with a corresponding reduction in the apparent diffusion coefficient values This is directly related to the cellularity and viscosity of the pus contained within an abscess cavity . In contrast, high-grade gliomas and metastases with central necrosis have a low signal on DWI and high apparent diffusion coefficient values .Nonbacterial abscesses often do not show restricted diffusion.
The MR spectroscopy (MRS) pattern derived from the central

portion of an abscess appears to be fairly characteristic. Thus, MRS seems to contribute to distinguishing an abscess from a necrotic brain tumor and a tuberculoma
. In an untreated abscess, resonances may be seen corresponding to acetate (1.92 ppm), lactate (1.3 ppm), alanine (1.5 ppm), succinate (2.4 ppm), and pyruvate, as well as a complex peak at 0.9 ppm indicating amino acids valine, leucine, and isoleucine
.

Acetate, lactate, succinate, and pyruvate are metabolic end products arising from microorganisms
. Acetate and succinate are not seen in association with necrotic tumors and are therefore fairly specific markers for pyogenic abscesses. However, these two resonances are not consistently identified in all abscess cavities In vivo MRS does reveal an amino acid peak (valine, leucine, and isoleucine) at 0.9 ppm, which can be found in all abscesses but not in necrotic/cystic tumors .

The central portion of a necrotic/cystic tumor often reveals only a lactate resonance peak. Thus, the presence of amino acid inverted peak at 0.9 ppm seems to be a reliable indicator of a pyogenic abscess
MRS can also be of some use in the etiologic classification of brain abscesses because different MR spectra can be obtained from specific underlying agents .
It could be possible to differentiate an anaerobic from a pyogenic brain abscess, as well as from aerobic and sterile lesions. The selective presence of succinate and acetate in the anaerobic abscess is probably the result of the involvement of alternative anaerobic pathways for energy demands, enhancing glycolysis and the fermentative pathways for energy generation .
The spectra of S. aureus abscesses do not demonstrate increased peaks of succinate and acetate or amino acid resonance. Resonances of lipids and lactates dominate the MR spectra of such lesions.

32.----c
Cysticercosis is one of the most common parasitic infections worldwide involving the central nervous system.
Neurocysticercosis is probably the most common cause of late-onset epilepsy in developing countries Neurocysticercosis is caused by the encysted larval stage of the pork tapeworm, Taenia solium.
Calcification, the end stage of neurocysticercosis.
Four patterns of intracranial involvement have been described according to lesion location : parenchymal, subarachnoid, intraventricular, and mixed.
The parenchymal is the most common type and is located in cerebral hemispheres and basal ganglia as a result of greater vascular supply to these regions.
Four pathologic stages are described in neurocysticercosis — vesicular, colloidal vesicular,

granular nodular, and nodular calcified (involution).

An eccentric scolex can be seen within the cyst. Because of the bright CSF signal on T2-weighted images that may obscure the scolex, the mural nodule is best seen on proton density or FLAIR images.

33.---a

The major pathologic features that characterize AD are senile plaques, neurofibrillary tangles, decreased synaptic density, neuron loss, and cerebral atrophy.

Neurofibrillary tangles consist of pathologic aggregates of tau protein--- component of the microtubule system is tau protein
It is well established that the neurofibrillary pathology of AD begins in the transentorhinal area and progresses to the hippocampus, to paralimbic and adjacent medial-basal temporal cortex, to neocortical association areas, and lastly to primary sensory-motor and visual areas
The second pathologic lesion associated with AD is the senile (neuritic) plaque. Neuritic plaque consists of a dense central β-amyloid core with inflammatory cells and dystrophic neurites in its periphery.

34.----e

There is variable enhancement after intravenous administration of gadolinium, and variable restricted diffusion. In contrast to the imaging of acute stroke, parenchyma that shows restricted diffusion in the setting of acute WE does not indicate irreversible cytotoxic edema.

35.---b

NF2 are prone to develop neoplasia not of the astrocyte and neuron but rather from other cells

36.—d

The hypervascular neoplastic nodule is usually located in a superficial subpial location. The hypervascular tumor nodule usually, but not always, presents with tubular flow voids.
Most hemangioblastomas do not bleed

37.---e

Neuroimaging studies in classical lissencephaly demonstrate a smooth brain with vertically oriented sylvian fissures. The cerebrum has been described as a figure eight as the result of the narrowing in the midportion by the sylvian fissures.

Patients with LIS1 abnormalities tend to have more severe agyria over the parietooccipital region with pachygyria frontally, whereas those with XLIS mutations have more pronounced agyria frontally.

38-.—c

Enhancement is not typical. In contradistinction to arachnoid cysts, after intrathecal injection, contrast typically insinuates itself into the interstices of the epidermoid.

Strands of tissue with soft tissue intensity are occasionally present in epidermoids, and their identification may help in differentiating them from arachnoid cystst.

On DWI, epidermoids exhibit high

signal because of the restriction of water molecules within the epidermoid resulting from their interaction with protein macromolecules. By contrast, the freely diffusing water molecules within an arachnoid cyst are of low signal intensity on DWI.

39.--a
Several criteria help to differentiate neural tumors and neurofibroma.Neural tumors tend to be more anteriorly located within the spinal canal, whereas spinal meningiomas have a posterolateral location except when they are located in the cervical region, where they are more likely to be anterior . Frequently, neurofibromas are multiple, whereas meningiomas tend to be solitary. Nerve sheath tumors are not attached to the dura and therefore have more mobility than meningiomas. Finally, neural tumors can have a central area of decreased signal on T2-weighted images not seen with meningiomas

40.---e
The medulloblastoma is the most frequent tumour seeding CSF spaces, representing 48% of the cases

41.----e
Spinal subarachnoid hemorrhage is common and has been noted in nearly one third of patients at presentation.
The intradural location of the shunt, constant involvement of arteries supplying the spinal cord, typical location ventral to the cord, and lack of intervening nidus are angioarchitectural features that differentiate SCAVF from both SDAVF and SCAVM.

.42.—e
Truncal asymmetry is induced by asymmetric expression of signaling molecules . Activin β and activin receptor II are expressed only on the right of Hensen's node. The snail-related gene (cSR-1) is enriched in the right lateral plate mesoderm. CWnt-8c and follistatin are expressed on the right. SHH is initially expressed on both sides of Hensen's node but later becomes restricted to the left side. The nodal-related gene (cNR-1) s expressed asymmetrically within left lateral plate mesoderm and just to the left of Hensen's node. The mouse gene lefty is expressed in left lateral plate mesoderm. HNF-3β and PTC (a possible SHH receptor) are expressed on the left. Ectopic expression of SHH on the right and activin on the left alters the expression of asymmetric genes and randomizes handedness . Retinoic acid controls the expression of these genes during left-right patterning

43.—b
Dual Dural-Arachnoid Tubes (Pang Type I)
Single Dural-Arachnoid Tube (Pang Type II)

44.—a
Nelson syndrome is caused by ACTH hypersecretion.

45.---a
In contrast to craniopharyngiomas, germinomas are more homogeneous and only rarely have cystic components.

Central diabetes insipidus with either an enlarged stalk, decreased growth hormone secretion, or elevated serum human chorionic gonadotropin-β is suspicious for an occult germinoma

46.---d

Calcification and hemorrhage are not common features of chiasmatic and hypothalamic Glioma but cysts are seen, particularly in the larger hypothalamic tumors. Contrast enhancement occurs in about half of all cases. Because of their known propensity to invade the brain along the optic radiations, T2-weighted images of the entire brain are necessary. This pattern of tumor extension is readily evident as hyperintensity on the T2-weighted image; however, patients with neurofibromatosis can present a problem in differential diagnosis. This relates to a high incidence of benign cerebral hamartomas and/or atypical glial cell rests in neurofibromatosis that can mimic glioma. These both appear as areas of high signal intensity on T2 weighting within the optic pathways. Lack of interval growth and possibly the absence of contrast enhancement are more supportive of hamartomas, whereas confinement to the optic pathways, enhancement, and significant mass effect suggests tumor extension.

47.----d

OPGs in patients with NF1 are isointense to brain on T1-weighted images and iso- to hyperintense on T2-weighted images. In some cases, T2-weighted MR demonstrates central isointensity along the affected optic nerve with surrounding hyperintensity corresponding to the arachnoidal gliomatosis. These tumors show with variable enhancement and are often nonenhancing

OPGs in patients without NF1 tend to be more heterogeneous in signal intensity owing to the presence of cysts and exhibit greater T2 hyperintensity than OPGs in NF1 patients. The solid portions of these tumors usually enhance intensely.

48.---b

The *anthropological base line* is drawn from the lower margin of the orbit to the superior border of the external auditory meatus (EAM) known as Reid's or Frankfurt line

49.---d

Commonly calcified lesions----
Oligodendrogliomas (90%)
Choroid plexus tumours
Ependymoma
Central neurocytoma
Meningioma
Craniopharyngioma
Teratoma
Teratoma
Commonly haemorrhagic lesions---
GBM (grade 4 glioma)
Oligodendroglioma
Metastases
Melonoma

50.----b

Germinoma show marked, homogeneous contrast enhancement and virtually never calcify.

51.---e
The commonest cause of ACA infarcts is vasospasm following subarachnoid haemorrhage.
. Brainstem infarcts are commonly due to occlusion of short perforating vessels. A combination of infratentorial, thalamic and occipital infarcts suggests an occlusion of distal basilar artery, or 'top of the basilar' syndrome. Multiple infarcts in different arterial territories suggest a cardiac rather than a carotid source of emboli, or haemodynamic strokes due to hypotension if the distribution conforms to the arterial border zones.

52.----a
Around 90 per cent of intracranial aneurysms arise from the carotid circulation, the remaining 10 per cent from vertebral or basilar arteries[86]. The anterior and posterior communicating arteries give rise to approximately one-third each of all intracranial aneurysms, with another 20 per cent from middle cerebral arteries and 5 per cent from the basilar termination. The remainder arises from other vessel origins and bifurcations.
Aneurysms of the posterior communicating artery can present with isolated third nerve palsy

53.---e
54.---e
The anterior spinal artery is the most important of supply because it supplies the major portion of the cord substance, including the motor cells of the anterior horns. It gives off tiny sulcocommissural arteries that run into the cord; they are not visible at angiography unless pathologically enlarged.

55-.---c
The central sulcus is seen in most infants by 27 weeks

56.----e
Dermal sinus is typically seen in the lumbosacral region

57.---e
58.---e
Onyx is a new non-adhesive liquid embolic agent which consists of a mixture of ethyl-vinyl alcohol polymer (EVOH), dimethyl sul-occlufoxide (DMSO) as a solvent and tantalum to render it radiopaque. In contrast to NBCA, it solidifies slowly, minimises the danger of insitu gluing of a microcatheter. Onyx has been used for cerebral arteriovenous malformations (AVMS) and giant cerebral aneurysms in which other forms of endovascular or surgical treatment are difficult

59.----e
Medulloblastoma is a tumour that is unlikely to calcify.

60.-----a
Causes of large head in infancy
Hydrocephalus
Subdural effusions
Normal (sometimes familial)
Migrational abnormalities (see below)
Lipidoses
Spongy degeneration
Alexander's disease
Tuberous sclerosis

61.---d
Azygous ACA is rare anomaly

62.---e
The presence of peripheral or mixed venous drainage pattern and the presence of angiomatous change (the tresence of dilated cortical vessels derived from arteries not usually expected to supply the territory occupied by an AVM.
The cumulative risk of hemorrhage from a parenchymal AVM is estimated at 25 to 4% per year.

63.---c
The most common primary septal tumour is central neurocytoma

64.---a
Neurocysticercosis is the most common parasitic CNS infection worldwide. Nodular or microring enhancement is common at granular nodular stage

65.---a
Ependymal cyst and Choroid plexus cysts are other neuroepithelial cyst

66.---e
Aspergillosis reach CNS by hematogenous route

67.---a
Leigh disease show low density areas in the putamina and caudate nuclei on NECT.It does not show enhancement

68.---e

69---a
Multiple sclerosis of spinal cord preferentially involve the dorsolateral cord

70.---b
Detachable balloons are one of the oldest mechanical devices and can be either of silicone or latex. They are used to occlude large vessels or large fistulas such as a carotico-cavernous fistula

71.-----b
The most commonly used endovascular approach is arterial embolisation using a permanent fluid agent such as NBCA

72..----d
Histiocytosis produce sclerotic margin in contrast to malignant lesions

73.---e
Pick's disease, account for about 15% of demented patients. SPECT studies show symmetrical reduction in rCBF in both frontal lobes inially
The typical defect of AD is a reduction of flow in the posterior parietal and temporal
Areas. This pattern of abnormality is highly specific in discriminating between AD and normals, and a little less specific in distinguishing between AD and other demential, but still highly characteristic.

74.---c
Fourth ventricle is compressed and displced anteriorly in descending transtentorial herniation

75.---e

76.---d

77.---d
Dural tail noted in 60% of cases

78.---d
Choroid plexus tumour is a uncommon cause of ependymal enhancement

79.---d
The affected cerebral white matter typically shows three zones.The central necrotic zone is seen as a low signal region on T1W1 and homogenously very hyperintense on T2W.the intermediate zone of active demyelination and

inflammation enhances following contrast administrationthe peripheral area shows no enhancement .

80.----e
81.---e
82-.---c

Syringomyelia is seen in 30%to 60% of all patints and in 60% to 90% in symptomatic patients

83.—d

There are also specific inherited hypomyelination disorders that may be detected on MRI as a myelination pattern which is immature for the child's age. These include Pelizaeus Merzbacher disease, in which T2-weighted imaging often shows more severe hypomyelination compared to T1-weighted imaging

Macrocephaly is a useful clinical pointer to diseases such as megalencephalic leukodystrophy with subcortical cysts (MLC), Canavan's and Alexander's leukoencephalopathies, glutaric aciduria type I, GM2 gangliosidosis and l-2 hydroxyglutaric aciduria. Imaging features of X-linked adrenoleukodystrophy (ALD) are of low attenuation on CT and T2-weighted hyperintensity on MRI in the posterior central white matter, specifically the splenium and peritrigonal white matter progressing to the corticospinal tracts and visual and auditory pathways. The regions of T2 signal abnormality show increased diffusion. The leading edge of the demyelination enhances, where there is active inflammation and disruption of the blood–brain barrier.

84.----e

The predominant involvement of the cerebral hemipheres with relative sparing of the posterior fossa structures is a pattern that favours hypoxic–ischaemic injury over other causes of global brain injury at term, such as perinatal/neonatal infection.
The injuries attributed to partial hypoxic ischaemia are seen in a parasagittal distribution, typically involving a combination of cortex and subcortical white matter, and most often across the frontoparietal regions.
 Whilst usually bilateral, this pattern is not uncommonly asymmetric. A characteristic region of involvement is the posterior part of the Sylvian fissures. More characteristically, the greatest injury occurs at the base of the gyri, within the depths of the sulci, resulting in focal atrophy in these areas and a pattern recognized as ulegyria.

85.----c

Carotid stenting is generally performed under local anaesthesia

86.----b

Intervention in neonate is technically difficult and hazardous .

87-.---b
88.---c

Cerebellar blood flow is usually used as a reference point for assessing cortical regional flow. Crossed cerebellar diaschisis describes the phenomenon in which cerebral infarction leads to diminished perfusion in the contralateral cerebellar